Foundations of

NURSING RESEARCH

FOURTH EDITION

Rose Marie Nieswiadomy, PhD, RN
Professor Emerita
Texas Woman's University
College of Nursing

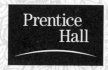

Prentice Hall

Upper Saddle River, New Jersey

Library of Congress Cataloging-in-Publication Data

Nieswiadomy, Rose Marie.
    Foundations of nursing research / Rose Marie Nieswiadomy—4th ed.
        p.   cm.
    Includes bibliographical references and index.
    ISBN 0–13–033991–1
    1. Nursing—Research—Methodology.   I. Title: Nursing research.   II. Title.
    [DNLM: 1. Nursing Research.—methods.   2. Data Collection.   3. Research design. WY
  20.5 N676f2001]
  RT81.5.N54 2001
  610.73′07′2—dc21

                                                                    2001035907

Notice: The author and the publisher of this volume have taken care to make certain that the doses of drugs and schedules of treatment are correct and compatible with the standards generally accepted at the time of publication. Nevertheless, as new information becomes available, changes in treatment and in the use of drugs become necessary. The reader is advised to carefully consult the instruction and information material included in the package insert of each drug or therapeutic agent before administration. This advice is especially important when using, administering, or recommending new or infrequently used drugs. The author and publisher disclaim all responsibility for any liability, loss, injury, or damage incurred as a consequence, directly or indirectly, of the use and application of any of the contents of this volume.

Publisher: Julie Alexander
Executive Editor: Maura Connor
Marketing Manager: Nicole Benson
Editorial Assistant: Beth Romph/Sladjana Repic
Managing Editor for Production: Patrick Walsh
Director of Manufacturing and Production: Bruce Johnson
Production Editor: Bruce Hobart, Pine Tree Composition
Manufacturing Buyer: Patrick Brown
Design Director: Cheryl Asherman
Design Coordinator: Maria Guglielmo
Cover Designer: Gary J. Sella
Composition: Pine Tree Composition
Printing and Binding: R.R. Donnelley & Sons, Harrisonburg, VA

Pearson Education Ltd., *London*
Pearson Education Australia Pty. Limited, *Sydney*
Pearson Education Singapore, Pte. Ltd.
Pearson Education North Asia Ltd., *Hong Kong*
Pearson Education Canada, Ltd., *Toronto*
Pearson Educación de Mexico, S.A. de C.V.
Pearson Education—Japan, *Tokyo*
Pearson Education Malaysia, Ptd. Ltd.
Pearson Education, Upper Saddle River, *New Jersey*

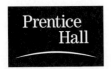

10 9 8 7 6 5 4 3 2 1
ISBN 0-13-033991-1

*To my husband, Ben, our four children,
and our seven grandchildren for helping me to
discover the really important things in life*

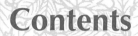

Contents

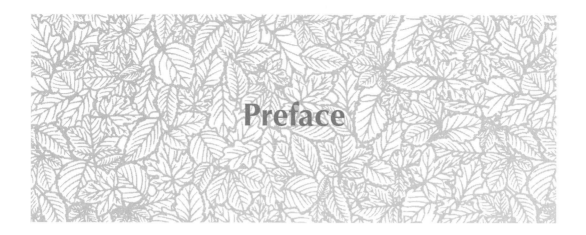

Preface

My primary purpose for writing the fourth edition of this book continues to be promoting interest in research, particularly research conducted by nurses. I firmly believe that research is essential to the growth of the nursing profession. Nursing research improves patient care and demonstrates that nurses are key members of the health care team. Research results show that nurses are not only caring but efficient providers of health care.

As a reader of this book, you are not expected to become proficient in critiquing research reports or to be able to conduct research independently. My goals for writing this book will have been achieved if you:

- are more enthusiastic about nursing research
- have gained knowledge about the research process
- possess beginning skills necessary to evaluate research findings
- are motivated to use research findings in your practice
- have the desire to conduct your own research studies in the future.

For those of you who are just beginning your careers in nursing, the future of the profession depends on you.

This book is intended primarily for individuals with little research experience, particularly undergraduate nursing students. However, many students in graduate programs have used this text to gain a better understanding of nursing research. They have commented that this text explains the research process clearly and succinctly. It is my hope that practicing nurses will also use this book as they evaluate study findings for use in practice and as they begin to conduct their own studies.

FEATURES OF THE BOOK

The informal writing style has been maintained in this fourth edition of the text. The book is even more learner-friendly than the previous three editions. In the past, readers have made many positive comments about the writing style. Students have said that they often feel as if they are talking with me, the author. Please interact with me as you read this text. You can nod in agreement, frown in disagreement, or shake your head in disbelief if you do not understand the material. Regardless of your responses, please *react!* Get involved. This is the best way to learn about research.

The exercises at the end of the chapters are meant to help you get excited about research. Because most of you will not be conducting research while you are learning about the research process, exercises in class will help to simulate what it would be like if you were actually carrying out the steps of a study.

Material is presented in a very concrete manner. This book presents approximately 60 excerpts from recent studies published by nurses to illustrate various aspects of research. New terms are highlighted and defined the first time they are discussed. At the end of Chapters 3 through 15, a section is devoted to critiquing the specific step of the research process that each chapter addresses. Also, a set of critiquing questions is highlighted in a box for easy access. Each chapter concludes with a summary of the content presented in the chapter.

Two distinctive features of the book are the Get Involved Activities and the Self-Tests at the end of each chapter. Readers tell me that they like to see how well they perform on the self-tests. Answers to all questions are provided at the back of the book.

A new feature of the text is the inclusion of *Research on the Web*. This feature appears in each chapter, encouraging readers to go to the free Companion Website at www.prenhall.com/nieswiadomy to access the interactive, chapter-specific modules. Each module consists of a variety of critical thinking and other exercises, links to other online resources regarding nursing research, and objectives.

Instructors adopting this textbook have free access to the online Syllabus Manager™ feature of the Companion Website, www.prenhall.com/nieswiadomy. It offers a whole host of features that facilitate the students' use of the Companion Website, and allows faculty to post syllabi, course information, and assignments online for their students. Finally, online course management companions for **Foundations of Nursing Research, 4th Edition** are available for schools using Blackboard, Course Compass, or WebCT course management systems. The online course management solutions feature interactive modules and an electronic test bank for teaching this course content through distance learning. For more information and a demonstration of Syllabus Manager™ or Prentice Hall's online course companions, please contact your Prentice Hall Sales Representative.

Tell yourself that learning about nursing research can be interesting, fun, and exciting. Have a happy journey!

Rose Marie Nieswiadomy, PhD, RN

Acknowledgments

There are many people to thank as the fourth edition of this book is published. It is hard to believe that this is actually the fourth edition. When I first decided to write a research textbook in 1985, I never dreamed that I would be writing a fourth edition. The need for this type of book is evident by its continued use in this country and other English-speaking countries throughout the world.

I, once again, owe a debt of gratitude to the instructors who have chosen this book as the primary text for their research courses and to other instructors who have recommended it as a reference source for their students.

Kudos go to all of the students who have given this textbook good reviews. I have received many of their comments about how learner-friendly the book is and how it is one of the few textbooks that they have read from cover to cover. Of course, it helps that this textbook does not weigh 20 pounds, as do some of their other textbooks!

I am grateful that master's and doctoral level students also use this book. They tell me that this text presents the research process very clearly. When they review this book they achieve a greater recall and understanding of research.

Practicing nurses also receive my heartfelt thanks for having the courage to pick up a research textbook. It demonstrates their awareness of the importance of nursing research.

Connie Maxwell, librarian at Texas Woman's University, critiqued the chapter on the review of the literature. With her help, this chapter has been updated and revised extensively.

Many people at Prentice Hall Health deserve my thanks, especially Maura Connor, Executive Editor, who made the decision to publish another edition of this textbook. I am also very grateful to Beth Romph, Editorial Assistant, for her encouraging e-mails as the book material was being prepared.

My family, again, deserves much credit for my accomplishments. They have been very understanding as I have worked on book revisions. There were only three grandchildren at the time of the first edition. Now seven grandchildren keep our family gatherings lively. I am a "workaholic," but my family members have helped me to remember what is *really* important in life.

In the last two editions, I presented a way to pronounce my last name. I hope it was helpful to those readers, and I will present it again for you. The name is of Polish derivation. The i's are silent, and the accent is on the first syllable. The name is pronounced like: Ness' wah dough me. I might mention that some members of my husband's family pronounce the name differently, particularly those members who speak Polish. I apologize to them for my attempt to simplify the pronunciation of this difficult name.

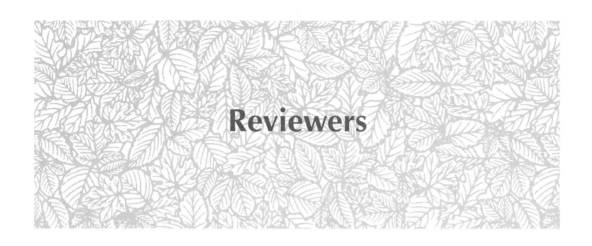

Reviewers

Marsha Bennett, DNS, APRN
Health Sciences Center HIV Outpatient
 Program Clinic
Louisiana State University
New Orleans, LA

L. Ellen Fineout-Overholt, PhD, RN
School of Nursing
University of Rochester
Rochester, NY

Barbara Holtzclaw, PhD, RN, FAAN
School of Nursing, Office of Nursing
 Research
University of Texas Health Sciences
 Center
San Antonio, TX

Jaya Jambunathan, PhD, RN
School of Nursing
University of Wisconsin
Oshkosh, WI

Doris Milton, PhD, RN
School of Nursing
University of Phoenix
Phoenix, AZ

Kay Palmer, MSN, RN, CRRN
School of Nursing
Old Dominion University
Norfolk, VA

Nancy A. Sowan, PhD, RN
School of Nursing
University of Vermont
Burlington, VT

Brenda Talley, PhD, RN, CNAA
School of Nursing
Georgia Southern University
Statesboro, GA

PART I

Introduction to Nursing Research

CHAPTER 1

Development of Nursing Research

❈ OBJECTIVES

On completion of this chapter, you will be prepared to:

1. Define nursing research
2. Identify sources of nursing knowledge
3. Describe scientific research
4. Compare two broad purposes for conducting research
5. Discuss four goals for conducting nursing research
6. Compare qualitative and quantitative research
7. Recognize the importance of outcomes research
8. Contrast the various roles of nurses in research
9. Recall some of the historic events in the development of nursing research
10. Determine priority areas for nursing research
11. Explain the significance of the National Institute of Nursing Research

✺ NEW TERMS DEFINED IN THIS CHAPTER

applied research
basic research
clinical nursing research
empirical data

nursing research
outcomes research
qualitative research
quantitative research

What is nursing research? If you were to walk outside right now and ask the first 10 people who passed by to answer this question, you probably would receive some strange answers. Most people are unaware that nurses conduct research.

Nursing research is frequently viewed as part of medical research. This appears to hold true even for highly educated members of society. A friend of mine (who has a master's degree in another field) described nursing research as "research that has to do with discovering new medications and treatments that are used, and things like that." I tried to explain to her that nursing research concerns nursing and things nurses do that are different from the actions of other disciplines. This does not mean that a nurse should not be involved in a study in which new drugs are being tested. But this type of study would be a medical rather than a nursing study. Nurses may be involved in interdisciplinary research, but to qualify as nursing research, a study should concern the unique realm of nursing.

The National League for Nursing (NLN) has recommended that all baccalaureate programs include research content in their curriculums. Florence Downs, editor of *Nursing Research,* wrote in 1996 that it has been a number of years since anyone has debated the need for research content in undergraduate curriculums. It is a given. However, she mentioned that she has received complaints from instructors stating that articles in *Nursing Research* contain "too many statistics and too many variables" and that most articles are too difficult for students to evaluate. Downs wrote that the days are over when we examined one variable at a time. She stated that research investigations and the reports of them have, indeed, become more complicated. However, she contended that nurses need to be able to understand research findings and the effects of these findings on practice. Downs further contended that this goal cannot be accomplished in a single research course.

IMPORTANCE OF NURSING RESEARCH

I'm sure you are trying to convince yourself that nursing research is important (or you wouldn't be reading this textbook!). You may be trying to meet the educational requirements for a baccalaureate degree or, as a registered nurse, someone has convinced you that you need more knowledge about research.

In the research classes that I teach, I try to do a "hard sell" on the first day of class. Sometimes the folded arms and facial expressions of students indicate that they are not convinced of the importance of learning about research. I try to help them understand that research knowledge will help them to be an excellent nurse. They are challenged to constantly question every intervention they perform or see performed. Questions to ask include: Am I performing this intervention because someone told me to or maybe even because this is the intervention that has *always* been used? What evidence exists that this is the most effective intervention for the problem? If an intervention is not based on research evidence, there is no way to determine that this intervention is the optimum one. I hope that your instructor or you, yourself, will not have to do a "hard sell" to convince you that research is of utmost importance to the nursing profession. I *promise* that your efforts to learn about nursing research will be rewarded in your nursing career in the future.

DEFINITIONS OF NURSING RESEARCH

There is some discrepancy among authors about the definition of nursing research. Polit and Hungler (1999) have broadly defined nursing research as "a systematic search for and validation of knowledge about issues of importance to the nursing profession" (p. 3). Burns and Grove (1997) defined nursing research as being concerned with knowledge that directly and indirectly influences clinical nursing practice. Several authors have defined nursing research in a narrower sense to indicate only research that concerns nursing care. Hott and Budin (1999) have written that in the strictest sense nursing research is concerned with nursing practice. Research in nursing education and research in nursing administration are seen as important, but these two types of research would be labeled as educational research in nursing and nursing administration research. Wilson and Hutchinson (1996) differentiated between nursing research and research in nursing. They indicated that nursing research is concerned with clinical problems, whereas research in nursing is the broader study of the nursing profession and includes historical, ethical, and political studies.

In this book, the term **nursing research** is defined as the systematic, objective process of analyzing phenomena of importance to nursing. Using this definition, nursing research includes all studies concerning nursing practice, nursing education, and nursing administration. Also, studies concerning nurses themselves are included in the broad category of nursing research. The term **clinical nursing research** will be used to indicate nursing research that involves clients or studies that have the potential for affecting the care of clients, such as studies with animals or with "normal" subjects.

To learn about nursing research and how to conduct research, it is important to gain an understanding of what scientific research is all about and why this method of gaining knowledge is valuable to nurses. The scientific method is only one source of nursing knowledge; however, it is generally considered to be the most reliable source of knowledge.

SOURCES OF NURSING KNOWLEDGE

Nurses have relied on several sources of knowledge to guide nursing practice. A great storehouse of knowledge for nurses has been tradition. Tradition involves the handing down of knowledge from one generation to another and leads to actions that occur because "we've always done it that way."

Another source of knowledge for nurses has been found in authority. Experts or authorities in a given field often provide knowledge for other people. In the past, nurses looked to physicians for a great deal of their practice knowledge. It has only been in recent years that nurses have begun to build a unique body of nursing knowledge.

Nurses have also used trial and error as a means of discovering knowledge. If one approach did not work, another one was used. Finally, when a certain approach was found to be effective, the trial-and-error process ceased. Frequently, the reasons behind the failure or success of a certain method were not determined. The goal was: "If it works, we'll use it."

The most objective and reliable source of nursing knowledge is obtained through disciplined research, according to Polit and Hungler (1999). They stated that research obtains knowledge that, although fallible, tends to be more reliable than knowledge obtained through tradition, authority, or experience.

SCIENTIFIC RESEARCH

Traditional scientific research is characterized by several features. The researcher uses systematic, orderly, and objective methods of seeking information. The scientific method uses **empirical data,** which are data gathered through the sense organs. Information is gained in the form of data or facts that are obtained in an unbiased manner from some aspect of the real world. The researcher tries to exercise as much control as possible over the research situation to minimize biased results. Various means of exercising such control will be discussed throughout this book. The researcher's opinions and personal biases should not influence the findings of a study.

There are many similarities between scientific research and the problem-solving approach that is familiar to all nurses. Both processes involve identifying a problem area, establishing a plan, collecting data, and evaluating the data. The purposes of these two activities are, however, quite different. Problem solving attempts to seek a solution to a problem that exists for a person or for persons in a given setting. The purpose of scientific research is much broader. It seeks to obtain knowledge that can be generalized to other people and to other settings. For example, the nursing staff might be concerned about the best approach to teaching Mrs. Smith, a blind patient, how to operate an insulin pump. This would be an example of an immediate problem that needs a solution. Scientific research, on the other hand, would be concerned with the best approach to use in teaching blind people, in general, how to operate insulin pumps. Scientific research is concerned with the ability to generalize research results.

PURPOSES OF NURSING RESEARCH

Research may be classified, according to the general purpose of the study, as basic and applied research. **Basic research** is concerned with generating new knowledge, while **applied research** is concerned with using knowledge to solve immediate problems. Basic research is also referred to as pure research.

The purpose of basic research according to Kerlinger (1986) is to test theory. Basic research is also used to generate new theories. Whether basic research seeks to generate or develop theories, immediate application of the results usually does not occur. In fact, years may pass before the social usefulness of the results of the research is determined or acknowledged. Basic research often uses laboratory animals as subjects.

McCarthy (2000) studied rats to determine factors that might influence food intake and gastric emptying when an infection is present. Interleukin-6 (IL-6) and tumor necrosis factor (TNF) were injected into a group of rats. Injection of TNF reduced food intake but did not affect gastric emptying. Injection of IL-6 reduced both food intake and gastric emptying. The researcher suggested that these findings may be helpful in the development of nutrition interventions for people with infections.

Applied research is directed toward generating knowledge that can be used in the near future. It is often conducted to seek solutions to immediate problems (Kerlinger, 1986; Polit & Hungler, 1999). It appears that the majority of nursing studies have been examples of applied research. Most of the studies cited in this text are examples of applied research.

The distinction between basic and applied research is really not as clear-cut as it may seem. Sometimes the findings of basic research are applied rather quickly in the clinical setting, whereas the findings of applied research actually lead to basic studies. A distinction between the two may be meaningless because of the overlap between the types. Many studies contain elements of both basic and applied research because theory is being tested that will have immediate implications for nursing. The distinction between basic and applied research may have more to do with financial support for the project than with the purpose of the study. In this sense, basic research may imply that the researcher is provided support to work on a particular project without having to indicate the immediate practical usefulness of the findings.

In the past, researchers in academic institutions have had the freedom to conduct basic research. Siegfried (1996) stated that science "has thrived on curiosity-driven research on topics chosen by individual researchers without immediate regard for practical applications" (p. 7D). He wrote that this system has produced understanding of human life and the universe. He contended that "saving money has begun to matter more than saving society, and science's financial fishbowl is shrinking" (p. 7D). Because of a decrease in government funding for basic research, investigators are seeking private funding. With private funding come special interest groups. Siegfried expressed the fear that science's previous tradition of academic freedom may shift to a private world of objectives and quality control.

Although nursing research is generally of the applied type, nurses are also finding it more difficult to receive funding for their research. To advance their likelihood of receiving funding in the managed care environment, Vessey (1996) called for nurse researchers to negotiate partnerships with managed care executives. She asserted that nurses need to demonstrate to these executives that by optimizing the health of individuals, the financial health of the corporation will be optimized as well. Baldwin and Nail (2000) contended that funding might depend on an investigator's ability to link his or her study to an organization's strategic goals.

GOALS FOR CONDUCTING NURSING RESEARCH

The importance of nursing research cannot be stressed enough. Some of the goals for conducting research are to produce (a) evidence-based nursing practice, (b) credibility of the nursing profession, (c) accountability for nursing practice, and (d) documentation of the cost-effectiveness of nursing care.

EVIDENCE-BASED NURSING PRACTICE

The major reason for conducting nursing research is to foster optimum care for clients. In the previous editions of this textbook, this section was titled "Improvements in Nursing Care." However, a decision was made to change the title because the term *evidence-based practice* is very popular today and is probably a term with which you are all familiar.

Evidence-based practice may be based on factors other than research findings, such as patient preferences and the expertise of clinicians; however, the aim of evidence-based practice is to provide the best possible care based on the best available research. O'Mathúna (2000) pointed out that critical pathways, clinical practice guidelines, and outcomes assessments are aspects of this trend. Books and articles are being written, and conferences are being held on evidence-based practice. The Sarah Cole Hirsh Institute for Best Nursing Practices Based on Evidence was established at the Frances Payne Bolton School of Nursing in 1998. Youngblut and Brooten (2000) expressed the hope that the recent emphasis on evidence-based practice in nursing and medicine will lead clinicians to look to the latest research finding to make practice improvements.

The nursing profession exists to provide a service to society, and this service should be based on accurate knowledge. Research has been determined to be the most reliable means of obtaining knowledge. As was previously mentioned, there are other means of acquiring knowledge, such as through tradition, authority, and trial and error. The scientific method, however, has been determined to be the most objective, systematic way of obtaining knowledge.

CREDIBILITY OF THE NURSING PROFESSION

In the past, nursing has frequently been thought of as a vocation rather than a profession. In fact, the struggle to gain professional status has been long and difficult. One of the criteria for a profession is the existence of a body of knowledge that is distinct from that of other disciplines. Nursing has traditionally borrowed knowledge from the natural and social sciences, and only in recent years have nurses concentrated on establishing a unique body of knowledge that would allow nursing to be clearly identified as a distinct profession. The most valid means of developing this knowledge base is scientific research. Through research, nurses can determine what it is that they do and how they do it that distinguishes them from other groups in the health care field.

Nurses must demonstrate to the general public that nursing makes a difference in the health status of people. If nurses cannot show what it is that is unique about their services, there will be no demand for these services.

ACCOUNTABILITY FOR NURSING PRACTICE

As nurses have become more independent in making decisions about the care of clients, their independence has brought about a greater need for accountability. There is an old saying that every privilege is accompanied by a corresponding duty. The privilege of being independent practitioners brings with it the duty of being accountable to those who are recipients of our care. Although nurses have generally been glad to achieve some degree of independence from the medical profession, in some ways life was easier when physicians were considered to be responsible for all aspects of health care. At that time, if a nurse made a medication error, the physician (and sometimes the hospital) was held responsible. The idea of a lawsuit being brought against a nurse was almost unthinkable. The general public has gained more knowledge of health care, and expectations of nurses as providers of care have increased.

To be accountable for their practice, nurses must have sound rationale for their actions, based on knowledge that is gained through scientific research. Nurses have the responsibility of keeping their knowledge base current, and one of the best sources of current knowledge is the research literature. The ability to critique research articles and determine findings that are appropriate for practice is a skill that is needed by all nurses.

DOCUMENTATION OF THE COST-EFFECTIVENESS OF NURSING CARE

Because of nursing's humanistic and altruistic tradition, it has been difficult for nurses to consider the cost-effectiveness of nursing care. The goal has been to help people achieve or maintain health, regardless of cost. But the reality of the health care picture has forced nurses to think in monetary terms. Some nurses are acquiring additional education in business and finance to help them better understand the financial aspects of health care. With the increased cost of health care, all disciplines within the health care field have been called on to demonstrate their value in a dollar and cents fashion.

Consumers have become more cognizant of the cost of health care and are asking for explanations of services they receive. These consumers need to be made aware of the importance of nursing care in relation to maintaining the health of well clients and in promoting the recovery and rehabilitation of ill clients.

Nursing services can consume a large percentage of a hospital's budget. With prospective payment systems determining the amount of reimbursements that hospitals receive, nursing care services are being closely examined. It is not difficult to determine that hospitals could cut costs by curtailing nursing services. If nursing care can be demonstrated to be cost-effective, hospitals will look to other sources for "cutting the fat." If effective nursing care can allow clients to leave hospitals in better condition and in less time than predicted, hospitals will make more profit or, in the case of nonprofit hospitals, lower their operating budgets. Unfortunately, only a small percentage of a hospital's budget is allocated for nursing research.

Many studies in the literature demonstrate the cost-effectiveness of nursing care. Ventura et al. (1985) conducted a study to examine the cost savings of nursing interventions with patients with peripheral vascular disease (PVD). The experimental group of patients was involved in health-promoting behaviors that involved increased exercise, improved foot care, and reduced smoking. It was determined that these patients required significantly fewer PVD-related hospitalizations and reported lower health care costs than the control group of patients. Inpatient hospitalization cost averaged $130 for patients in the experimental group and $2477 for the control group patients over a 20-week period.

Brooten et al. (1986) studied early hospital discharge and home follow-up care of very-low-birth-weight infants. They found that follow-up care by a nurse specialist is safe and cost-effective. This type of care potentially decreases iatrogenic illness and hospital-acquired infections, enhances parent-infant interaction, and significantly reduces hospital costs for care.

The cost of primary nursing and team nursing was examined by Gardner (1991). Primary nursing was found to both directly and indirectly reduce costs, when compared to team nursing.

Ferguson (1996) discussed the cost-effectiveness of a nurse practitioner-managed health care unit that was implemented in a meat packing/rendering plant in the northern United States. During the first 5 years (1988–1992) a net savings of over $1.3 million was realized in the cost of workers' compensation alone.

Rudy et al. (1996) reported on a study of chronically critically ill patients who were placed in a special care unit (SCU) or in an intensive care unit (ICU). They found significant cost savings for the SCU group. The average cost of delivering care in the SCU was $5000 less per patient than in the ICU.

The cost-savings of telephone nursing (TN) was reported by Greenberg (2000). Her study took place in a pediatric outpatient clinic setting in the Southwest. Results of 90 calls (25% of the calls for 1 month) were examined. The dollar savings for 1 month was estimated to be $2360. This figure was determined by subtracting the dollars ($2216) spent on actual outcomes from the dollars ($4576) that would have been spent based on outcomes without TN.

QUANTITATIVE AND QUALITATIVE RESEARCH

Nurse researchers conduct both quantitative and qualitative studies. **Quantitative research** is concerned with objectivity, tight controls over the research situation, and the ability to generalize findings. **Qualitative research** is concerned with the subjective meaning of an experience to an individual.

In the past, nurse researchers have primarily conducted quantitative research. Quantitative research has been the traditional scientific approach used by many of the other disciplines. Some people do not consider qualitative research to be scientific. Others view quantitative research as "hard science" and qualitative research as "soft science." Still others view both research approaches as scientific.

The number of researchers who are conducting qualitative research has increased. In 1985, Madeleine Leininger wrote that there were approximately 50 qualitative nurse researchers. Although the exact number of nurses conducting qualitative research today is not known, the numbers have increased dramatically.

Consider patients who are experiencing chronic pain. Quantitative research would be concerned with the level of pain that these people were experiencing, and qualitative research would be concerned with what it means to be living with chronic pain.

Quantitative research designs are presented in Chapter 8, and qualitative designs are covered in Chapter 9.

OUTCOMES RESEARCH

Just as evidence-based practice has become a popular term, outcomes research is a new buzzword that you will hear frequently. I like to think that nursing research has always been interested in outcomes, we just didn't give it that label.

Outcomes research focuses on measurable outcomes of interventions with certain patient populations. The increased interest in this type of studies is tied in with the high cost of health care. Health care policymakers, such as managed care organizations, want to know if the care that is being provided is cost-effective. Consumers also want to know if the services that they purchase will improve their health. Therefore, outcomes become very important.

Outcomes research has been placed in a separate category because the types of designs, methods, and sampling procedures used in these studies may be somewhat different from those used in the traditional quantitative or qualitative studies. For example, rather than exercising tight control over the sample, the goal might be to deliberately include a wide range of patients with varying levels of health status and comorbidities to determine how effective an intervention or treatment might be for this varied group of people. As outcomes research continues to emerge, you will want to seek further information in the latest clinical and research journals.

ROLES OF NURSES IN RESEARCH

The roles of nurses in research according to level of educational preparation were identified by the ANA's Council of Nurse Researchers in 1981 (Table 1–1). The guidelines have been revised slightly during the last 10 years. These guidelines, in the form of a position statement, can be found on the following Web site: http://www.nursingworld.org/readroom/position/research

The latest revisions of the guidelines have included postdoctoral preparation. Postdoctoral study involves agreements between novice researchers, usually with recent doctorates, and established investigators. These seasoned investigators agree to mentor the novices for a period of 2 or 3 years. Private and federal funding is available for postdoctoral preparation.

Overall, there are many roles that nurses can assume in association with research projects. Some of these include the following:

1. Principal investigator
2. Member of a research team
3. Identifier of researchable problems
4. Evaluator of research findings
5. User of research findings

6. Patient/client advocate during studies
7. Subject in studies

PRINCIPAL INVESTIGATOR

Nurses can and should serve as principal investigators in scientific investigations. To be a principal investigator, special research preparation is necessary. It might be possible for a beginning researcher to conduct a small-scale survey study, but preparation beyond the baccalaureate level is necessary for independent investigator status in most nursing research studies.

MEMBER OF A RESEARCH TEAM

Nurses can serve as members of a research team. They may act as data collectors or administer the experimental intervention of the study. As nurses increasingly participate in research, it is possible that interest and enthusiasm to conduct their own investigations may grow. In 1982, Rittenmeyer wrote that research will become a higher priority as knowledge of the benefits of research increases. She predicted that by 1990 research would be part of the nurse's normal workload. Unfortunately, the 20th century closed without her prediction coming true.

IDENTIFIER OF RESEARCHABLE PROBLEMS

All nurses, from associate degree to doctoral level prepared, have the responsibility of trying to identify areas of needed research (Table 1–1). Nurses at the bedside are particularly well situated to identify patient-related researchable problems.

EVALUATOR OF RESEARCH FINDINGS

Every nurse should be involved in the evaluation of research findings. As research consumers, nurses have the obligation to become familiar with research findings and determine the usefulness of these findings in the practice area. Beginning researchers should critique research articles, first with the help of an experienced researcher and eventually on their own, through the use of knowledge gained in a structured research course (either in their basic nursing education program or in a continuing education course). The evaluation of research is not an easy task. This book will help you acquire some of the skills needed to critique research articles and reports.

As evidence of the expectation that all nurses know how to evaluate research articles, Rankin and Esteves published an article in the *American Journal of Nursing* on critiquing research (1996). The reader could apply for continuing education hours by completing and returning the accompanying questionnaire. The article began by stating that many nurses do not feel confident that they can evaluate research articles. However, the authors cautioned against relying on the mass media to tell us what is important. Media discussions of research frequently lack the objectivity needed by nurses to determine if findings are appropriate for use in nursing practice.

TABLE 1–1. Investigative Functions of a Nurse at Various Educational Levels

Associate Degree in Nursing
1. Demonstrates awareness of the value or relevance of research in nursing.
2. Assists in identifying problem areas in nursing practice.
3. Assists in collection of data within an established structured format.

Baccalaureate in Nursing
1. Reads, interprets, and evaluates research for applicability to nursing practice.
2. Identifies nursing problems that need to be investigated and participates in the implementation of scientific studies.
3. Uses nursing practice as a means of gathering data for refining and extending practice.
4. Applies established findings of nursing and other health-related research to nursing practice.
5. Shares research findings with colleagues.

Master's Degree in Nursing
1. Analyzes and reformulates nursing practice problems so that scientific knowledge and scientific methods can be used to find solutions.
2. Enhances the quality and clinical relevance of nursing research by providing expertise in clinical problems and by providing knowledge about the way in which these clinical services are delivered.
3. Facilitates investigations of problems in clinical settings through such activities as contributing to a climate supportive of investigative activities, collaborating with others in investigations, and enhancing nursing's access to clients and data.
4. Conducts investigations for the purpose of monitoring the quality of the practice of nursing in a clinical setting.
5. Assists others to apply scientific knowledge in nursing practice.

Doctoral Degree in Nursing or a Related Discipline
1. Provides leadership for the integration of scientific knowledge with other sources of knowledge for the advancement of practice.
2. Conducts investigations to evaluate the contribution of nursing activities to the well-being of clients.
3. Develops methods to monitor the quality of the practice of nursing in a clinical setting and to evaluate contributions of nursing activities to the well-being of clients.

Graduate of a Research-Oriented Doctoral Program
1. Develops theoretical explanations of phenomena relevant to nursing by empirical research and analytic processes.
2. Uses analytical and empirical methods to discover ways to modify or extend existing scientific knowledge so that it is relevant to nursing.
3. Develops methods for scientific inquiry of phenomena relevant to nursing.

Reprinted with permission from *Guidelines for the Investigative Function of Nurses,* Washington DC: American Nurses Association, 1981.

USER OF RESEARCH FINDINGS

Through the years, nurses have tended to carry out nursing procedures and provide nursing care "the way we've always done it." Change is difficult to bring about, but research findings have no value if they are not put into use. After evaluating research findings, nurses should use relevant findings in their practice. The primary goal of nursing research, as has been mentioned, is the improved care of clients. However, nurses must be judicious in their use of research findings. The results of one small study conducted with a sample of 15 volunteers would not provide sufficient evidence for a change in nursing practice.

PATIENT/CLIENT ADVOCATE DURING STUDIES

All nurses have the responsibility to act as patient/client advocates when their patients/clients are involved in research. This advocacy involves making sure that the ethical aspects of research are upheld. Nurses might help answer questions and explain a study to potential participants before the study begins. They also might be available during the study to answer questions or provide support to study participants.

SUBJECT IN STUDIES

Nurses also can act as subjects in research. Many nurses (including myself) are involved in a long-term survey study, the Nurses' Health Study, which is being conducted by researchers at Harvard Medical School. The study was designed to examine some of the health risks that pose a special threat to women. Nurses were chosen as subjects, according to Frank Speizer, the principal investigator, because the study called for "a sophisticated group of individuals who could report exposure and diseases more accurately than the general population" ("Massive Nurses Health Study," 1983, p. 998). The study was begun in 1976 and was originally intended to last for 4 years, but additional funding has been received and the study has continued for more than 25 years. In 1989, a new cohort of younger nurses was added to the study in what is called Nurses' Health Study II. More than 300 publications have resulted from the data obtained in these studies.

HISTORY OF NURSING RESEARCH

Nursing research has been slow to develop in this country as well as in the rest of the world. Some of this slow growth is related to the development of nursing education. Despite her skill in independent scientific investigation, Florence Nightingale derived the foundation for modern nursing education from the military tradition, which emphasized the concept of authority. The authoritarian system of training was a deterrent to the development of inquiring minds (Simmons & Henderson, 1964). Schools of nursing throughout the world have been influenced by British nursing education and have continued to rely on tradition and authority, as did British schools.

Nursing research was able to develop and expand only as nurses received advanced educational preparation. The growth of nursing research seems to be directly related to the educational levels of nurses. Although the first university-based nursing program in the United States was begun in 1909, the number of such programs increased very slowly. In the early part of the 20th century, nurse leaders were more concerned with increasing the number of nurses and establishing hospital-affiliated nursing schools than with establishing university programs.

Because nurses were not prepared to conduct research, many of the early nursing studies were conducted by members of other disciplines. Beginning with the 1923 study, whose final report was titled the Goldmark Report, nonnurses became involved in studying nurses and nursing. Sociologists were particularly interested in the "learning, living, and working" experienced by nurses (Abdellah & Levine, 1965, p. 4). Research conducted by sociologists and behavioral scientists added to their respective bodies of knowledge but did not necessarily expand nursing's body of knowledge (Henderson, 1956).

As nurses received advanced educational preparation and became qualified to conduct research, many of the studies they carried out were in nursing education because most nurses, before 1950, received their advanced degrees in education. However, even during the early half of this century, the need for clinical nursing research was evident. In an article in the *American Journal of Nursing* in 1927, Marvin proposed many research questions involving procedures. What was the safest, simplest, quickest method of preparing a hypodermic? How long should the hands be scrubbed, by what method, and with what kind and strength of soap? By the 1950s, interest in nursing care studies began to rise. During the 1970s, particularly the last 5 years of that decade, practice-related research expanded rapidly.

Although Florence Nightingale recommended clinical nursing research in the mid-1800s, her advice was not followed by most nurses until over 100 years later. Some of the studies that she recommended, such as those concerning environmental health hazards, are being conducted today. Only recently has Nightingale come to be appreciated for the truly extraordinary woman that she was. If nurses had begun sooner to follow the example of their first leader, nursing would be much further along in establishing a body of nursing knowledge. However, there is reason for optimism at this time. Both the number and the quality of nursing studies have increased dramatically.

There are many noteworthy events in the historical development of nursing research. Some of the more important events are highlighted.

- *1850s:* Florence Nightingale studied nursing care during the Crimean War. She called for research that focused on nursing practice. Nightingale admonished nurses to develop the habit of systematically making and recording observations. She recorded observations in a systematic way and used statistics to clearly illustrate her findings.

- *1902:* Lavinia Dock reported a school nurse "experiment" that was begun by Lillian Wald. Nurses gave free care to schoolchildren and visited the homes of sick children.

- *1906:* Adelaide Nutting conducted a survey of the educational status of nursing.

- *1909:* The first university-based nursing program was established at the University of Minnesota.

- *1923:* A well-known study of nursing and nursing education was conducted by the Committee for the Study of Nursing Education and funded by the Rockefeller Foundation. This study is frequently referred to as the Goldmark Report. The study recommended advanced educational preparation for teachers, administrators, and public health nurses and was instrumental in the establishment of early collegiate nursing schools at Yale, Vanderbilt, and Western Reserve.

- *1924:* The first doctoral program for nurses was established in 1924 at Teachers College, Columbia University. The Ed.D. degree was offered to nurses preparing to teach at the college level.

- *1927:* Jean Broadhurst and her colleagues reported a research investigation on hand-washing procedures.

  Edith S. Bryan became the first nurse to earn a doctoral degree when she received a Ph.D. in psychology and counseling from Johns Hopkins University.

- *1928:* Ethel Johns and Blanche Pfefferkorn published a study concerning the activities in which nurses were involved. This study was one of the first of many studies that focused on nurses.

- *1932:* Elizabeth Ryan and Virginia B. Miller investigated thermometer-disinfecting techniques.

- *1936:* Sigma Theta Tau, National Honor Society for Nursing, began funding nursing research.

- *1948:* Esther Lucille Brown, a social anthropologist, published her famous study on nursing education. Titled *Nursing for the Future,* this study called for nursing education to take place in university settings. One of the major recommendations of this study was that hospitals should hire enough permanent staff so that nursing students would not be required to staff these institutions. The Brown Report, as the study was called, recommended research in nursing and pointed to the need for nurse educators to be involved in research.

  Doris Schwartz documented the effectiveness of nursing care for inducing sleep in patients and for decreasing their intake of medications.

- *1949:* The Division of Nursing Resources was organized within the U.S. Public Health Service.

  Esta H. McNett demonstrated the usefulness of masks in preventing the spread of tuberculosis.

- *1952:* The first issue of *Nursing Research* was published.

- *1953:* The Institute of Research and Service in Nursing Education was founded at Teachers College, Columbia University. This unit had a full-time staff involved in the study of nursing and nursing education.

- *1955:* The American Nurses Foundation was established with the goal of promoting high-level wellness and the improvement of patient care. This foundation provides funds for nursing research.

  The Nursing Research Grants and Fellowship Programs were established by the U.S. Public Health Service.

- *1957:* The first unit directed primarily toward research in nursing practice was established at the Department of Nursing of the Walter Reed Army Institute of Research.

The Western Council for Higher Education in Nursing (WCHEN) sponsored a nursing research conference at the University of Colorado.

- *1962:* The federally supported Nurse Scientist Graduate Training Grants Programs were begun.

- *1963:* Lydia Hall published her 5-year study of chronically ill patients who were cared for at the Loeb Center in New York.

- *1970:* The National Commission for the Study of Nursing and Nursing Education, established by the American Nurses Association (ANA) and the National League for Nursing (NLN), published the results of a 3-year study on nursing. The report, titled *An Abstract for Action,* was popularly called the Lysaught Report, after Jerome Lysaught, director of the project. One of the recommendations of the report was that research be financed in both nursing practice and nursing education.

A center for nursing research was established at Wayne State University.

- *1972:* The ANA established a Department of Nursing Research.

- *1974:* At its national convention, the ANA delineated nursing practice as the area to which nursing research should be directed in the next decade.

- *1976:* The Commission on Nursing Research of the ANA recommended that research preparation be included in undergraduate, graduate, and continuing education programs.

- *1977:* The Veterans Administration began employing nurse researchers.

- *1978:* The first issue of *Research in Nursing and Health* was published.

- *1979:* The first issue of *Western Journal of Nursing Research* was published.

- *1980:* The Commission on Nursing Research of the ANA set up a list of research priorities for the 1980s.

- *1982:* Eleven volumes were published of the work of the Conduct and Utilization of Research in Nursing (CURN) project.

- *1983:* The first Center for Nursing Research was established. It encompassed the American Nurses Foundation and the American Academy of Nursing.

- *1986:* The National Center for Nursing Research (NCNR) was established within the National Institutes of Health.

- *1987:* Dr. Ada Hinshaw, Director of the NCNR called for nursing organizations to identify their research priorities.

- *1988:* The National Center for Nursing Research convened the first Conference on Research Priorities (CORP #1) to establish research priorities through 1994.

The first issues of *Applied Nursing Research* and *Nursing Science Quarterly* were published.

- *1992:* The first issue of *Clinical Nursing Research* was published.

- *1993:* The National Institute of Nursing Research (NINR) was established within the National Institutes of Health. This organization replaced the NCNR.

The second Conference on Research Priorities (CORP #2) was held to establish research priorities for 1995–1999.

- *1994:* The first issue of *Qualitative Nursing Research* was published.
- *1997:* The International Council of Nurses convened a group of experts to establish world-wide nursing research priorities.
- *1999:* The first issue of *Biological Research for Nursing* was published.
- *2001:* The budget for NINR reached almost $90 million.

RESEARCH PRIORITIES FOR THE FUTURE

Professional nursing organizations and individual nurse leaders are united in identifying the need for research that will help to build a scientific knowledge base for nursing practice. In 1980, the ANA Commission on Nursing Research identified priorities for nursing research. These priorities included research concerned with health promotion and preventive health practices for all age groups, health care needs of high-risk groups, life satisfaction of individuals and families, and the development of cost-effective health care systems.

In 1985, the ANA Cabinet on Nursing Research identified 10 priority areas. These included: (a) to promote health, well-being, and the ability to care for oneself among all age, social, and cultural groups; (b) to minimize or prevent behaviorally and environmentally induced health problems that compromise the quality of life and reduce productivity; and (c) to minimize the negative effects of new health technologies on the adaptive abilities of individuals and families experiencing acute or chronic health problems.

In November 1987, Dr. Ada Sue Hinshaw, director of the National Center for Nursing Research (NCNR) invited nursing organizations to identify their research priorities. Since that time, many nursing organizations have conducted surveys of their membership to determine research priorities.

Research priorities for people with Alzheimer's disease were identified at a research conference held in 1988 (Duffey, Hepburn, Christensen, & Brugge-Wiger, 1989). The top priority was given to research on the management of physical problems (i.e., incontinence of bowel and bladder, falls, sleep disturbance, gait disturbance, maintenance of adequate nutrition). Management of disruptive behaviors (i.e., agitation, wandering) was listed as the second priority.

Priorities for acquired immunodeficiency syndrome (AIDS) research were identified by a panel of 104 nurse experts in the field of human immunodeficiency virus (HIV)/AIDS (Benedict, 1990). Pain and symptom management were ranked the highest priority. Maintaining wellness ranked second. The third priority was identified as educational strategies for at-risk groups. Sowell (2000) reported on a more recent study of nurses in AIDS care. A Delphi survey was conducted with 700 nurses who were members of the Association of Nurses in AIDS Care (ANAC). Some of the priorities identified in this study were symptom management, community-level HIV education and prevention, quality of life issues in chronic HIV disease, HIV prevention focusing on individual or specific group behavior, and research related to adherence to drug therapy.

The National Association of Orthopaedic Nurses identified a list of priorities in 1990 (Salmond, 1994). They used a Delphi technique to survey experts in the field. Some of the highest ratings were given to preventing confusion in elderly patients post-hip fracture, determining the most effective safety measures to use with the patient with acute confu-sional state, and differentiating pain responses according to diagnoses, ages, and pain management interventions. In 1997, Sedlak, Ross, Arslanian, and Taggart (1998) repli-cated the 1990 study. Their respondents expressed the need for more research on pain and patient complications, such as deep vein thrombosis (DVT). The authors expressed some concern about this particular priority because of the large amount of published research on DVT. Sedlak et al. called for an ongoing and wider dissemination of research results.

In 1995, a list of research priorities was published by the Oncology Nursing Society (ONS) (Stetz, Haberman, Holcombe, & Jones, 1995). These priorities were generated by sending questionnaires to a random sample of ONS members. Responses were received from 789 (36% response rate). The top five priorities were pain, prevention activities, quality of life, risk reduction/screening, and ethical issues.

In 1999, Pullen, Tuck, and Wallace published a list of priorities in mental health nursing. These priorities were obtained by examining the published literature from 1990 to 1996. No specific mental health nursing agenda was found. Six broad categories were identified: support, holism, mental health nursing practice, quality care outcomes, mental health etiology, and mental health delivery systems. These authors cautioned that as nurs-ing promotes evidence-based practice, there is a need for clear research priorities. They called for mental health nursing experts and organizations to propose a national-interna-tional mental health research agenda.

Although clinical nursing research is essential for the profession, other types of re-search are also needed. Grier (1982) decried that patient care research had become the "sacred cow" for nursing research. Brown, Tanner, and Padrick (1984) have written that research regarding nurse characteristics, nursing education, and nursing administration should not be abandoned because these factors affect the care that nurses provide. Abdel-lah and Levine (1994) are two other authors who have called for studies other than clini-cal studies. They wrote that we need reliable tests to predict clinical performance by students and research on occupational choice in longitudinal studies. Fitzpatrick (1999) contended that nursing education research should receive the same recognition as clinical research. She mentioned the pressure in recent years to transform nursing educational pro-grams to meet changing health care needs and contended that any changes should be based on research.

Replication studies should be a high priority for nursing research. This is particularly true for clinical nursing research. Because of the small, nonrandom samples used in many studies, nurses need to conduct many similar studies on the same topic to allow for gener-alization of findings. Nursing studies have generally been one-of-a-kind, with few replica-tion or extension studies. It is rare that a single study is a sufficient foundation for making decisions about nursing practice (Martin, 1995).

NATIONAL INSTITUTE OF NURSING RESEARCH

The National Institute of Nursing Research (NINR) (www.nursingsociety.org) was officially established within the National Institutes of Health (NIH) on June 14, 1993. It replaced the National Center for Nursing Research (NCNR), which had been established in 1986. With the creation of the NINR, nursing research received a big boost in respectability. Funding for nursing research has increased a great deal. In 1986, the NCNR had a budget of $16 million. In 1995, the NINR received an appropriation of close to $50 million. By 2001, funding had been increased to almost $90 million.

Patricia Grady, Director of the NINR, considers the mission of this institute to be very challenging (Grady, 1996). According to Grady, the mission includes reducing the burden of illness and disability, improving health-related quality of life, and improving clinical environments. In testimony before the House Appropriations Subcommittee on March 2, 2000, Grady emphasized, "It is critical that nursing research grow to meet the present and future health care needs of Americans" (Grady, 2000, p. 127).

The NINR has convened two meetings held 5 years apart (1988 and 1993) titled "Conference on Research Priorities in Nursing Science." These conferences have been known as CORP #1 and CORP #2. The 1988 meeting set priorities for 1989 to 1994. Some of the high priority areas were low-birth-weight infants, HIV infection, and nursing informatics. The 1993 conference set priorities for 1995–1999. These priorities included research on living with chronic illness, interventions to promote immunocompetence, approaches to remediate cognitive impairment, and nursing interventions in HIV/AIDS.

In recent years, the decision was to made to include a wider variety of participants in planning research priorities (National Institute of Nursing Research, 2000a). Planning now involves more frequent meetings of smaller groups. These groups include nurse researchers, representatives of other NIH Institutes, and experts from the multidisciplinary community of scientists and health care professionals.

In 2000, the NINR joined with more than 50 societies that represent the behavioral and social sciences to usher in the "Decade of Behavior: 2000-2010." This broad-based research and public policy initiative focuses on improving health, education, and safety (National Institute of Nursing Research, 2000b). This goal shall be achieved by (a) promoting the application of behavioral and social science research to major national challenges, (b) enhancing the ability of these sciences to address major societal challenges and formulating a strategy for training the next generation of scientists, and (c) educating the public, federal policy makers, and lawmakers on the value of the behavioral and social sciences. For more information on the Decade of Behavior visit the following Web site: http://www.decadeofbehavior.org

SUMMARY

Nursing research is defined as the systematic, objective process of analyzing phenomena of importance to nursing. It includes studies concerning nursing practice, nursing education, nursing administration, and nurses themselves. **Clinical nursing research** is research that has the potential for affecting the care of clients.

Nursing knowledge has come from tradition, authority, trial and error, and scientific research. Scientific research uses **empirical data** (data gathered through the senses) and is a systematic, orderly, and objective method of seeking information.

Basic research, which is also called pure research, is concerned with generating new knowledge; **applied research** seeks solutions to immediate problems. Most nursing studies have been applied research. Many studies, however, contain elements of both basic and applied research.

The most important goals for conducting nursing research are the production of evidence-based nursing practice, credibility of the nursing profession, accountability for nursing practice, and documentation of the cost-effectiveness of nursing care.

Quantitative research is concerned with objectivity, tight controls over the research situation, and the ability to generalize findings. **Qualitative research** is concerned with the subjective meaning of an experience to an individual. **Outcomes research** focuses on measurable outcomes of interventions with certain patient populations.

Nurses can act as principal investigators, members of research teams, identifiers of researchable problems, evaluators of research findings, users of research findings, client advocates during studies, and subjects in research.

Because nurses were not prepared to conduct research, many of the early nursing studies were conducted by members of other disciplines. Some of these studies, such as the Goldmark Report in 1923 and the Brown Report in 1948, contributed important information about nursing and nursing education. As nurses began to receive advanced degrees, these degrees were generally in the field of education. Many of the studies conducted by the first nurse researchers in this country were therefore in the area of nursing education. Although Florence Nightingale recommended clinical nursing research in the mid-1800s, this type of research was scarce until the 1970s.

Many nursing organizations have identified clinical nursing research priorities for the future. The National Institute of Nursing is being provided with increased funds for nursing research.

NURSING RESEARCH ON THE WEB

For additional online resources, research activities, and exercises, go to www.prenhall. com/nieswiadomy. Select Chapter 1 from the drop down menu.

✄ GET INVOLVED ACTIVITIES

1. Divide into two debate teams. One team will be **for** the issue "Nearly all nursing research should be *clinical* research." The other team will be **against** the issue.

2. The fifth function or expectation of baccalaureate-prepared nurses that was identified by the ANA is "Shares research findings with colleagues." Think of five methods of carrying out this expectation, either at school or at work.

3. Express to your peers your greatest fears about critiquing research articles.

4. Share with your colleagues how you will decide if you should use research findings in your practice.

5. A philanthropist puts a note on the bulletin board at your school or work setting. She wrote that she is willing to fund a $200,000 nursing study in the name of her deceased mother who was cared for by "wonderful nurses." She is asking for suggestions. What **one** study would you suggest?

✖ SELF-TEST

Circle the letter before the *best* answer.

1. The most objective means of obtaining nursing knowledge is through:
   A. trial and error.
   B. tradition.
   C. scientific research.
   D. authority.

2. Which of the following statements concerning nursing research is true?
   A. The scientific base for nursing practice expanded greatly in the first half of this century.
   B. The majority of nursing studies before 1950 focused on clinical problems.
   C. Many studies have focused on nurses themselves.
   D. The first nursing investigations were conducted in the United States.

3. The major reason for conducting nursing research is to:
   A. improve nursing care for clients.
   B. promote the growth of the nursing profession.
   C. document the cost-effectiveness of nursing care.
   D. ensure accountability for nursing practice.

4. Which of the following is generally true concerning the knowledge base for nursing?
   A. Most of the knowledge that has been used by nurses was developed by nurses.
   B. Most of the knowledge that has been used by nurses was developed by members of other disciplines.
   C. Nurses have used knowledge developed by nurses and by members of other disciplines in fairly even proportions.

5. Which of the following roles of the nurse in research is *least* appropriate for the beginning researcher?
   A. principal investigator
   B. evaluator of research findings
   C. user of research findings
   D. participant in studies
   E. identifier of researchable problems

6. As nurses first began to receive advanced educational preparation and became qualified to conduct research, many of their studies concerned:
   A. nursing education.
   B. characteristics of nurses.
   C. nursing administration.
   D. nursing care.

7. The emphasis on clinical nursing research expanded rapidly in the:
   A. 1930s.
   B. 1940s.

C. 1950s.

D. 1960s.

E. 1970s.

8. The first journal devoted primarily to the publication of nursing research was:

A. *Nursing Research.*

B. *Research in Nursing and Health.*

C. *Applied Nursing Research.*

D. *American Journal of Nursing.*

9. Nursing leaders have called for research focusing on which of the following topics?

A. quality of life

B. wound healing

C. living with chronic illness

D. cognitive impairment

E. all of the above

10. Which of the following agencies is most influential, at the present time, in funding nursing research?

A. American Nurses Association

B. National Center for Nursing Research

C. National Institute of Nursing Research

D. Sigma Theta Tau International, Honor Society for Nursing

✖ REFERENCES

Abdellah, F. G., & Levine, E. (1965). *Better patient care through nursing research.* New York: Macmillan.

Abdellah, F. G., & Levine, E. (1994). *Preparing nursing research for the 21st century.* New York: Springer.

American Nurses' Association Commission on Nursing Research (1980). Generating a scientific basis for nursing practice: Research priorities for the 1980s. *Nursing Research, 29,* 219.

Baldwin, K. M., & Nail, L. M. (2000). Opportunities and challenges in clinical nursing research. *Journal of Nursing Scholarship, 32,* 163–166.

Benedict, S. (1990). Nursing research priorities related to HIV/AIDS. *Oncology Nursing Forum, 17,* 571–573.

Broadhurst, J. (1927). Hand brush suggestions for visiting nurses. *Public Health Nursing, 19,* 487–489.

Brooten, D., Kumar, S., Brown, L. P., Butts, P., Finkler, S. A., Bakewell-Sachs, S., Gibbons, A., & Delivoria-Papadopoulos, M. (1986). A randomized clinical trial of early hospital discharge and home follow-up of very-low-birth-weight infants. *New England Journal of Medicine, 315,* 934–939.

Brown, E. (1948). *Nursing for the future.* New York: Russell Sage.

Brown, J., Tanner, C., & Padrick, K. (1984). Nursing's search for scientific knowledge. *Nursing Research, 33,* 26–32.

Burns, N., & Grove, S. (1997). *The practice of nursing research: Conduct, critique and utilization* (3rd ed.). Philadelphia: Saunders.

Committee for the Study of Nursing Education. (1923). *Nursing and nursing education in the United States.* New York: Macmillan.

Dock, L. (1902). School nurse experiment in New York. *American Journal of Nursing, 3,* 108–110.

Downs, F. S. (1996). Research as a survival technique (editorial). *Nursing Research, 45,* 323.

Duffey, L., Hepburn, K., Christensen, R., & Brugge-Wiger, P. (1989). A research agenda in care for patients with Alzheimer's disease. *Image: Journal of Nursing Scholarship, 21,* 254–257.

Ferguson, L. A. (1996). Enhancing health care to underserved populations. *AAOHN Journal, 44,* 332–335.

Fitzpatrick, J. J. (1999). Lateness is not greatness. *Nursing and Health Care Perspectives, 20,* 231.

Gardner, K. (1991). A summary of findings of a five-year comparison study of primary and team nursing. *Nursing Research, 40,* 113–117.

Grady, P. A. (1996). Landmark anniversary for nursing research at the National Institutes of Health. *Image: Journal of Nursing Scholarship, 28,* 4–5.

Grady, P. A. (2000). News from NINR. *Nursing Outlook, 48,* 127.

Greenberg, M. E. (2000). Telephone nursing: Evidence of client and organizational benefits. *Nursing Economics, 18,* 117–123.

Grier, M. (1982). Editorial. *Research in Nursing and Health, 5,* 111.

Hall, L. (1963). A center for nursing. *Nursing Outlook, 11,* 805–806.

Henderson, V. (1956). Research in nursing practice—when? *Nursing Research, 4,* 99.

Hott, J. R., & Budin, W. C. (1999). *Notter's essentials of nursing research* (6th ed.). New York: Springer.

Johns, E., & Pfefferkorn, B. (1928). *An activity analysis of nursing.* New York: Committee on the Grading of Nursing Schools.

Kerlinger, F. (1986). *Foundations of behavioral research* (3rd ed.). New York: Holt, Rinehart & Winston.

Leininger, M. M. (1985). *Qualitative research methods in nursing.* Orlando, FL: Grune & Stratton.

Lysaught, J. (1970). *An abstract for action.* New York: McGraw-Hill.

Martin, P. A. (1995). More replication studies needed. *Applied Nursing Research, 8,* 102–103.

Marvin, M. (1927). Research in nursing. *American Journal of Nursing, 27,* 331–335.

Massive nurses' health study in seventh year, reports first findings on disease links in women (1983). *American Journal of Nursing, 83,* 998–999.

McCarthy, D. O. (2000). Tumor necrosis factor alpha and Interleukin-6 have differential effects on food intake and gastric emptying in fasted rats. *Research in Nursing & Health, 23,* 222–228.

McNett, E. (1949). The face mask in tuberculosis. *American Journal of Nursing, 49,* 32–36.

O'Mathúna, D. P. (2000). Evidence-based practice and reviews of therapeutic touch. *Journal of Nursing Scholarship, 32,* 279–285.

National Institute of Nursing Research (2000a). *Mission statement. Retrieved October 12, 2000 from the World Wide Web: http//www.nih.gov/ninr/a_mission.html*

National Institute of Nursing Research. (2000b). *NINR and the "Decade of Behavior" Initiative.* Retrieved September 24, 2000 from the World Wide Web: http://www.nih.gov.ninr/press/decade.html

Polit, D. F., & Hungler, B. E. (1999). *Nursing research: Principles and methods* (6th ed.). Philadelphia: Lippincott.

Rankin, M. & Esteves, M. D. (1996). How to assess a research study. *American Journal of Nursing, 96,* 33–36.

Pullen, L., Tuck, I., & Wallace, D. C. (1999). Research priorities in mental health nursing. *Issues in Mental Health Nursing, 20,* 217–227.

Rittenmeyer, P. (1982). The evolution of nursing research. *Western Journal of Nursing Research, 4,* 223–225.

Rudy, E. B., Daly, B. J., Douglas, S., Montenegro, H. D., Song, R., & Dyer, M. A. (1996). Patient outcomes for the chronically critically ill: Special care unit versus intensive care unit. *Nursing Research, 44,* 324–331.

Ryan, E., & Miller, V. (1932). Disinfection of clinical thermometers: Bacteriological study and estimated costs. *American Journal of Nursing, 32,* 197–206.

Salmond, S. W. (1994). Orthopaedic nursing research priorities: A delphi study. *Orthopaedic Nursing, 13,* 31–45.

Schwartz, D. R. (1948). Nursing care can be measured. *American Journal of Nursing, 48,* 149.

Sedlak, C., Ross, D., Arslanian, C., & Taggart, H. (1998). Orthopaedic nursing research priorities: A replication and extension. *Orthopaedic Nursing, 17*(2), 51–58.

Siegfried, T. (1996, September 9). Shift to private funds means changes in scientific culture. *The Dallas Morning News,* p. 7D.

Simmons, L. W., & Henderson, V. (1964). *Nursing research—A survey and assessment.* New York: Appleton-Century-Crofts.

Sowell, R. L. (2000). Identifying HIV/AIDS research priorities for the next millennium: A Delphi study with nurses in AIDS care. *Journal of the Association of Nurses in AIDS Care, 11*(3), 42–52.

Stetz, K. M., Haberman, M. R., Holcombe, J., & Jones, L. S. (1995). 1994 Oncology Nursing Society research priorities survey. *Oncology Nursing Forum, 22,* 785–789.

Ventura, M., Young, D., Feldman, M., Pastore, P., Pikula, S., & Yates, M. (1985). Cost savings as an indicator of successful nursing intervention. *Nursing Research, 34,* 50–53.

Vessey, J. (1996). The bottom line. *Nursing Research, 45,* 67.

Youngblut, J. M., & Brooten, D. (2000). Moving research into practice: A new partner. *Nursing Outlook, 48*(2), 55–56.

Wilson, H. S., & Hutchinson, S. A. (1996). *Consumer's guide to nursing research.* Albany, NY: Delmar.

CHAPTER 2

An Overview of Quantitative Research

OUTLINE

Steps in Quantitative Research
- Identify the Problem
- Determine the Purpose of the Study
- Review the Literature
- Develop a Theoretical/Conceptual Framework
- Identify the Study Assumptions
- Acknowledge the Limitations of the Study
- Formulate the Hypothesis or Research Question
- Define Study Variables/Terms
- Select the Research Design
- Identify the Population
- Select the Sample
- Conduct a Pilot Study
- Collect the Data
- Organize the Data for Analysis
- Analyze the Data
- Interpret the Findings
- Communicate the Findings

Summary
Nursing Research on the Web
Get Involved Activities
Self-test

OBJECTIVES

On completion of this chapter, you will be prepared to:

1. List the steps in conducting quantitative research
2. Discuss the steps in quantitative research

NEW TERMS DEFINED IN THIS CHAPTER

accessible population
assumptions
data
dependent variable
hypothesis
independent variable
limitations
operational definition
pilot study
population
research design
sample
target population
variable

What is nursing research? How do you do it? This chapter will help answer some of your questions about quantitative nursing research. At this point, try to get a general, overall picture of this type of research. Most quantitative studies follow the same steps. As you progress through this book, these steps will become clearer. Each of the steps in conducting a quantitative study will be elaborated on in other chapters. Chapter 9 discusses qualitative research designs. The steps in conducting qualitative research are more variable and depend on the type of qualitative design that is being used.

STEPS IN QUANTITATIVE RESEARCH

Nearly every author refers to the formulation of the research problem as the first step and the communication of research results as the final step in scientific quantitative research. There is some variation in the other steps. Some authors combine several steps into one step, which accounts for the smaller numbers of steps identified by some sources. Both Dempsey and Dempsey (2000) and Wilson and Hutchinson (1996) identified 10 steps. Burns and Grove (1997) listed 13 steps. Polit and Hungler (1999) identified 16 steps. This text presents 17 steps.

There can be some overlapping of the steps in the research process and some shifting back and forth between the steps. In general, however, the scientific research process proceeds in an orderly fashion and consists of the steps identified in Table 2–1.

TABLE 2–1. Steps in the Research Process

Identify the problem
Determine the purpose of the study
Review the literature
Develop a theoretical/conceptual framework
Identify the study assumptions
Acknowledge the limitations of the study
Formulate the hypothesis or research question
Define study variables/terms
Select the research design
Identify the population
Select the sample
Conduct a pilot study
Collect the data
Organize the data for analysis
Analyze the data
Interpret the findings
Communicate the findings

IDENTIFY THE PROBLEM

The first step, and one of the most important steps, in the research process is to clearly identify the problem that will be studied. Generally, a broad topic area is selected, and then the topic is narrowed down to a specific one-sentence statement of the problem. This step of the research process may be the most difficult of all and may take a great deal of time. Martin (1994) contended that a "good" problem statement helps the researcher to move through the steps of the research process. The identification of nursing research problems is discussed in Chapter 4.

Study problems can be identified from personal experiences, from literature sources, from previous research, or through the testing of theories. The problem should be of interest to the researcher and be significant to nursing.

The problem of the study is best stated as a question. Questions demand answers. The problem statement should specify the population and the variables that are being studied. A **variable** is a characteristic or attribute that differs among the persons, objects, events, and so forth that are being studied (e.g., age, blood type). An example of a problem statement might be: Is there a correlation between body image and self-esteem levels of women who have experienced a mastectomy?

DETERMINE THE PURPOSE OF THE STUDY

Although the term *purpose* is often used interchangeably with *problem,* a distinction can be made between these two terms. The problem statement addresses *what* will be studied; the purpose furnishes *why* the study is being done. There must be a sound rationale or justification for every research project. Some studies are viewed as inconsequential and wasteful of time and money. The researcher must make explicit the expectations for the use of the study results. If the purpose of a study is clearly presented and justified, the researcher will be much more likely to receive approval for the study and also will be more likely to obtain subjects for the study.

Consider the problem statement concerning body image and self-esteem levels of women who have undergone a mastectomy. A study to examine these variables might have the following purpose: to develop a better understanding of the difficulties experienced by women after loss of a body part that is closely associated with their feminine identity.

REVIEW THE LITERATURE

Research should build on previous knowledge. Before beginning a quantitative study, it is important to determine what knowledge exists of the study topic. There are few topics about which there is no existing knowledge base. There are many routes of access to the published literature. Literature sources can be located through the library card catalog, indexes, abstracts, and computer-assisted searches. Material on reviewing the literature is presented in Chapter 5.

Besides determining the extent of the existing knowledge related to the study topic, the review of the literature will also help to develop a theoretical or conceptual framework for a study. Finally, the review of the literature can help the researcher plan study methods. Instruments or tools may be discovered that can be used to measure the study variables. The researcher will be able to profit from the successes and failures of other researchers.

One visit to the library or one session of surfing the Web is not sufficient for a good review of the literature. The review should be continued during the course of the investigation until the time of data collection. This ensures the researcher that she or he has as much information as possible and the most up-to-date information on the study topic.

Occasionally, the initial review of the literature may actually precede the identification of the problem. The problem area may be determined from the suggestions or recommendations of researchers who have conducted previous studies in the area of interest.

DEVELOP A THEORETICAL/CONCEPTUAL FRAMEWORK

The goal of research is to develop scientific knowledge. Research and theory are intertwined. Research can test theories as well as help to develop and refine theories. Thus, theoretical frameworks are a valuable part of scientific research (see Chapter 6). The theoretical or conceptual framework will assist in the selection of the study variables and in defining them. The framework also will direct the hypothesis(es) and the interpretation of the findings. In an editorial in *Nursing Research,* Downs (1994) stated that a "study that lacks a theoretical rationale lacks substance and fails to answer the 'so what' question" (p. 195).

Some research of a purely descriptive nature may not require a theoretical framework. Most nursing studies can profit, however, from the identification of a framework for the study. An examination of recently published nursing studies shows that increasing numbers of these studies are based on a clearly identified theoretical framework. Research that is conducted within the context of a theoretical framework, compared to research that is not theory based, is more valuable in providing understanding and knowledge that can be used in the future. Research without theory provides a set of isolated facts.

Nursing has been viewed as an applied science and has relied on the theories of other disciplines. Nurse researchers are developing theories and beginning to build a body of nursing knowledge (see Chapter 6). Because the process is slow, nurses continue to use many theories from other disciplines.

IDENTIFY THE STUDY ASSUMPTIONS

Assumptions are beliefs that are held to be true but have not necessarily been proven. Each scientific investigation is based on assumptions. These assumptions should be stated explicitly. Frequently, however, the assumptions are implicit. This means that the study was based on certain assumptions but the researcher did not openly acknowledge or list these assumptions. Study assumptions influence the questions that are asked, the data that are gathered, the methods used to gather the data, and the interpretation of the data (Myers, 1982).

Assumptions are of three types: (a) universal assumptions, (b) assumptions based on theory or research findings, and (c) assumptions that are necessary to carry out the study. Universal assumptions are beliefs that are assumed to be true by a large percentage of society; for example, all human beings need love. Assumptions also may be derived from theory or previous research. If a study is based on a certain theory, the assumptions of that theory become the assumptions of the study that is based on that particular theory. In addition, the results of previous studies can form the basis for assumptions in the present research investigation. Finally, certain commonsense assumptions must be made to carry out a study. For example, if an investigator were conducting a study to examine behaviors of fathers toward their children, it would be necessary to assume that the men in the study were actually the fathers of the children in the study.

Let us consider an example in which nurses are trying to determine the most appropriate means to teach patients to operate an insulin pump. A universal assumption might be that uncontrolled diabetes is a threat to the physical well-being of individuals. An assumption based on research might be that the insulin pump is an effective means of delivering medication to diabetics. Finally, a commonsense assumption might be made that the subjects are interested in controlling their diabetes and that they have the mental capacity to understand the material that is being taught.

ACKNOWLEDGE THE LIMITATIONS OF THE STUDY

The researcher should try to identify study limitations or weaknesses. **Limitations** are uncontrolled variables that may affect study results and limit the generalizability of the findings. In nearly every nursing study, there are variables over which the researcher either has no control or chooses not to exercise control. These variables are called extraneous variables. For example, the educational level of subjects would be a study limitation if the researcher could not control this variable and thought that it might influence the study results. In experimental studies, uncontrolled variables are referred to as threats to internal and external validity (see Chapter 8).

The researcher should openly acknowledge the limitations of a study as much as possible before data are collected. Other limitations may occur while the study is in progress (such as malfunctions of equipment and subject dropout). The limitations must be considered when the conclusions of a study are formulated and when recommendations are made for future research.

FORMULATE THE HYPOTHESIS OR RESEARCH QUESTION

A researcher's expectation about the results of a study is expressed in a hypothesis. A **hypothesis** predicts the relationship between two or more variables. Whereas the problem statement asks a question, the hypothesis furnishes the predicted answer to the question. The hypothesis contains the population and variables, just as the problem statement does. In addition, the hypothesis proposes the relationship between the independent and the dependent variables. In experimental studies, the **independent variable** is the "cause" or the variable that is thought to influence the dependent variable. The **dependent variable** is the "effect" or the variable that is influenced by the researcher's manipulation (control) of the independent variable. A hypothesis must be testable or verifiable empirically, which means that it must be capable of being tested in the "real world" by observations gathered through the senses.

Consider the problem statement: Is there a correlation between body image and self-esteem levels of women who have experienced a mastectomy? After the review of the literature on the topic, a theory might be discovered that predicts that a positive relationship exists between body image and self-esteem levels. The following hypothesis might then be formulated: The more positive the body image of women who have experienced a mastectomy, the higher is their self-esteem level. This type of hypothesis is referred to as a directional research hypothesis. It contains the direction of the researcher's expectations for the study results.

Although the null hypothesis (which predicts that no relationship exists between variables) is tested statistically, the directional research hypothesis is the preferred type for nursing studies. This type of hypothesis is derived from the theoretical/conceptual framework for the study and, therefore, should indicate the expected relationship between variables.

Experimental, comparative, and correlational studies call for hypotheses. In exploratory studies and some descriptive studies, a hypothesis is not needed. In those studies that do not require hypotheses, the research is guided by research questions that are a further elaboration of the problem statement. For example, the problem statement might be: What are the adjustment behaviors of family members when the husband/father has experienced a myocardial infarction? The research questions might be: Do family members become closer or more distant in their interpersonal relationships with each other? What is the greatest adjustment difficulty reported by family members? Do different families report similar adjustment problems?

DEFINE STUDY VARIABLES/TERMS

The variables and terms contained in the study hypotheses or research questions need to be defined so that their meaning is clear to the researcher and to the reader of a research report. The definitions are usually dictionary definitions or theoretical definitions obtained from literature sources. In addition to a dictionary or theoretical definition, a variable should be operationally defined. An **operational definition** indicates how a variable will be observed or measured. Operational definitions frequently include the instrument that will be used to measure the variables. If anxiety were being measured, the theoretical definition might be taken from a certain theorist's description of anxiety. The operational definition would then be indicated by the identification of the tool or behavior that would be used to measure anxiety.

The operational definition allows replication of a study. If a researcher would like to replicate a study, using another group of subjects or another setting, it would be necessary to know exactly how the variables were measured in the previous study.

Besides defining the variables in a hypothesis or research question, the population for the study should be delimited or narrowed down to the specific group that will be studied. If the population in the hypothesis was identified as myocardial infarction patients, this group could be further defined as men between the ages of 35 and 55 years who have experienced a first myocardial infarction and who are patients in a large teaching hospital in the northeastern United States.

SELECT THE RESEARCH DESIGN

The **research design** is the plan for how the study will be conducted. It is concerned with the type of data that will be collected and the means used to obtain these data. For example, the researcher must decide if the study will examine cause-and-effect relationships or describe only existing situations. The researcher chooses the design that is most appropriate to test the study hypothesis(es) or answer the research question(s).

Research designs can be categorized as quantitative or qualitative. They also can be categorized as experimental or nonexperimental. Experimental designs can be further divided into true experimental, quasiexperimental, and preexperimental designs. Nonexperimental designs include survey studies, correlational studies, comparative studies, and methodological studies. Research designs are discussed in Chapters 8 and 9.

In experimental research, the investigator plays an active role and has more control over the research situation than in a nonexperimental study. More control can be exercised over the extraneous variables that might influence research results. In experimental nursing studies, a nursing intervention is usually introduced. The nurse researcher manipulates this variable by deciding who will and will not receive an intervention. Frequently, one group will receive the usual intervention, while another group will receive some new intervention that is hoped to be more effective. In nonexperimental research, the investigator collects data without actively manipulating any variable. It is appropriate to discuss cause-and-effect relationships only when experimental designs are used. It is sometimes difficult, however, because of ethical reasons to conduct experimental research with human beings. For this reason, many nursing research investigations have been of the nonexperimental type.

IDENTIFY THE POPULATION

The **population** is a complete set of individuals or objects that possess some common characteristic of interest to the researcher. The researcher must specify the broad population or group of interest as well as the actual population that is available for the study. The first type of population is identified as the target population, and the second type is called the accessible population (see Chapter 10). The **target population,** also called the universe, is made up of the group of people or objects to which the researcher wishes to generalize the findings of a study. The **accessible population** is that group that is actually available for study by the researcher. The term **population** does not always mean that human beings will be studied. A nurse researcher might study a population of charts or a population of blood pressure readings, for example.

By identifying the population, the researcher makes clear the group to which the study results can be applied. Scientific research is concerned with generalizing research results to other subjects and other settings. Populations are always of interest in scientific research even when only a small group of subjects is being studied. Otherwise, the research becomes problem solving.

Although the researcher would like to assert that the study results apply to a wide target population, this population must be similar to the accessible population for such an assertion to be made. For example, the accessible population might be pregnant women in one clinic setting. These women are primigravidas and their ages vary from 25 to 35 years. The target population would be 25- to 35-year-old primigravidas.

SELECT THE SAMPLE

Although researchers are always interested in populations, usually a subgroup of the population, called a **sample,** is studied. The sample is chosen to represent the population and is used to make generalizations about the population. Obtaining data from an entire population is costly and time consuming, and it may even be impossible, at times, to contact or locate every member of a given population. If the sample is carefully selected, the researcher can make claims about the population with a certain degree of confidence. The method of selecting the sample will determine how representative the sample is of the population.

Probability samples are those chosen by a random selection process in which each member of the population has a chance of being in the sample. There are several different types of probability sampling methods. These will be discussed in Chapter 10. If nonprobability sampling is used, the researcher has less confidence that the sample is representative of the population. The investigator cannot estimate the probability that each element of the population has a chance of being selected for the sample, and the possibility of a biased sample is great. The researcher must make the determination of which sampling method to use after considering the advantages and disadvantages of the various types of probability and nonprobability sampling methods.

Because nursing research is generally conducted with human beings, subjects' rights must be considered and the proper permissions secured before subjects are approached to participate in a study. All research with humans must involve voluntary participation of the subjects. Even in nursing studies that use a random selection process, the sample may not be truly random, unless all selected subjects actually agree to participate in the study.

CONDUCT A PILOT STUDY

It is advisable to conduct a pilot study before the study subjects are approached and the actual study is carried out. A **pilot study** involves a miniature, trial version of the planned study. People are selected for the pilot study who are similar in characteristics to the sample that will be used for the actual study. Tulman and Fawcett (1996) wrote that a pilot study can be called "primary prevention." They contended that a pilot study can prevent the researcher from conducting a large-scale study that might be an expensive disaster. Many researchers have discovered this truth when it is too late!

According to Jairath, Hogerny, and Parsons (2000), there are several reasons for conducting a pilot study. The major objectives are to examine issues related to the design, sample size, data collection procedures, and data analysis approaches.

A pilot study can be used to test a new instrument or to evaluate an existing instrument that has been altered. The researcher may think that the questionnaire is so simple that a 10-year-old could fill it out, but may find out in a pilot study that 30-year-olds have great difficulty in understanding several of the questions. The pilot study also can be used to evaluate the study procedures and, in general, help to get the "bugs" out before the actual study is conducted. Factors can be examined, such as how long it will take to conduct the data collection and how subjects can be expected to respond to the data collection methods.

After the pilot study is conducted, necessary revisions should be made. It may be advisable to carry out another pilot study if changes have been made in the instrument(s) or in the research procedures.

COLLECT THE DATA

The **data** are the pieces of information or facts that are collected in scientific investigations. Although the data-collection step of the research process may be very time consuming, it is sometimes considered to be the most exciting part of research.

The variable or variables in a study must be measured. This is carried out through the data-collection procedures. Data collection should be a systematic process. Questions that must be answered are these: What data will be collected? How will the data be collected? Who will collect the data? Where will the data be collected? When will the data be collected?

A multitude of data-collection methods are available to nurse researchers. The choice of methods is determined by the study hypothesis(es) or the research question(s), the design of the study, and the amount of knowledge that is available about the study topic. Many research projects use more than one data-collection method. Some of these methods and the various instruments appropriate for nurse researchers are discussed in Chapters 11 and 12.

ORGANIZE THE DATA FOR ANALYSIS

After the data are collected, it is necessary to organize the data for tabulation and evaluation. This task can be overwhelming at times. Actually, this step of the research process should have been planned long before the data were collected. The researcher should have prepared dummy tables and graphs that could then be filled in with the data once they are obtained.

If questionnaires have been used, it will be necessary to determine if they have been completed correctly. Decisions will have to be made about missing data. If interviews have been tape recorded, the tapes will have to be analyzed and data then placed in some kind of written form.

A statistician should be consulted in the early phase of the research process, as well as in the data analysis phase of the study. Just as plans for organizing the data should be made before data collection begins, plans for analyzing the data also should be made before obtaining the data. It is frustrating for a statistician to be approached by a researcher with a mound of data and the plea "What shall I do with this stuff?" The statistician can help to determine what data are needed for a study and what statistical procedures will be appropriate to analyze the data.

ANALYZE THE DATA

This stage of the research process may make some of you cringe, for you can quickly ascertain that statistics may be involved. After reviewing statistical concepts in Chapters 13 and 14, you will realize that an understanding of difficult mathematical principles is not necessary to conduct research or evaluate research results.

In this day of computers, data analysis has been greatly simplified. When data had to be analyzed by hand or even when pocket calculators became available, data analysis was very time consuming. Now, a researcher can sit at a computer terminal and input large amounts of data and receive the results of the analysis almost instantaneously.

INTERPRET THE FINDINGS

After the data are analyzed, the findings should be interpreted in light of the study hypothesis(es) or research question(s). If a hypothesis was tested, a determination is made as to whether the data support the research hypothesis. Also, the framework for the study is discussed in light of the findings. If the data support the research hypothesis, then the theoretical or conceptual framework is also supported. Conversely, if the research hypothesis is not supported, the framework for the study is also not supported. Of course, the researcher should discuss any problems incurred in the course of the study or any limitations of the design that may have influenced the study results.

The results of the present study are compared with those of previous studies that investigated the same or similar variables; the researcher thus is able to contribute to the existing body of knowledge on the study topic.

After the findings are interpreted, the researcher should indicate the implications for nursing. A consideration is made of changes that might be called for in nursing practice, nursing education, or nursing administration as a result of the study findings. Finally, recommendations for future research are proposed.

COMMUNICATE THE FINDINGS

The final step in the research process, and the most important one for nursing, is the communication of the study findings. No matter how significant the findings may be, they are of little value to the rest of the nursing profession if the researcher fails to disseminate these results to other colleagues. The results of many nursing studies never get published or shared with other nurses.

Research findings can be communicated through many different mediums. The best method of reaching a large number of nurses is through publication in research journals such as *Applied Nursing Research, Biological Research for Nursing, Clinical Nursing Research, Journal of Advanced Nursing, Nursing Research, Research in Nursing and Health,* and *Western Journal of Nursing Research.* Research results also may be published in clinical journals such as *Heart & Lung* and *Journal of Obstetric, Gynecologic, and Neonatal Nursing.* Additional journals are listed in Chapter 16. Nurses should also present their research results in person to colleagues at national, regional, state, and local gatherings of nurses.

An exciting method of presenting research results at meetings is through poster sessions. Attractive posters are prepared that describe the major areas of the research, such as the problem statement, hypotheses, and findings. Posters, as a communication medium, permit many study results to be disseminated to interested research consumers. The number of oral presentations that can be attended in a given day is quite limited, but many research posters can be viewed in a short time. Generally, the investigator is present at least part of the time that the poster session is being held to answer questions about the study.

SUMMARY

In general, quantitative research proceeds in an orderly fashion. First, the researcher identifies the problem to be studied and the purpose of the study. The problem statement specifies the population and the variables that are being studied. A **variable** is a characteristic or attribute that differs among the persons, objects, or events that are being studied.

The literature is reviewed to determine the existing knowledge on the study topic. A theoretical/conceptual framework is developed to guide the research. The **assumptions** on which the study is based are clearly identified, and the **limitations** or weaknesses of the study are acknowledged.

Next, the researcher states the study expectations in the form of a **hypothesis.** The hypothesis links the **independent variable** (cause) with the **dependent variable** (effect).

The variables and terms in the study hypotheses or research questions need to be defined. In addition to a dictionary or a theoretical definition, a variable should be operationally defined. An **operational definition** indicates how a variable will be measured. The **research design** is the plan for how the study will be conducted. A design is selected that is most appropriate to test the study hypothesis(es) or answer the research question(s). Research designs can be classified as quantitative or qualitative. They also can be classified as experimental or nonexperimental.

The **population** or group of interest is identified. A **target population** is a group to which the researcher wishes to generalize the study findings. An **accessible population** is the group that is actually available for study by the researcher. The **sample** is a subgroup that is chosen to represent the population.

It is advisable to conduct a **pilot study,** or miniature, trial version of a study, before the actual data are collected. **Data** are the pieces of information that are collected during the study. After data are collected, they are organized, analyzed, and interpreted. Finally, the last phase of a study involves the communication of the results.

NURSING RESEARCH ON THE WEB

For additional online resources, research activities, and exercises, go to www.prenhall. com/nieswiadomy. Select Chapter 2 from the drop down menu.

✖ GET INVOLVED ACTIVITIES

1. Divide into two teams and debate the value of adding another step to the research process. This step would be called Utilization of Research Findings. One team would support adding this step by taking the position that it is the responsibility of the researcher to see that research findings are implemented. The other team would oppose adding this step to the research process by supporting the position that implementation of research is the responsibility of other people at a later time.

2. Develop a research proposal, using all of the steps outlined in this chapter. Start with a problem statement. The topic can be something humorous that is specific to your class, such as, "Is there a difference between the number of times a week that married students eat out compared to single students?" Proceed through the rest of the steps of the research process. You may want to collect data, have some student or students analyze it, and bring the results to class the next class period. Using a trivial topic like this may make the research process seem less formidable.

3. Determine an appropriate publication source that could be used to communicate the results of a study topic that the class decides on or to communicate the results of the study that the class has proposed in Activity 2.

4. Select a research article that will be read by the entire group. Determine how many steps of the research process can be clearly identified in the article.

✖ SELF-TEST

Circle the letter before the *best* answer.

1. All authors agree on the following number of steps in conducting quantitative research:
   A. 10
   B. 15
   C. 17
   D. none of the above

2. Which of the following answers is true concerning quantitative research?
   A. The steps always proceed in the same way in each study.
   B. There may be some shifting back and forth between the steps.
   C. The most important step is to identify the study hypotheses.
   D. The steps are never carried out in an orderly fashion.

3. One of main purposes of conducting a review of the literature before carrying out a research project is to:
   A. determine existing knowledge on the topic.
   B. help select an optimum sample size.
   C. discover an instrument for data collection that has been used many times.
   D. prevent duplication of research.

4. Assumptions are:
   A. beliefs that are thought to be true but have not necessarily been proven.
   B. false beliefs held by the researcher.
   C. expectations for study results.
   D. none of the above

5. The plan for how a study will be conducted is called the:
   A. design.
   B. hypothesis.
   C. data-collection method.
   D. research process.

6. The small group selected from a larger group to participate in a study is known as the:
   A. study population.
   B. sample population.
   C. sample.
   D. element.

7. At what point in the research process should a statistician be consulted?
   A. early in the research project
   B. immediately before data are collected
   C. after data have been collected
   D. before the data have been analyzed

8. To obtain the desired data in a study, which of the following types of definitions is most essential?

   A. theoretical
   B. dictionary
   C. conceptual
   D. operational

9. The final step of the research process for the researcher is to:

   A. collect the data.
   B. analyze the data.
   C. interpret the findings.
   D. communicate the findings.

10. Which of the following communication mediums could be used to present research findings?

   A. books
   B. journals
   C. research seminars
   D. poster sessions
   E. all of the above

✖ REFERENCES

Burns, N., & Grove, S. (1997). *The practice of nursing research: Conduct, critique, and utilization* (3rd ed.). Philadelphia: Saunders.

Dempsey, P. A., & Dempsey, A. D. (2000). *Using nursing research: Process, critical evaluation, and utilization* (5th ed.). Philadelphia: Lippincott.

Downs, F. S. (1994). Hitching the research wagon to theory (editorial). *Nursing Research, 45,* 195.

Jairath, N., Hogerney, M., & Parsons, C. (2000). The role of the pilot study: A case illustration from cardiac nursing research. *Applied Nursing Research, 13,* 92-96.

Martin, P. A. (1994). The utility of the research problem statement. *Applied Nursing Research, 7,* 47–49.

Myers, S. (1982). The search for assumptions. *Western Journal of Nursing Research, 4,* 91–97.

Polit, D. F., & Hungler, B. P. (1999). *Nursing research: Principles and methods* (6th ed.). Philadelphia: Lippincott.

Tulman, L., & Fawcett, J. (1996). Lessons learned from a pilot study of biobehavioral correlates of functional status in women with breast cancer. *Nursing Research, 45,* 356–358.

Wilson, H. S., & Hutchinson, S. A. (1996). *The consumer's guide to nursing research.* Albany, NY: Delmar.

CHAPTER 3

Ethical Issues in Nursing Research

�֍ OUTLINE

**Development of Ethical Codes
and Guidelines**
Research Guidelines for Nurses
Misconduct in Research
Elements of Informed Consent
- Researcher Is Identified and Credentials
  Presented
- Subject Selection Process Is Described
- Purpose of Study Is Described
- Study Procedures Are Discussed
- Potential Risks Are Described
- Potential Benefits Are Described
- Compensation, if Any, Is Discussed
- Alternative Procedures, if Any,
  Are Disclosed

- Anonymity or Confidentiality Is Assured
- Right to Refuse to Participate
  or to Withdraw from Study Without
  Penalty Is Assured
- Offer to Answer All Questions Is Made
- Means of Obtaining Study Results
  Is Presented

Documentation of Informed Consent
The Nurse Researcher as a Patient Advocate
Critiquing the Ethical Aspects of a Study
Summary
Nursing Research on the Web
Get Involved Activities
Self-test

✖ OBJECTIVES

On completion of this chapter, you will be prepared to:

1. Discuss some of the unethical studies that have been documented in the literature
2. Trace the development of ethical codes and guidelines
3. Appreciate the role of institutional review boards
4. Identify the elements of informed consent
5. Recognize unethical research
6. Act as a patient advocate during research investigations
7. Critique the ethical aspects of a study

✖ NEW TERMS DEFINED IN THIS CHAPTER

anonymity
confidentiality
informed consent

How long does it take for body parts to freeze when people are kept naked outdoors in subfreezing temperatures? What signs and symptoms are seen when people are kept in tanks of ice water for 3 hours? These questions were asked by "researchers" in Germany in the early 1940s. They were trying to determine the most effective means of treating German Air Force pilots who had been exposed to cold conditions. The "subjects" for these experiments were prisoners in the German concentration camps.

During 1942 and 1943, prisoners' wounds were deliberately infected with bacteria. Infection was aggravated by the forcing of wood shavings and ground glass into the wounds. Sulfanilamide was then given to these prisoners to determine the effectiveness of this drug. Some subjects died and others suffered serious injury. Between June and September 1944, photographs and body measurements were taken on 112 Jewish prisoners. Then they were killed, and their skeletons were defleshed. One purpose of this study was to determine if photographs from live human beings could be used to predict skeletal size. The skeleton collection was to be displayed at the Reich University of Strasbourg (Nuremberg Military Tribunals, 1949).

How could such atrocities be committed in the name of science? Some of these studies were based on the rationale that the victims were not "real" people like the Germans. The German race was viewed as superior, and it was believed that this race would one day rule the world.

Widespread knowledge about unethical research conducted in Germany was obtained immediately after World War II. Only recently, however, has the public become informed about the atrocities committed in Japan during that same period. It appears that a conspiracy between the United States government leaders and the Japanese prevented this material from being made public (Shearer, 1982). To obtain the results of the Japanese experiments, immunity was granted to Shiro Ishii, commander of the Japanese biological warfare unit, and his subordinates. The silence was first broken in 1975 when a Japanese film producer, Haruko Yoshinaga, tracked down 35 people involved in the incidents. Japanese and American writers then began demanding information from the Pentagon under the Freedom of Information Act. Shearer (1982) revealed some of these horrible experiments:

1. Infecting women prisoners with syphilis, having them impregnated by male prisoners, then dissecting the live babies and mothers.
2. Draining the blood from prisoners' veins and substituting horse blood.
3. Exploding gas gangrene bombs next to prisoners tied to stakes.
4. Vivisecting prisoners to compile data on the human endurance of pain (p. 10).

In 1995, six former members of the Japanese biological warfare unit published a book to tell about the atrocities that they had seen committed or had heard about ("Japanese Book Details Scientific Atrocities," 1996). The book is titled *The Truth About Unit 731.*

Because the United States is a country with a strong Judeo-Christian background, it may seem unlikely that such heinous research could ever be conducted in this country. But the following examples of research were, in fact, carried out in the United States.

To test the effectiveness of mercury in treating syphilis, the United States Public Health Service began a study in 1932 in Macon County, Alabama. The 891 subjects were Black male farmers over 25 years of age. Of this group, 412 had active cases of syphilis; 275 had syphilis that was supposedly cured by mercury, arsenic, and bismuth; and 204, who were used as a control group, had no diagnosis of syphilis. Those subjects with active cases were given *no* treatment. Subjects were given periodic checkups, treatment for other medical conditions, a yearly cash payment, and burial expenses (Lasagna, 1975). Even after penicillin was discovered, it appears that these subjects were still given no treatment. This unethical study became public knowledge 40 years after it was begun.

It is common knowledge that smallpox is no longer a threat to the world. Few people remember, or even know, that Edward Jenner deliberately exposed an 8-year-old child to cowpox to try out his new vaccine for smallpox (Hayter, 1979). During the 1960s and 1970s, a group of mentally retarded children in Willowbrook, New York, were deliberately exposed to infectious hepatitis (Krugman, Giles, & Hammond, 1971). In July 1963, doctors at the Jewish Chronic Disease Hospital in Brooklyn, New York, injected live cancer cells into 22 elderly patients. The study was designed to measure patients' ability to reject foreign cells. The patients were told that they were being given skin tests (Katz, 1972).

In Los Angeles, California, between 1989 and 1991 approximately 900 children, who were mostly Black or Hispanic, were given an experimental measles vaccine called EZ ("Measles Mistake," 1996). The researchers never told the parents about the experiment because the vaccine was unlicensed. Kaiser Permanente and the Centers for Disease Control and Prevention (CDC), sponsors of the study, said that the drug was safe but agreed that they should have notified parents about the status of the drug.

A similar situation occurred in 1991 at the Standing Rock Sioux Reservation in the Dakotas ("Parents Say Government Quiet," 1996). A group of American Indian children were given a vaccine for hepatitis A. Parents were never told that their children were part of a research project and that the vaccine had not been approved at that time. The study was sponsored by the CDC and the Indian Health Service.

DEVELOPMENT OF ETHICAL CODES AND GUIDELINES

The need for ethical guidelines becomes clear after reading these accounts of unethical research projects. The development of appropriate guidelines is not simple. Ethics is concerned with rules and principles of human behavior. Because human behavior is a very complex phenomenon, rules to govern the actions of human beings are difficult to formulate. Studies of recorded history show that people have always been interested in this topic. The biblical Ten Commandments is an example of a code of conduct that has endured throughout the centuries. Ethical principles frequently change with time and the development of new knowledge.

The present ethical standards used in nursing research, and in research conducted by other disciplines, are based on the guidelines developed after World War II. The atrocities committed in the German prison camps led to the Nuremberg Trials after the war. The 1947 Nuremberg Code resulted from the revelations of unethical human behavior that occurred during the war. This code is concerned with several criteria for research including the following:

1. Researcher must inform subjects about the study.
2. Research must be for the good of society.
3. Research must be based on animal experiments, if possible.
4. Researcher must try to avoid injury to research subjects.
5. Researcher must be qualified to conduct research.
6. Subjects or the researcher can stop the study if problems occur.

Many other ethical codes have been developed since the development of the Nuremberg Code. Groups of professionals, such as anthropologists, sociologists, and psychologists, have developed codes for their members. Various governmental agencies have also developed guidelines. The United Nations developed a declaration on human rights in 1949. The United States Department of Health, Education and Welfare (HEW) (now the Department of Health and Human Services, DHHS) published guidelines in 1971. These have been revised several times. Also, special guidelines exist for research with vulnerable groups such as children, the mentally retarded, and prisoners. Any institution that receives federal money for research must abide by the DHHS guidelines or risk losing federal money.

The federal government guidelines resulted in the creation of Institutional Review Boards (IRBs). These review boards are given various names such as Human Research Committee, Human Subjects Committee, and Committee for the Protection of Human Subjects. Every agency that receives federal money for research must have an IRB to review research proposals. The federal government, through the Office of Protection from Research Risk (OPRR), oversees IRBs.

Agencies may also have other research committees that review research proposals. Some institutions have nursing research committees that are specifically concerned with nursing research in that particular institution. Because research policies and procedures vary from agency to agency, the researcher should become informed about the requirements of specific institutions that will be used for data collection.

RESEARCH GUIDELINES FOR NURSES

In 1968, the American Nurses Association Research and Studies Commission published a set of guidelines for nursing research. These guidelines were revised in 1975 and 1985 and are titled *Human Rights Guidelines for Nurses in Clinical and Other Research.* These revised guidelines address the rights of the research subject and the nurses involved in research. Subjects must be protected from harm, their privacy should be ensured, and their dignity preserved. Nurses who are asked to participate in research should be fully informed about the research, and nurses should be included on the IRBs that review research proposals.

MISCONDUCT IN RESEARCH

Although findings of scientific misconduct are not common, the federal government's Office of Research Integrity (ORI) in the DHHS investigates approximately 200 cases a year of suspected misconduct by researchers who have received federal funding. Four or five cases of misconduct are uncovered each year through these investigations.

Recently, a federal investigation revealed that an immunologist at the University of Texas Southwestern Medical Center in Dallas had falsified data for at least 5 years in his study of arthritis (Ambrose, 2000). The report revealed that by adding a radioactive chemical to laboratory vials, he was able to manipulate results of cytotoxic T-lymphocyte assays in rats without actually conducting the assays. Although, the researcher denied the charges, he agreed to refrain from seeking any federal research grants until 2005.

Since 1993, nursing research studies have been cited by the ORI several times. This information is published in the NIH Guide and is available online (http://www.nih.gov/grants/guide/notice-files).

Olsen and Mahrenholz (2000) reported on ethical problems discovered in 157 nursing research protocols submitted to one School of Nursing's Institutional Review Board (IRB). Revisions were required for 46.5% of the protocols and 8.3% were not approved. Problems were found in the informed consent process in 43.3% of the protocols. The authors suggested that nurse researchers need to be particularly attentive to issues of coercion and deceptive language in informed consent documents.

A recent issue facing nurse researchers concerns sources of funding. Private foundations and the federal government provide much of the money for nursing research projects. However, many nurse researchers are turning to industry as another source of funding. In this day of managed care, corporations may be interested in certain projects that may match their companies' interests and products, particularly in the area of health promotion, which is of prime importance to nursing. Erlen (2000) cautioned that "conflicts of interest" might occur when nurse researchers accept funds and enter into financial relationships with industry.

ELEMENTS OF INFORMED CONSENT

The principal means for ensuring that the rights of research subjects are protected is through informed consent. **Informed consent** concerns subjects participation in research in which they have full understanding of the study before the study begins. The major elements of informed consent are the following:

1. Researcher is identified and credentials presented.
2. Subject selection process is described.
3. Purpose of study is described.
4. Study procedures are discussed.
5. Potential risks are described.
6. Potential benefits are described.
7. Compensation, if any, is discussed.
8. Alternative procedures, if any, are disclosed.
9. Anonymity or confidentiality is assured.
10. Right to refuse to participate or to withdraw from study without penalty is assured.
11. Offer to answer all questions is made.
12. Means of obtaining study results is presented.

RESEARCHER IS IDENTIFIED AND CREDENTIALS PRESENTED

The researcher must identify himself or herself and present qualifications to conduct the study. If a sponsor or sponsoring agency is involved, subjects should be given this information. Frequently, a sentence such as the following will be included in the study explanation: "I am a nursing student at _____ University and am conducting a research study as part of the requirements for _____."

Nurse researchers in clinical practice must take extra precautions to inform clients that they are acting in their capacity as researchers and not as nurses. Potential subjects may not be able to differentiate when the nurse is acting as a caregiver or as a researcher.

SUBJECT SELECTION PROCESS IS DESCRIBED

It should be noted that the use of the term *research subjects* is decreasing. Today you also may see in the literature the terms *participants, respondents,* and *informants.* The term *subjects* is still used often in this text because it remains prominent in the literature. Also, *subjects' rights* is a very important issue. The term *informants' rights* just does not seem to carry the same meaning. An informant sounds more like someone who is providing information to the police department!

One of the primary goals of all researchers is to choose an unbiased sample. Sampling procedures to enhance the selection of such a sample are discussed in Chapter 10; the focus here is placed on the ethical nature of selecting a sample.

The subjects should be told how they were chosen to participate in the study. If subjects were randomly selected, they should be provided with this information. If they must meet certain criteria to be eligible, these criteria should be presented early in the request for their participation.

As most of you know, most research has been conducted with white males. This practice can no longer continue. Women have traditionally not been included in research. The rationale has been that women's biological rhythms might "mess up the results."

There is evidence of some increase in the use of women in studies. Larson (1994) examined 754 research protocols that were approved at one tertiary care center during 1989 and 1990. Most of the studies (81.4%) included both men and women. However, the elderly, the poor, and ethnic minorities were excluded without identifiable justification.

Public Law 103-4, passed in 1993, requires that researchers recruit women and minorities for their studies. In 1994 NIH officials revised their gender and minority inclusion policy to meet the requirements of this law (the policy was revised again in 2000). Researchers applying to the NIH for funding are required to include plans for the recruitment of women, men, and ethnic or racial groups. Harden and McFarland (2000) wrote that adequate gender and minority representation is "crucial to ensure that the research has relevance to all segments of the diverse U.S. population" (p. 86).

Inequities in the health of different groups of Americans has become a top priority for the Department of Health and Human Services (DHHS) and the National Institutes of Health (NIH). In April 2000, the NIH's Office on Research on Minority Health released a new Web site that contains information about an initiative to focus on minority health (http://www.1.od.nih.gov/ORMH/). The NIH has called for every Institute to submit a strategic plan that address health inequities.

The National Institute of Nursing Research (NINR) has committed more than 20% of its funding for the last 3 years to minority health issues (Grady, 2000). Health disparity research was one of the five research targeted areas for 2001. According to Dr. Patricia Grady, Director of NINR, particular emphasis has been placed on self-management of diabetes, which is a condition that affects disproportionate numbers of African Americans, Hispanics, and Native Americans.

PURPOSE OF STUDY IS DESCRIBED

The purpose or objectives of the study should be clearly presented. The material should be in the preferred language of the potential subject and at the subject's reading level, for all printed material.

The researcher should be honest and open in presenting the purpose of the study. It is not always necessary, however, to describe the entire nature of the study. For example, if a study was being conducted to determine the difference in patients' satisfaction with nursing care given under a primary nursing or team nursing approach, subjects might be told that the study was examining patients' satisfaction with the type of nursing care that they were receiving. It would not be necessary to describe primary nursing and team nursing to the potential subjects. Ask yourself what information you would want to receive or would want a close relative to receive to make an informed decision about participation in a study.

STUDY PROCEDURES ARE DISCUSSED

All aspects of the study should be fully explained. This includes telling the potential subjects when and where the study will take place. The researcher must stress the subjects' time involvement and all activities that the subjects must perform. This aspect of informed consent is particularly important in experimental studies where people will participate in or receive some type of treatment. Sometimes a "cover story" is presented to subjects rather than the true explanation of the study. Deliberate deception of this sort is unethical. Even if subjects are later told of the deception, the use of false information is unethical.

One study (Milgram, 1963) was conducted to examine obedience to authority. The study was done in a laboratory setting and was described to potential subjects as a learning experiment. Subjects were told to administer electrical shocks when the "learners" gave incorrect responses. The "learners" were actually actors. These actors, who were out of sight, groaned and screamed during the experiment. In all, 26 of the subjects, or 65% of the group, continued to administer shocks throughout the experiment, even when they thought they were administering lethal shocks. Responses of discomfort among the subjects who were administering the supposed electrical shocks included sweating, trembling, and stuttering. One subject had a convulsive seizure. This study demonstrates severe deception by the researcher.

If it is necessary to withhold information about a study from potential subjects, they must be informed of this before the study, and a debriefing session must be held afterward. This debriefing session will be used to ensure that participants understand the reasons and justification for the procedures used in the study. It is the researcher's responsibility to ensure that there are no more than minimal risks involved in the study and that the subjects' rights are protected in all other areas.

In a study where it is not desirable to fully inform subjects before it begins, subjects have the right to be fully informed at the conclusion of the study and be given an opportunity to withdraw consent to include their data in the study results. Many researchers prefer not to conduct studies in which the researcher is not completely candid with subjects before the beginning of the study.

POTENTIAL RISKS ARE DESCRIBED

Subjects must be told of any possible discomforts, either physical or psychological, that might occur as a result of participation. Any invasion of privacy must also be discussed. It is difficult at times for the researcher to identify all of the potential risk factors because of the variations in human responses to different situations. The investigator is obligated to try to identify all possible risks that would surely influence the subjects' decision to participate. Many questions arise about what constitutes a risk. If a study is being conducted in which healthy volunteers will be involved in mild exercise, should these subjects be informed explicitly that they could experience a "heart attack" or a "stroke" during the exercise? The researcher might scare off all prospective subjects! Consultation with experts in the research area should be held and then discretion exercised in presenting risks to potential subjects. One of the roles of IRBs is to assess the adequacy of consent forms.

POTENTIAL BENEFITS ARE DESCRIBED

The Nuremberg Code set the requirement that research must be for the good of society. All research, even basic research that is conducted primarily to obtain new knowledge, must have the potential for benefiting society. A study that is conducted to satisfy the researcher's curiosity would be unethical.

In describing benefits to potential subjects, the investigator should describe both those applicable to the people involved in the study as well as how the results could benefit others. In a study (Simpson, 1985) involving the use of play therapy before physical examinations of preschool-aged children, the mothers of the potential subjects were told that the potential benefits included possible reductions in anxiety of the children during the physical examinations, better cooperation during the procedures, and, therefore, more accurate results from the examinations. Mothers also were told that these results would help nurses in the future to better prepare preschool-aged children for physical examinations. A copy of the consent form for this study is found in Appendix A.

COMPENSATION, IF ANY, IS DISCUSSED

Monetary compensation or any other type of compensation should be described to potential subjects. Any time compensation is being provided in a study, the possibility exists that biased results may be obtained. Subjects may try to "perform" in a manner that will fulfill the researcher's expectations. Nevertheless, researchers frequently use small monetary incentives as enticements for potential subjects. One good example of this is seen in the various types of market research that are conducted around the country. To control for biased responses, participants are usually not told which of the comparison products is the focus of the study. In nursing research, the researcher should avoid monetary compensation, if possible. Subject "compensation" should come from those items listed under "potential benefits." The researcher should cover the cost of such items as laboratory tests and travel expenses for the subjects.

Occasionally, the nurse researcher is obligated to offer services in the event that potential risks materialize into actual risks. In one study, a researcher presented an anxiety management seminar to nurses to help them control anxiety in their work settings. One of the risks involved a potential rise in anxiety levels, rather than the intended decrease in anxiety, as a result of attending the anxiety seminar. The researcher informed subjects that she was experienced in psychotherapy and would be available if their anxiety levels rose during the study.

ALTERNATIVE PROCEDURES, IF ANY, ARE DISCLOSED

Potential subjects should be informed of any alternative procedures that may be followed, such as "You may fill out the questionnaire here or take it home." Moreover, they must be given an explanation of alternative procedures or treatments that may be received by others. For example, a control group of subjects in an experimental study must be made aware that other subjects will be receiving some type of treatment. If potential subjects have a choice of groups, this option must be presented to them. The "Hawthorne effect" (see Chapter 8) can bring about changes in subjects because they are aware that they are participants in a study. For this reason, it is becoming increasingly common to provide some type of alternative activity for the control group to make them feel they are participants. Frequently, as part of the explanation given before the study, the researcher will tell the control group that the experimental treatment will be available to them on completion of the study. If the control group is really a comparison group, in that these subjects are receiving some alternative treatment such as the traditional treatment, the subjects in the experimental group could also be offered this alternative treatment at the conclusion of the study.

ANONYMITY OR CONFIDENTIALITY IS ASSURED

The terms anonymity and confidentiality may be confused. **Anonymity** occurs when no one, including the researcher, can link subjects with the data they provide. If subjects can be linked to data, the researcher has the obligation to address confidentiality. **Confidentiality** involves protection of the subjects' identities by the researcher. In many studies, it is not possible to maintain anonymity. The researcher will usually come face-to-face with subjects in an experimental study. To maintain confidentiality, data are frequently coded and subjects' names and code numbers are kept in a separate location accessible only to the researcher or members of the research team. Any list that links subject names with data should be destroyed at the conclusion of the study.

To ensure anonymity or confidentiality, subjects and the site where the study was conducted should be described in general terms in the description of the sample and the setting. If either the subjects or the study location can be identified by this general description, confidentiality has been violated. For example, the setting might be identified as a 1000-bed psychiatric institution in a small southwestern city. If there is only one such institution in that area, you have identified the institution as surely as if you had included the name. Identity of hospitals, schools, and other institutions should be kept confidential, unless these agencies have given permission to be identified in the study.

Confidentiality can be ensured by the deletion of any identifying information that would allow subject identification. Subjects should always be assured that they are free to omit information from their responses if they believe the data will identify them in any way. If subjects are being assured of anonymity, which is frequently done in survey research, instructions should clearly inform subjects to refrain from including their names or other identifying information on the questionnaires.

RIGHT TO REFUSE TO PARTICIPATE OR TO WITHDRAW FROM STUDY WITHOUT PENALTY IS ASSURED

All participation in nursing research *must* be voluntary. Even if a random sampling procedure is used to obtain participants, these people must be given the opportunity to decide if they wish to participate. No form of coercion should be involved. There must be no penalty involved for nonparticipation. For example, patient care should not be affected by patients' participation or nonparticipation in a study. Students' grades in a course should not be influenced by research participation.

Beginning researchers frequently have difficulty separating the role of researcher from practitioner. A nurse might decide to conduct a study in which his or her "own" patients will be the subjects, or the patients' charts will be used for data collection. In such an instance, the researcher must approach the research setting as if he or she were a complete stranger. If research is being conducted, permission must be obtained to use patients' records, even if the nurse has full access to these records in clinical practice.

Potential research subjects must be informed that they may withdraw from a study at any time and for any reason. This is particularly important in experimental studies in which a treatment is involved.

OFFER TO ANSWER ALL QUESTIONS IS MADE

Potential subjects must always be given the opportunity to ask questions about the study. It is almost impossible for the researcher to include every aspect of the study in a verbal or written explanation. Subjects frequently have questions about the study, and they should have the opportunity to ask them during the verbal explanation of the study. The researcher is obligated to be available (by phone or mail) if questions arise at a later time or if subjects have questions when reading the written explanation of a study.

MEANS OF OBTAINING STUDY RESULTS IS PRESENTED

Many potential research subjects are concerned with the use of study findings. Will their employers get a copy of the results? Will the study be published? How can they find out the results? Although the researcher probably does not know for sure if the study results will ever be published, the researcher's publication plans (and desires) must be indicated. Research subjects should always be given the opportunity to obtain the study results. This does not mean that a copy must be sent to all participants. In fact, many participants are not interested in the results. It is appropriate, therefore, for the researcher to place some of the responsibility for obtaining results on the study subjects. A comment such as the following may be included in the consent information: "A copy of the study results may be obtained by writing or calling the researcher." Of course, this would necessitate the inclusion of an address or phone number where the researcher could be reached at the conclusion of the study. The approximate date when results will be available should also be provided.

DOCUMENTATION OF INFORMED CONSENT

The researcher must document that informed consent was obtained. If self-report questionnaires are used, a statement should be included on the questionnaire, in capital letters, similar to the following: RETURN OF THIS QUESTIONNAIRE WILL INDICATE YOUR CONSENT TO PARTICIPATE IN THIS STUDY. In other types of studies, consent is obtained in written form, stating that the subject has willingly given permission and is aware of the risks and benefits. Oral permission may be obtained, but must be witnessed by a third person. If the subject is a minor or is not able to give informed consent because of mental or physical disability, the consent of a legally authorized representative, such as a child's parent, must be obtained. As previously mentioned, an example of a consent form is shown in Appendix A.

All information on a consent form must be understandable to the subject or the subject's representative. This means that the oral or written explanation must be in the subject's native language or preferred language and be at the subject's reading level. Nurses are aware that many forms signed by patients have not represented informed consent. Nurses must ensure that this practice is rectified.

In 1995, a White House appointed advisory committee asked 1800 randomly selected patients if they were involved in a medical research project ("One-fourth of medical research subjects," 1995). Of the 412 who were actually research subjects, 99 said they had never been a participant in a research study. Sixteen of these people had even signed consent forms.

THE NURSE RESEARCHER AS A PATIENT ADVOCATE

The nurse researcher has the responsibility to protect the privacy and dignity of the people involved in the research and protect them from harm. Even if study subjects willingly and knowingly agree to participate in a study involving undue physical risks, psychological risks, or both, the researcher has an obligation to refrain from conducting such research. The nurse researcher must assume responsibility for study conditions and avoid undue physical or psychological risks to the subjects.

Certain special groups of people are considered particularly vulnerable research subjects because they are either unable to give informed consent or the likelihood of coercion to participate is strong. These groups include children, geriatric clients, prisoners, people with AIDS, the homeless, and unconscious or sedated patients. Special precautions must be taken to ensure that the study has a low risk potential for these vulnerable people.

CRITIQUING THE ETHICAL ASPECTS OF A STUDY

It may be difficult to critique the ethical aspects of a research report. There is usually little space given to this part of the study. Most journal articles contain one or two sentences that mention that subjects' rights were protected and that informed consent was obtained. It is understandable that little is printed about the ethical issues of the study. Much of this information would be repeated in each study that is published. However, the reader of a research report may be able to make some determination of the ethical nature of the study. For example, if it is stated that permission to conduct the study was obtained from an IRB, confidence is greater that subjects' rights were protected. Also, if the study has been funded, there is some assurance that the researcher had to provide evidence of protection of subjects' rights before funds were awarded. Guidelines for critiquing the ethical aspects of a study are presented in Box 3–1.

SUMMARY

Many unethical studies were conducted during World War II, particularly in the prison camps in Germany. Unethical research studies have also been revealed here in the United States.

Because of the public outcry against the atrocities committed in Germany in the 1940s, the Nuremberg Code was developed in 1947. This code calls for voluntary subjects and qualified researchers. Other ethical codes have been formulated since World War II. Many professional groups have developed codes for their members.

The federal government developed research guidelines in the early 1970s, and these guidelines have been revised several times. The original guidelines called for the creation of Institutional Review Boards (IRBs) to be established in all agencies that receive federal money for research. IRBs review research proposals and set standards for research conducted in their agencies.

Box 3–1. Guidelines for Critiquing the Ethical Aspects of a Study

1. Was the study approved by an Institutional Review Board (IRB)?
2. Was informed consent obtained from subjects?
3. Is there information about provisions for anonymity or confidentiality?
4. Were vulnerable subjects used?
5. Does it appear that subjects might have been coerced into acting as subjects?
6. Is it evident that the benefits of participation in the study outweighed the risks involved?
7. Were subjects provided the opportunity to ask questions about the study and told how to contact the researcher if other questions arose?
8. Were the subjects told how they could get the results of the study?

In 1968, the American Nurses Association developed a set of guidelines for nursing research. These guidelines, titled *Human Rights Guidelines for Nurses in Clinical and Other Research,* were revised in 1975 and 1985.

The principal means for ensuring the rights of research subjects is through informed consent. **Informed consent** means that subjects agree to participate in studies about which they have complete understanding of the study before the study begins. The major elements of informed consent concern the researcher's qualifications, subject selection process, purpose of the study, study procedures, potential risks and benefits to subjects, compensation, alternative procedures, anonymity and confidentiality, right to refuse to participate, offer to answer questions, and means of obtaining study results.

Anonymity means that no one can identify the subjects in a study. **Confidentiality** means that the researcher will protect the subjects' identities.

The nurse researcher must act as a patient advocate. This advocacy involves protecting patients' privacy and dignity and ensuring that there are no undue physical or psychological risks to subjects. Particular attention should be given to the rights of certain vulnerable groups, such as children, geriatric clients, prisoners, and unconscious or sedated patients.

NURSING RESEARCH ON THE WEB

For additional online resources, research activities, and exercises, go to www.prenhall.com/nieswiadomy. Select Chapter 3 from the drop down menu.

GET INVOLVED ACTIVITIES

1. Before your next class, peruse the newspapers or periodicals to see if there is any report of an unethical study.
2. Ask your colleagues at work or your family or friends to tell you about some unethical research that they have seen or heard about.
3. Please read the following explanation of a study and try to determine if all of the elements of informed consent are present. Use the 12 elements of informed consent presented in this chapter as your criteria.

Students,

You are being invited to participate in a research project concerning assertiveness levels and locus of control. Participation in this project is strictly voluntary, and your grade in this class will not be influenced by your failure to participate in this study. You may choose to write a short research paper to earn the equivalent class credit.

Your participation in this study will require approximately 30 minutes of class time and will involve completion of two questionnaires. There are no risks involved in this study other than the uncomfortable feelings that may arise when reading the questions. There are several potential benefits of participating in this study. You may learn more about yourself and also learn about the research process. Additionally, the knowledge gained from this study will help nurse educators to predict assertiveness levels and locus of control levels of nursing students in the future.

Answers will remain anonymous. Please do not put your name or any identifying information on the questionnaires. If you have any questions, please feel free to ask them. Results will be available on completion of the study.

✖ SELF-TEST

Circle the letter before the *best* answer.

1. A questionnaire is being used to gather data on the study sample. Identification numbers on the corner of the questionnaires correspond to the researcher's master list of names and numbers. Respondents are assured that this information will not be shared with anyone. The researcher is trying to provide:
    A. informed consent.
    B. anonymity.
    C. data security.
    D. confidentiality.

2. Anonymity is the name given to the procedure that ensures subjects that their responses:
    A. cannot be identified by anyone.
    B. will not be shared with anyone.
    C. will be destroyed at the end of the study.
    D. will be kept under lock and key.

3. If an individual volunteers to participate in a study, he or she is always guaranteed that which of the following will be done?
    A. Anonymity will be provided.
    B. Confidentiality will be provided.
    C. Informed consent will be obtained.
    D. Protection from psychological stress will be assured.

4. Which of the following statements is true concerning a research proposal that is being submitted for review at an agency that receives federal money for research?
    A. Anonymity must be guaranteed in the study proposal.
    B. The proposal must be reviewed by the institution's Institutional Review Board (IRB).
    C. The nursing research committee must approve the proposal.
    D. Subject consent must be received before the proposal is reviewed.

5. Which of the following is "least" likely to be provided for subjects?
    A. informed consent
    B. anonymity
    C. confidentiality
    D. privacy

Write T (True) or F (False) beside the following statements:

_____ 6. Once a subject signs an informed consent form, he or she is agreeing to remain in the study until it is completed.

_____ 7. All study subjects *must* be guaranteed anonymity.

_____ 8. Access to the results of a study in which they have participated is the right of all participants.

_____ 9. In a study in which confidentiality is guaranteed, anonymity is usually guaranteed also.

_____10. A subject in a survey study is more likely to be guaranteed anonymity than is a subject in an experimental study.

✖ REFERENCES

Ambrose, S. G. (2000, October 18). UT Southwestern scientist falsified research, inquiry says. *The Dallas Morning News,* p. 27A.

American Nurses Association (1985). *Human rights guidelines for nurses in clinical and other research* (Code No. D-46 5M). Kansas City, MO: The Association.

Erlen, J. A. (2000). 'Conflict of interest': An ethical dilemma for the nurse researcher. *Orthopoedic Nursing, 19,* 74–77.

Grady, P. (2000). NINR and health disparities. *Nursing Outlook, 48,* 150.

Harden, J. T., & McFarland, G. (2000). Avoiding gender and minority barriers to NIH funding. *Journal of Nursing Scholarship, 32,* 83–86.

Hayter, J. (1979). Issues related to human subjects. In F. Downs & J. Fleming (Eds.), *Issues in nursing research* (pp. 107–147). New York: Appleton-Century-Crofts.

Japanese book details scientific atrocities (1996, February 5). *The Dallas Morning News,* p. 24A.

Katz, K. (1972). *Experimentation with human beings.* New York: Russell Sage.

Krugman, S., Giles, J., & Hammond, J. (1971). Viral hepatitis, type B (MS-2 strain): Studies on active immunization. *Journal of the American Medical Association, 217,* 41–45.

Larson, E. (1994). Exclusion of certain groups from clinical research. *Image: Journal of Nursing Scholarship, 26,* 185–190.

Lasagna, L. (1975). *The VD epidemic: How it started, where it's going, and what to do about it.* Philadelphia: Temple University Press.

Measles mistake (1996, June 20). *USA Today,* p. 1D.

Milgram, S. (1963). Behavioral study of obedience. *Journal of Abnormal and Social Psychology, 67,* 371–378.

Nuremberg Military Tribunals. (1949). *Trials of war criminals before the Nuremberg Military Tribunals under Control Council Law No. 10* (Publication No. 1949–841584, Vol. 2). Washington, DC: U.S. Government Printing Office.

Olsen, D. P., & Mahrenholz, D. (2000). IRB-identified ethical issues in nursing research. *Journal of Professional Nursing, 16,* 140–148.

One-fourth of medical-research subjects unaware they're involved, survey says (1995, June 24). *The Dallas Morning News,* p. 8A.

Parents say government quiet on vaccine testing (1996, December 22). *The Dallas Morning News,* p. 6A.

Shearer, L. (1982, October 17). Now it can be told. *The Dallas Morning News,* pp. 10–11.

Simpson, M. (1985). *Therapeutic play and cooperation of preschoolers during physical examinations.* Unpublished master's thesis, Texas Woman's University, Denton.

PART II

Preliminary Steps in the Research Process

CHAPTER 4

Identifying Nursing Research Problems

✖ OBJECTIVES

On completion of this chapter, you will be prepared to:

1. Identify sources of nursing research problems
2. Distinguish between the problem and purpose of a study
3. Determine factors to be considered when choosing an appropriate topic for a research study
4. List the criteria to be considered when writing a problem statement
5. Discuss the format for writing a problem statement
6. Write problem statements for nursing studies
7. Critique problem statements in research reports and articles

✖ NEW TERMS DEFINED IN THIS CHAPTER

bivariate study
multivariate study

replication study
univariate study

How does a nurse determine what to study? Some nurse researchers have a clearly identified research problem area from the beginning of their research projects, but this usually is not the case. It is difficult to narrow down the broad problem area to a feasible study. A mistake of beginning researchers (and some experienced ones) is to try to examine too much in one study. The belief seems to be "If a little data are good, a lot of data are even better." It would be much more beneficial to nursing for a researcher to conduct a well-designed, small study rather than a poorly designed large study.

Many beginning researchers believe that all the important nursing research has already been conducted. This is not true. Most of the studies that have been conducted have raised further questions that need answers. Sharts-Hopko (2000) called for nurses to identify the problems or issues that come up repeatedly in their practice areas. She asked nurses to consider problems that take up staff time or cause frustration to staff.

The number of potential nursing studies is infinite. In the first chapter you read about some research priorities that have been identified by various nursing leaders and nursing organizations. The excuse of "I can't think of anything to study" is not an acceptable reason for failing to conduct research.

The first step and one of the most important requirements of the research process is to be able to clearly delineate the study area and state the research problem concisely. This is also one of the most difficult tasks of the researcher, especially for the beginning researcher. Many hours may be spent on this part of the research project, and the problem statement may be written and rewritten many times. Occasionally, you may decide you like the first one the best, after all! A clearly stated research problem will give direction to the study. It also will help the research consumer. It is difficult to evaluate a research article if there is no clear statement of the study problem.

One of the expectations of undergraduate nursing students is that they will be able to identify research problems (see Table 1–1). Therefore, this chapter will help you determine how to identify a researchable problem and how to write a clear and concise problem statement. Also, information will be provided on how to critique the problem statements in research articles.

SOURCES OF NURSING RESEARCH PROBLEMS

The sources for generating appropriate nursing research problems are numerous. Four of the most important ones will be discussed: (a) personal experiences, (b) literature sources, (c) existing theories, and (d) previous research.

PERSONAL EXPERIENCES

There probably is not a nurse or nursing student among us who has not observed something in nursing practice that was a source of concern. You may have wondered why nurses dislike working with clients with a history of alcoholism or why some nurses seem to make patients feel like criminals when pain medications are requested. You may also have experienced a nagging doubt about why a procedure is done in a certain manner. On the positive side, you may have observed that clients who are allowed unrestricted visiting hours seem to adjust better to hospitalization and that allowing patients to select special foods from a hospital menu seems to decrease their complaints about hospital food. Thus, from your personal experiences and observations you may identify a topic for study.

LITERATURE SOURCES

The existing nursing literature is an excellent source of ideas for research. Nearly every study that has been published concludes with recommendations for further studies. Unpublished theses and dissertations also contain suggestions for studies. Turn to the last page of the final chapter, and you probably will find the researcher's suggestions and pleas for needed research. Responses to these suggestions could positively influence the direction of nursing research.

The call for future research is not limited to recommendations at the end of published and unpublished studies. Contemporary nursing leaders continually plead for nursing research in articles and books. Many speakers at nursing conventions and conferences address the need for specific areas of nursing research. Priorities for nursing research were discussed in Chapter 1.

EXISTING THEORIES

One type of research that is desperately needed in nursing tests existing theories. Research is a process of theory development and testing. Nurses use many theories from other disciplines in their practice. Are these theories always appropriate for nursing? For example, is change theory as applicable in a hospital as it is in a manufacturing company? Are learning theories as predictive of the behavior of sick people as they are for the behavior of well people?

If an existing theory is used in developing a researchable problem, a specific propositional statement or statements from the theory must be isolated. Generally, an entire theory is not tested; only a part or parts of the theory are subjected to testing in the clinical situation. For example, a learning principle from Rogers' (1969) theory might be chosen to be tested in a patient education program. This learning principle would be transformed into a propositional statement. Later a hypothesis would be formulated from the propositional statement. For example, Rogers says that learning is facilitated when the student participates responsibly in the learning process. He calls for students to contract with the teacher as to what the student should do in the pursuit of knowledge. The researcher would then ask, "Given this proposition from Rogers' theory, what hypothesis or research question would be needed to study this proposition?"

The testing of an existing theory, or deductive research, is greatly needed in nursing. Most researchers, however, begin with a problem that has personal relevance in their immediate work environment. This is understandable because the motivation to conduct research is usually higher if the researcher feels some personal involvement and interest in the results of the study.

PREVIOUS RESEARCH

One disadvantage in using personal experiences as the source of research problems is that this practice frequently leads to a large number of small, unrelated studies with limited generalizability of study results. Although "doing your own thing" is important in the motivation of researchers to conduct studies, the nursing profession needs researchers who are willing to replicate or repeat other studies. A body of knowledge should be developed on sound foundations of research findings. If nursing practice is to be guided by research, the results of studies must be verified. Hypotheses must be tested and retested on adequate sample sizes. Replication studies, therefore, are needed. **Replication studies** involve repeating a study with all the essential elements of the original study held intact. Different samples and settings may be used. Replication studies in nursing have not been numerous, and the lack of these studies has hindered the development of a cumulative body of nursing knowledge.

For some reason, the idea of replication seems to carry a negative connotation. Students have asked, "Can a person 'copy' someone else's study? Isn't that like cheating?" During the formative years in educational settings, the dire consequences of plagiarism are continually stressed. It is quite possible that nurses' reluctance to replicate studies is related to this earlier socialization process.

The value of replication studies needs to be stressed to beginning researchers and to experienced researchers, as well. A researcher who avoids replication studies needs to ask the question, "Would I have more confidence in the results of a single study conducted with 30 subjects in one setting or the results of several similar studies using many subjects in different settings?"

In addition to exact replication studies, investigations are needed that address the shortcomings of previous research. Different instruments may be used, refinements may be made in the experimental treatments, or more appropriate outcome measures may be identified. A search of the literature in 2000 revealed few replications studies during the past 10 years.

Ienatsch (1999) surveyed 42 Texas registered nurses (RNs) about their knowledge, attitudes, treatment practices, and health behaviors regarding blood cholesterol. The nurses completed a 48-item questionnaire developed by the National Heart, Lung, and Blood Institute. This study replicated a survey of 206 New York City RNs. The Texas nurses expressed enthusiasm for counseling clients regarding cholesterol management. However, only one eighth of them strongly agreed that they were prepared to counsel clients. Statistical analysis revealed no significant differences in most responses concerning cholesterol between the Texas and New York nurse samples.

DIFFERENCE BETWEEN THE PROBLEM AND THE PURPOSE OF THE STUDY

Frequently, the problem or research question and the purpose of the study are seen as synonymous. These two aspects of a study are really quite different. The problem statement of a study contains *what* will be examined by the researcher, or the content of the study, whereas the purpose statement of the study contains *why* the study will be conducted. The following two statements demonstrate the difference between the purpose and the problem of a study.

Problem of the Study. Before their first interactions with psychiatric clients, is there a difference in the anxiety levels of nursing students who have read their clients' charts before interacting with these clients and those who have not read their clients' charts before interacting with these clients?

Purpose of the Study. To determine a means of facilitating nursing students' first interactions with clients in the psychiatric setting.

As can be seen, the problem statement clearly indicates that nursing students' anxiety levels will be measured on their first day in a psychiatric setting. Comparisons will be made between students who read charts and those who do not read charts before interacting with psychiatric clients. The purpose of the study is to help nursing instructors determine ways to control students' anxiety levels in psychiatric settings.

RESEARCH PROBLEM CONSIDERATIONS

Many factors should be considered when trying to decide if a certain topic is appropriate for a scientific investigation. Some of these factors include ethical issues, significance of the study for nursing, personal motivation of the researcher, qualifications of the researcher, and feasibility of the study.

ETHICAL ISSUES

One of the most important considerations in a study concerns the ethical aspects of the project. Everyone is familiar with the terrible atrocities of World War II in which prisoners were subjected to many types of inhumane treatment under the guise of research. Although ethical guidelines for research were developed after World War II, many unethical studies have been conducted since then and continue today. Some of these studies were discussed in Chapter 3.

It is the responsibility of researchers to guarantee, to the best of their ability, that their research is ethical. Investigators must be familiar with ethical guidelines of the federal government, professional organizations, and specific institutions where research is to be conducted.

SIGNIFICANCE TO NURSING

Every nursing study should have significance for nursing. This does not mean that the findings must have the capability of transforming the nursing profession and nursing practice. But if a common reaction to a study results is "so what?," it may well be a nonsignificant piece of research.

The researcher should ask questions such as these: Will clients or health care professionals benefit from the findings of this study? Will the body of nursing knowledge be increased as the result of this study? Can nurses use the results? If the answers to these questions are "yes," the problem has significance for nursing.

PERSONAL MOTIVATION

Personal motivation may not be the single-most important deciding factor in a researcher's decision to conduct a study, but it certainly ranks high on the priority list. If a person is not interested in the problem to be investigated, it will be difficult to work up enthusiasm for the project and conduct a worthwhile study.

Without personal interest, the research process may become tedious, and the study may never be completed. On the other hand, if a researcher is intrigued and curious about the problem, research can become fascinating. The steps can become a "treasure hunt." When the data are being prepared for analysis, the excitement grows and the adrenaline flows. At this stage in your understanding and familiarity with the research process, you may be having difficulty in believing this. But ask a nurse who has conducted research. Even if the study was conducted as a course requirement and enthusiasm was not great at the beginning of the project, it is quite likely that enthusiasm and curiosity increased as the study progressed.

Think of questions that have arisen during your clinical experiences. Also, you may have become intrigued by something you have read about in a professional journal or textbook. Many areas in nursing need further research. It is hoped that in the near future you will find an area that is not only significant to nursing but is of personal interest to you.

RESEARCHER QUALIFICATIONS

Not every nurse is qualified to conduct research. Caution must be exercised when research skills are not well developed. Inappropriate designs may be chosen and inadequate data-collection methods used.

Research is generally conducted by nurses who have received advanced educational preparation. However, beginning research skills should be learned at the undergraduate level. A class research project may be conducted in which students design a survey study and act as the subjects. Enthusiasm for research seems to rise during the course of a class project. If several sections of a research course are being taught during the same semester, students in the various sections can compare their results. A spirit of healthy competition may be fostered. If clinical research is planned, the beginning researcher should collaborate with a more experienced researcher, such as a faculty member or a clinical nurse specialist.

FEASIBILITY OF STUDY

Feasibility is an essential consideration of any research project. The researcher needs to be reasonably sure that the study can actually be carried out. Many questions need to be answered. How long will the project take? Are appropriate instruments available? Can subjects be obtained? What is the cost? Does the researcher have support for the project?

Time. A nurse might be interested in studying sibling relationships among quintuplets. Knowledge of the incidence of quintuplet births would certainly discourage anyone considering research on this particular population unless the researcher planned to make this a lifetime project! Time is always a factor to consider. It is wise to allow more time than seems to be needed because unexpected delays frequently occur.

Cost. All research projects cost money; some studies are much more expensive than others. The researcher must realistically consider the financial resources available. Many sources of outside funding exist but not nearly enough to cover all of the needed research. Some of the various sources of funding are discussed in Chapter 16.

Equipment and Supplies. "The best laid plans of mice and men oft times go astray," according to a line in Robert Burns' poem "To a Mouse." This saying is certainly true in the research situation. The researcher can devise a study that is significant to nursing and that appears to be feasible to conduct only to find that there is no equipment to accurately measure the research variables. Even if equipment is available, it may not be in proper working condition. All research projects require some type of resources. An accurate determination of the needed equipment and supplies should be made before the final decision is made to conduct a study.

Some questions that should be asked (and answered) before beginning a research project are these:

1. What equipment will be needed?
2. Is this equipment available and in proper working order?
3. Is there a qualified operator of the equipment?
4. Are the necessary supplies available, or can they be obtained?

Some of the more common pieces of equipment used in nursing research are physiological data-gathering devices such as thermometers and stethoscopes. Also, office equipment such as word processors and duplicating machines may be needed. Access to a computer may be essential if a large amount of data must be analyzed. If the researcher takes into consideration equipment and supplies in the early phases of a research project, there is less likelihood that the project will have to be revised or discarded later because of equipment or supply problems.

Administrative Support. Many research projects require administrative support. Nurses working in health care institutions, such as hospitals, may seek released time to conduct research or financial support for a proposed project. Research requires time, money, and supplies. The nurse researcher may find it very difficult to conduct research independently.

Faculty research expectations and support for research by faculty members vary among educational institutions. Not only is financial support helpful, but in many cases psychological support from the administration is even more helpful. Knowing that your superiors support your research efforts can be a powerful motivating force.

Peer Support. We never outgrow our need for peer support. Many research ideas have never been developed because potential researchers received no support for their ideas from their peers. A comment such as, "Why would you want to conduct a study like that?" could discourage a researcher from proceeding with a study. One of the best ways a nurse researcher can determine a researchable problem is through interactions and discussions with other nurses. This collegial relationship is important for the researcher, especially for the beginning researcher who has not yet developed confidence in his or her research skills. A climate of shared interest in nursing research is essential among the members of the nursing profession.

Availability of Subjects.   A researcher may believe that study subjects are readily available and are anxious to participate in a proposed study. Much to the researcher's surprise, this may not be the case. Potential subjects may not meet the study criteria, may be unwilling to participate, or may already be participating in other studies.

PROBLEM STATEMENT CRITERIA

The important criteria for a research problem statement are that it (a) is written in interrogative sentence form, (b) includes the population, (c) includes the variable(s), and (d) is empirically testable.

WRITTEN IN INTERROGATIVE SENTENCE FORM

The use of a question format to state the research problem seems to be the clearest way to identify the problem area of a study (Polit & Hungler, 1999). When questions are asked, answers are sought. If a declarative sentence is used to describe the problem area, the desire to seek an answer to the problem does not seem as clear-cut. Consider the following two ways of expressing the same study problem:

- *Declarative Form:* The problem of this study is to determine the relationship between the number of hours that baccalaureate nursing students have studied and their anxiety levels before the midterm examination.

- *Interrogative Form:* Is there a relationship between the number of hours that baccalaureate nursing students have studied and their anxiety levels before the midterm examination?

The question format does seem to demand an answer more than the declarative form. Kerlinger (1986) stated that a research problem is an interrogative sentence that asks "what relation exists between two or more variables" (p. 16). All research problem statements in this textbook will be written in the interrogative form. Many problem statements in the literature are written in the declarative form.

A research problem should always be stated in a complete and grammatically correct sentence. The problem statement should be stated in a manner that the research consumer can read, understand, and respond to. To get all necessary information into a problem statement, the sentence may become rather long. Students have made comments such as "You are asking me to write a run-on sentence" and "My English teacher would have given me a failing grade on a sentence like that." Although the problem statement may be long in some instances, it should always be grammatically correct. Otherwise, confusion will arise, and the research problem may be unclear.

INCLUDES THE POPULATION

The population should be delimited (narrowed down) to the main group of interest. A population such as "nurses," "students," or "patients" is too broad to be examined. It would be better to identify these populations as "neonatal intensive care unit nurses," "baccalaureate nursing students," and "patients with a recent diagnosis of diabetes." This narrowing down of the population in the problem statement still will not identify the specific study population. The specific population will need to be discussed in detail in another area of the research proposal or research report.

INCLUDES THE VARIABLE(S)

The problem statement should contain the variable(s) to be studied. One, two, or many variables may be examined in a study.

One-variable Studies.   When a study is of an exploratory nature and contains only one variable, it may be called a **univariate study.** An example of a problem statement for such a study might be: What sources of work stress are identified by thoracic intensive care unit nurses? The single variable in this question is "sources of work stress." It is considered a variable because it is expected that the reported sources of stress will vary among the different nurses surveyed. Single-variable, or univariate, studies are frequently the beginning step in a research project. In the example given here, sources of stress could be identified in the univariate study. Then another study might be conducted to determine if there is a correlation between the number of reported sources of stress and the nurses' desire to leave the thoracic intensive care unit as a place of employment. A further study might be conducted in which one of the common stressors was controlled to determine if the desire to leave thoracic intensive care nursing would differ among the experimental group compared with the control group. These last two study suggestions each focus on two variables.

Two-variable Studies.   Generally, nursing research is concerned with more than one variable. It would be interesting to know what sources of stress are identified by thoracic intensive care unit nurses, but it would be more important to know how these stressors affect these nurses and whether there is anything that could be done to decrease the stressors or reduce their impact on the nurses.

Research in nursing, as well as in other disciplines, is frequently concerned with two variables. When two variables are examined, the study can be called a **bivariate study.** Generally, one of the variables is called the independent and one the dependent variable. Consider the example concerning stress among nurses in the thoracic intensive care unit. The problem statement might be: Is there a correlation between the number of sources of stress reported by nurses in a thoracic intensive care unit and the nurses' desire to leave employment in the thoracic intensive care unit? In this question, the independent variable is the number of reported sources of stress, and the dependent variable is the desire to leave employment in the thoracic intensive care unit.

Also, consider the previous example of the study in which an attempt might be made to control or decrease one of the stressors identified by thoracic intensive care unit nurses, to determine if their desire to leave this area of employment would decrease. The identified stressor might be the nurses' unfamiliarity with the equipment in the unit. The research problem might be: Is the level of desire to leave thoracic intensive care unit nursing different between a group of thoracic nurses who have attended a workshop on thoracic intensive care unit equipment and a group of thoracic nurses who have not attended the workshop? Although the problem is wordy, it is better to repeat words than to create any misunderstanding about what is being compared. The independent variable in this problem statement is "attendance or nonattendance at a workshop on thoracic intensive care unit equipment," and the dependent variable is "desire to leave thoracic intensive care unit nursing."

Occasionally, in a correlational study, an independent and dependent variable are not identifiable because it is not possible to determine which variable is influencing the other. For example, if you were examining the relationship between students' scores on a psychology test and their scores on a math test, it would not be appropriate to identify one as the independent and one as the dependent variable. You would not be able to label one of these variables as the "cause" and the other variable as the "effect."

Multiple-variable Studies. Whenever more than two variables are examined in a study, the research can be considered as a multiple-variable or **multivariate study.** Multiple-variable research is becoming increasingly common in nursing. Frequently, it is the interaction of variables that is of interest. For example, a researcher might conduct a study to determine why clients do not take their medications as directed after they are discharged. Educational levels might be considered as the influential factor, and the researcher may believe that the patients with high levels of education will be more compliant with the medical regimen than patients with low levels of education. Quite likely the results of the study will not support this belief. Why? Many factors may be influencing the person's medication compliance behavior. People may consider themselves as "weak" and lacking control over their bodies if they have to take medications. The medicine may be viewed favorably or unfavorably by a relative of the client. The medication may be expensive. So, the likelihood exists that a variety of factors may be influencing the client's compliance behavior.

Why do nursing students pass or fail the national licensing examination? Is just one factor involved, such as grade point average? Or could many factors be influential, such as the amount of time studied, the motivation to be a nurse, and the amount of time slept the night before the examination?

EMPIRICALLY TESTABLE

Testable problem statements contain variables that can be measured by the researcher. For a problem statement to be empirically testable, empirical data must be available about the variable or variables of interest. As you remember, empirical data consist of data gathered through the sense organs. These data consist of observations that are made through hearing, sight, touch, taste, or smell. Additional equipment to aid our senses also may be used. This equipment might be thermometers, scales, or stethoscopes.

Ethical and value issues or "right" and "wrong" decisions are not appropriate for scientific research. Consider these research questions: Should patients be allowed to have an unlimited number of visitors? What is the best way to teach nursing students about the research process? These are not researchable questions. Scientific problems do not concern values or ethical issues. A good way to detect a value question is to look for words like "should" and "better." The two previous examples could be changed to testable problem statements in the following manner: "Is there a difference in the anxiety levels of patients between those who are allowed an unlimited number of visitors and those who are allowed visitors only at specified visiting hours?" and "Is there a difference between the final examination scores of nursing research students who are taught with a lecture method and those who are taught with a seminar method?"

It is also better to avoid words like "cause" and "effect." Rather than writing a problem statement that says, "What is the effect of room temperature on the oral temperature measurements of children?" instead ask "Is there a difference in the oral temperature measurements of a group of children in a room where the temperature is kept at 65°F in comparison to the oral temperature measurements of this same group of children when the room temperature is kept at 75°F?" Although investigators are interested in cause-and-effect relationships, causality is difficult to prove and, therefore, it is better to avoid using this word or similar words in the problem statement or hypothesis of a study.

PROBLEM STATEMENT FORMAT

The following material is presented to help you learn how to write problem statements. Do not consider these examples as the *only* way to write problem statements.

Problem statements for studies that examine more than one variable are usually written as correlational statements or comparative statements.

I. Correlational Statement

Format: Is there a correlation between **X** (independent variable) and **Y** (dependent variable) in the population?

Example: Is there a correlation between **anxiety** and **midterm examination scores** of baccalaureate nursing students?

II. Comparative Statement
A. Descriptive Study

Format: Is there a difference in **Y** (dependent variable) between people in the population who **have X** characteristic (independent variable) and those who **do not have X** characteristic?

Example: Is there a difference in **readiness to learn about preoperative teaching** between preoperative patients who **have high anxiety levels** compared with preoperative patients who **do not have high anxiety levels?**

B. Experimental Study

Format: Is there a difference in **Y** (dependent variable) between Group A who **received X** (independent variable) and Group B who **did not receive X?**

Example: Is there a difference in the **preoperative anxiety levels** of patients who were **taught relaxation techniques** compared to those patients who were **not taught relaxation techniques?**

Practice substituting other variables for the **X** and **Y** in the examples. You will soon be able to formulate problem statements with greater ease.

It may appear that there are two independent variables in the problem statements for the descriptive and experimental studies. In fact, there is only one independent variable in both of these problem statements, but there are two levels or subdivisions of the independent variable. In the descriptive study problem statement, the two levels of the independent variable are high anxiety and low anxiety. In the experimental study, the two levels of the independent variable are taught relaxation techniques and not taught relaxation techniques.

As you may have noticed, these problem statements are written in a neutral, nonpredictive form. The descriptive study problem statement could have been written this way: Are preoperative patients who have high anxiety levels less ready to learn about preoperative teaching than preoperative patients who have low anxiety levels? There are several reasons for leaving the problem statement neutral or nonpredictive. The researcher may have very little information about the study area or have little knowledge about the possible results of a study when the problem statement is written. It is advisable to conduct a review of the literature and then develop a theoretical or conceptual framework for the study. With this background, hypotheses can then be written that identify the expected study results. The prediction should be put in the hypothesis.

CRITIQUING THE PROBLEM STATEMENT

The initial task of the reader of a research article is to locate the problem statement or, as is frequently the case, the purpose statement. The problem statement should be presented at the beginning of a research report. It is often found in the abstract, but it also should be presented in the body of the article, usually at the end of the introductory section of the article. If the problem statement is not clearly stated, it will be difficult for the reader to proceed further in evaluating the study.

Once the problem statement is located, certain guidelines may be used in evaluating the statement. First, the reader should determine the ethical nature of the study. Next, the reader considers the significance of the problem area to nursing. The scope of the problem is also considered. Is the problem area too narrow or too broad? The researcher may be trying to study too many variables in one study.

The problem statement should be clear and concise. It should contain both the population and the variable(s) that will be studied. The possibility of gathering empirical data on the topic of interest should be evident. Questions to be asked while evaluating a problem statement are presented in Box 4–1.

Box 4–1. Guidelines for Critiquing the Problem Statement

1. Is the problem (purpose) statement clear?
2. Is the problem statement written in a single declarative or interrogatory sentence?
3. Are the study variables and the population included in the problem statement?
4. Does the problem statement indicate that empirical data could be gathered on the topic of interest?
5. Does the problem statement indicate that the study would be ethical?
6. Is the feasibility of the study apparent when reading the problem statement?
7. Is the significance of the study to nursing apparent in the problem statement?

SUMMARY

The selection of a research problem or research question is probably the most important and the most difficult step in the research process. Some of the most common sources for obtaining research ideas are personal experiences, literature sources, existing theories, and previous studies. Nurses need to conduct **replication studies** based on previous nursing research investigations.

Several criteria should be considered in determining a research problem. First, ethical issues must be considered. Second, the problem should be significant to nursing. Third, personal motivation to conduct the study should be present. Fourth, the researcher's qualifications must be considered. Finally, the feasibility of the study must be considered. How long will the project take? How much will it cost? Can needed equipment and supplies be obtained? Does the researcher have administrative and peer support for the project? Is a study population available?

The research problem statement should be written in the interrogative form, contain the population and the variables that are being studied, and be empirically testable. The use of a question format is a clear way to identify the problem area for a study. Questions demand answers. Another way to make a problem statement concise is by delimiting or narrowing down the population for the study. Also, the variables under study must be clearly identified. One, two, or many variables may be studied.

Studies may be referred to as **univariate, bivariate,** and **multivariate** studies, according to whether one, two, or many variables are being studied. There is an increasing emphasis on multivariate research because nursing is concerned with the relationships between many combinations of variables.

Testable problem statements contain variables that can be measured empirically. Empirical data consist of data gathered through the sense organs. Scientific research problems do not concern value or ethical issues.

The problem should be stated formally in writing before the next step of the research process is undertaken. Research problems that examine more than one variable are usually written in the form of a correlational statement or a comparative statement.

NURSING RESEARCH ON THE WEB

For additional online resources, research activities, and exercises, go to www.prenhall.com/nieswiadomy. Select Chapter 4 from the drop down menu.

✖ GET INVOLVED ACTIVITIES

1. Bring in research articles that contain problem statements/purpose statements. Have volunteers read their statements. Pick the "best" statement.

2. Rewrite some of the declarative problem statements/purpose statements that have been brought to class in the interrogatory problem statement format that you have learned.

3. Think of problems to address that are not appropriate to research (such as "Should all nurses carry malpractice insurance?").

4. Gather in groups of four to six students and practice writing problem statements in an interrogatory format. Place the problem statements on overhead transparencies and take turns presenting problem statements to the rest of the class.

✖ SELF-TEST

Evaluate the following problem statements. Select answer A, B, C, or D according to the presence of the necessary elements of an acceptable problem statement.

A. The population is missing.

B. The dependent variable is missing.

C. The independent variable is missing.

D. All elements are present.

_____ 1. Is there a correlation between fathers' heights and their sons' heights?

_____ 2. Is there a difference in the level of assertiveness between men and women?

_____ 3. Is there a difference in anxiety levels after a relaxation exercise?

_____ 4. Is there a correlation between exercise and weight loss?

_____ 5. Is there a relationship between the self-concept of baccalaureate nursing students and their level of career aspirations?

_____ 6. Is there a difference in pregnant women who attend prenatal classes and those who do not attend prenatal classes?

_____ 7. Is there a difference in the anxiety levels of preoperative patients after practicing relaxation exercises?

_____ 8. Is there a correlation between anxiety levels and pulse rates?

_____ 9. Is there a difference in people who have exercised and those who have not exercised?

_____ 10. Is there a difference in the birth weight of infants?

✻ REFERENCES

Ienatsch, G. (1999). Knowledge, attitudes, treatment practices, and health behaviors of nurses regarding blood cholesterol. *The Journal of Continuing Education in Nursing, 30,* 13–19.

Kerlinger, F. (1986). *Foundations of behavioral research* (3rd ed.). New York: Holt, Rinehart & Winston.

Polit, D. F., & Hungler, B. P. (1999). *Nursing research: Principles and methods* (6th ed.). Philadelphia: Lippincott.

Rogers, C. (1969). *Freedom to learn.* Columbus, OH: Charles E. Merrill.

Sharts-Hopko, N. C. (2000). *Journal of The Association of Nurses in AIDS Care, 11,* 86–88.

CHAPTER 5

Review of the Literature

✸ OUTLINE

✸ OBJECTIVES

On completion of this chapter, you will be prepared to:

1. Determine the purposes for the literature review
2. Recognize the need for becoming familiar with the library's services
3. Distinguish between primary and secondary sources in research literature
4. Discuss print resources that may be used in locating literature references
5. Discuss electronic sources that may be used in locating literature references
6. Compare and contrast print and electronic sources that are useful for nurses when conducting a literature review
7. Obtain references from online journals

8. Conduct a literature search on a given topic
9. Extract pertinent information from literature sources
10. Critique the literature review section of research articles

✖ NEW TERMS DEFINED IN THIS CHAPTER

abstracts
CD-ROMs
ejournals
ezines

indexes
primary source
secondary source

When revising this 4th edition of *Foundations of Nursing Research,* Chapter 5 was left to last. Can you guess why? First, I knew that this chapter would become outdated much quicker than the other 16 chapters, and second, I felt least qualified to write this chapter! I started hinting about my need for help to my librarian friend many months ago. So, with her help I have attempted to bring the information in this chapter up to date as of February 2001.

Information is presented on the purposes of a literature review, the use of the library, primary and secondary reference sources, print sources, electronic sources, online journals, and obtaining information from sources. Much more information will be presented concerning sources on the World Wide Web (WWW) than in previous editions of this textbook. Remember, however, that the Web is ever changing. A web site that you visit today may be totally different (or disappear) in a short period of time.

The material is presented as if you were preparing to conduct a literature review for a proposed study. However, the information may be used to conduct a review of the literature for any article that you might write or any project that you might conduct. The chapter closes with a section on how to critique the literature review section of a research article.

PURPOSES OF THE LITERATURE REVIEW

There are many purposes for reviewing the literature before conducting a research study. The most important one is to determine what is already known about the topic that you wish to study. Research is an ongoing process that builds on previous knowledge. Few topics are so rare that they have never been investigated.

Generally, the researcher begins the literature review with a study topic in mind. Occasionally, a literature source serves as the basis for the topic. Many published studies contain recommendations for future research; therefore, the idea for a study may actually be formed while reading a published study report. Regardless of the basis for the topic, existing knowledge of the topic must be determined by a review of the literature. A search is made to locate previous studies in that area. If previous research is found, the researcher must decide whether to replicate a study or examine another aspect of the problem. The review of the literature is necessary, therefore, to narrow the problem to be studied.

Once the researcher is familiar with the existing literature, a framework must be established in which to place the study results. This involves locating theoretical or conceptual formulations that will help guide the study. Research hypotheses or questions are based on the theoretical or conceptual framework of the study, and research findings are interpreted in light of the study framework. Therefore, the literature review will help locate a framework for the proposed study.

Another purpose of the review of the literature is to help plan the study methodology. Appropriate research methods and research tools for the study may be selected after reading the accounts of other studies. The researcher may be able to capitalize on the successes as well as the errors of other investigators.

Nurses in the United States are particularly fortunate because of the vast amount of published material in the field of nursing. When conducting a review of the literature, nurses may wish there were not so much material! However, nurses in many countries are envious of our resources because only a few nursing journals are published in their native language.

USE OF THE LIBRARY

As time passes, fewer and fewer nurses and nursing students are making use of libraries. Recently a student told me that she could not turn in her paper on time because she could not obtain, from the Internet, a 1980 reference in the *American Journal of Nursing*. I asked her if she had thought of going to the library. She said, "How would I find the reference there?" I determined that she had never used a hard copy of an index, such as the *Cumulative Index to Nursing and Allied Health* (CINAHL). This particular index (which we used to call the "Red Book") was the "bread and butter" of literature searches for most nurses in the past. After I told her about the CINAHL, she said, "But I would have to go to the library shelves and look for the article." We won't talk about the thoughts that were going through my mind!

In an editorial in *Journal of Nursing Education,* Pravikoff (2000) mentioned that she had talked about the library to two baccalaureate nursing students who would soon be graduating. They told her that they had yet to spend any time in the school library searching for information for research papers or care plans. They had retrieved their information from the World Wide Web.

Molly Dougherty, editor of *Nursing Research,* wrote that the downside of electronic publications might be that students and scientists are paying too much attention to the most immediately available information. She asserted, "If availability supercedes careful and comprehensive knowledge acquisition as the underpinning of inquiry, knowledge development may be jeopardized" (Dougherty, 1999, p. 239).

According to Hill and Stickell (2000) "Libraries are waging an internal war between books and bytes" (p. 10). Nearly all knowledge can now be translated into a worldwide language of bits and bytes. However, questions have arisen about the long-lasting preservation of digital material. Will it withstand the test of time as well as printed material? Hill and Stickell asked, "What will we think of digitization as a means of preservation 10 or 15 years from now?" (p. 10).

Even though the Internet and the Web are absolutely astounding in their ability to retrieve information, please don't give up your trips to the library! Libraries contain a wealth of information. If you are unfamiliar with a particular library, acquaint yourself with that library's facilities and holdings. Tour the library and consult the staff. Librarians are usually delighted to familiarize you with the use of the card catalog (generally online), the various indexes, computer-assisted searches, and other reference materials. The librarian also will inform you about such things as hours, photocopy services, checkout policies, and interlibrary loan materials available from other cooperating libraries.

PRIMARY AND SECONDARY SOURCES

Literature sources may be classified as primary or secondary sources. A **primary source** in the research literature is a description of a research study that was written by the original investigator(s). A **secondary source** in the research literature is a summary or description of a research study that was written by someone other than the study investigator(s).

Primary sources for studies are frequently found in journal articles. For example, the journal *Nursing Research* publishes research study results that have been written by the original investigator(s). Other journals that contain many primary sources for nursing studies include *Advances in Nursing Science, Applied Nursing Research, Biological Research for Nursing, Clinical Nursing Research, Nursing Science Quarterly, Research in Nursing and Health,* and *Western Journal of Nursing Research.* Many clinical journals, such as *Heart & Lung: The Journal of Acute and Critical Care* and *Pediatric Nursing,* also contain research reports. Additional journals are listed in Chapter 16.

If you are critiquing the "Review of the Literature" section of an article, it may be difficult for you to determine if the author is citing primary or secondary sources. The only information you have to rely on is contained in the reference list at the end of the article. One clue that a cited source is probably a primary one is that the article was published in a research journal. The only way to make a definite determination of the type of source would be to locate each reference.

If a theorist has been cited, the reference list should contain that theorist's name as the author of the cited material. If Maslow's theory is being discussed in the article you are critiquing, you should expect to see a reference that shows Maslow as the author.

The beginning researcher may be tempted to rely on secondary sources. Oftentimes, summaries of studies or theories are quicker to read and easier to understand than the original works. Secondary sources may provide valuable insight into the material, but it is the original or primary source that should be read, when possible, to check study findings and to draw conclusions about a research study. There is always a danger that the author of a secondary source may misinterpret information or leave out important information that might be valuable to the reader.

Try to begin your search with the most recent primary sources. These sources will frequently contain reference citations for earlier research reports that may be important for a study. Read the abstract or summary of the study to determine if the source should be read in depth.

PRINT SOURCES

Knowledge continually expands at a rapid pace, and the recording and storing of this knowledge create special problems. Even more important to the researcher is the process of locating specific pieces of knowledge. In the past, conducting a literature review was quite a task. Computers were not available; a hand search was the only method of obtaining information that had been published. Even though various search mechanisms have simplified the process, locating pertinent sources still can be a challenge. Fortunately, many sources are available to nurses. This section discusses the oldest type of resources—print sources.

Although print sources are being accessed less often than in the past, all nurses need to be familiar with them. Some literature can be obtained only through the print format because the information has not been included in an electronic form. For example, the electronic database for Cumulative Index to Nursing and Allied Health (CINAHL) contains no sources that were published before 1982. So, if you need information about an article published in 1980 in the *American Journal of Nursing,* you would need to consult the print version of CINAHL. Two types of print sources are indexes and abstracts.

INDEXES

Indexes contain reference materials on periodicals and some books. Printed indexes are library resources that provide assistance in obtaining journal articles and other publications relative to a topic of interest. There are a number of indexes of interest to nurses. Several of the more important ones are discussed in this section.

Cumulative Index to Nursing & Allied Health Literature. The *Cumulative Index to Nursing & Allied Health Literature* (CINAHL) is produced by CINAHL Information Systems in Glendale, California. This comprehensive index covers more than 1200 nursing and allied health journals. Some of the allied health fields are medical records, occupational therapy, physical therapy, and physician's assistant. The number of titles that is being added is increasing dramatically. For example, 102 titles were added in 1998.

The CINAHL was first published in 1956. There is a 5-year cumulation for 1956 to 1960, a 3-year cumulation for 1961 to 1963 and 1964 to 1966, and a 2-year cumulation for 1967 and 1968. The index has published a yearly cumulation since 1969. There are currently three quarterly issues (January-March, April-June, and July-September) and an annual multivolume hardbound cumulation, which also contains material from October through December of that year. A Subject Heading List volume is shipped with the January-March issue.

Since 1967, references may be located by either subject headings or authors. Before 1967, there was one alphabetical listing, and authors' names were interfiled with subject headings.

The title of the index was *Cumulative Index to Nursing Literature* until 1977, when the decision was made to include allied health literature. This change came about because of the trend toward a multidisciplinary approach to health care. The CINAHL also includes selected articles from biomedical journals included in *Index Medicus* and other selected journals. In addition, publications from the National League for Nursing, the American Nurses Association, and state nurses' associations are referenced in this index.

The *Cumulative Index to Nursing Literature* is the only index to periodical literature in nursing for the years from 1960 to 1965. Nursing literature from 1900 to 1959 is indexed in *Nursing Studies Index*. Since 1966, both CINAHL and the *International Nursing Index* (INI) have published references to nursing literature. CINAHL has been available since 1984 through electronic sources (magnetic tapes, CD-ROMs, and online).

International Nursing Index.   The *International Nursing Index* (INI) is produced by Lippincott Williams & Wilkins in cooperation with the National Library of Medicine. INI was first published in 1966. This index is published three times a year, with the third issue containing the annual cumulation.

The purpose of the INI is to provide comprehensive coverage of nursing literature from all over the world. English-language references appear first under any given topic. Then articles of other languages appear in alphabetical order. These references appear in brackets to indicate that they are not English references. More than 300 nursing journals are indexed. Also, significant articles from non-nursing journals are included. Although this index is primarily concerned with the coverage of nursing journals, it also contains listings of dissertations by nurses and publications of nursing organizations.

The index contains references according to subject headings and authors. The subject headings and format are similar to that found in *Index Medicus*. Some additional headings are included in INI that are specific to nursing. A nursing thesaurus is included in the annual cumulation. This thesaurus helps readers by providing nursing terms that are used as subject headings in the index. Medical terms, such as classifications of specific diseases, are not included in this thesaurus. The MeSH subject headings found in *Index Medicus* may be used to obtain medical headings that can be searched in INI. The MEDLINE database can be used to search INI.

There is a great deal of overlap between the INI and the CINAHL. Nearly all English language nursing journals are covered in both INI and CINAHL. The researcher in this country would probably prefer to use the CINAHL in a manual library search because all references are from English-language sources. Also, the inclusion of allied health literature provides coverage of additional material of interest to nurses.

Nursing Studies Index.   The *Nursing Studies Index* (NSI) was prepared at the Yale University School of Nursing under the direction of Virginia Henderson. This index provides an annotated guide to English language reports of studies and historical and biographical materials concerning nursing. Both a subject heading and author index are included. This index covers periodicals, books, and pamphlets. It provides the only index to nursing literature from 1900 to 1959.

The NSI was published in four volumes. Volume I, published in 1972, covers 1900 through 1929; Volume II, published in 1970, covers 1930 through 1949, Volume III, published in 1966, covers 1950 through 1956; and Volume IV, published in 1963, covers 1957 through 1959. The staff worked backward in time, starting with the most recent material, which was more easily located. We owe a debt of gratitude to the people who worked so diligently on this project to provide a reference source for nursing studies conducted in the first half of the century.

Index Medicus. Published monthly by the National Library of Medicine (NLM), *Index Medicus* (IM) is the most well-known index of medical literature. It covers all aspects of biomedicine and includes nursing and some other allied health fields. The first volume was published in 1879, and an annual cumulation began in 1960.

Index Medicus covers more than 3400 biomedical journals. Journals are listed in four sections: (a) alphabetical listing by abbreviated title, followed by full title; (b) alphabetical listing by full title, followed by abbreviated title; (c) alphabetical listing by subject field, and (d) alphabetical listing by country of publication. English-language articles are listed first in each topic section. Foreign-language articles follow and are enclosed in brackets to indicate that they are non-English citations. *Index Medicus* can be searched online through MEDLINE.

Hospital and Health Administration Index. The *Hospital and Health Administration Index* (formerly *Hospital Literature Index*) was published by the American Hospital Association from 1945 until 1999. It is now a service of the National Library of Medicine. It is published three times a year, with the third issue containing an annual cumulative index. This index provides subject and author access to more than 2200 journals and newsletters. These sources contain references to literature dealing with the nonclinical aspects of health care, such as health care planning and health care facility administration. This index can be searched through HealthSTAR, an online database of NLM.

ABSTRACTS

Abstracting services are published in many professional fields. **Abstracts** contain brief summaries of articles. Research abstracts contain the purpose, methods, and major findings of studies. By reading abstracts of studies, the researcher can determine if a copy of the entire research study should be obtained. Some of the abstracts of particular importance to nursing are discussed.

Nursing Research Abstracts. From 1960 to 1978, abstracts of research studies significant to nursing were published in the bimonthly issues of *Nursing Research.* Each November/December issue contained an author and subject guide to the abstracts that had been published during the previous year in *Nursing Research.*

Nursing Abstracts. A bimonthly abstracting service published by Nursing Abstracts Company, *Nursing Abstracts* has been published since 1979. This literatures source abstracts significant nursing studies that have appeared in many nursing journals.

Psychological Abstracts. The American Psychological Association has published *Psychological Abstracts* since 1927. These abstracts cover journals, technical reports, book chapters, and books in the field of psychology. Certain psychologically oriented articles from nursing journals are included. This abstracting service is published monthly and is cumulated semiannually. More than 1500 journals and technical reports are scanned each year to provide the material for *Psychological Abstracts.* Nursing journals that are scanned are *Advances in Nursing Science, Clinical Nursing Research, International*

Journal of Nursing Studies, Issues in Mental Health Nursing, and *Nursing Research.* These abstracts may be searched through the PsycINFO online database.

Dissertation Abstracts International. A comprehensive abstracting source for doctoral dissertations, *Dissertation Abstracts International* (DAI) has been published since 1938. DAI is published monthly and cumulated annually. Each month's edition of DAI contains approximately 5000 new entries. Entries are divided into three sections: Section A contains abstracts for the humanities and social sciences, Section B is designated for sciences and engineering, and Section C covers non-North American material. The authors of the dissertations write their own abstracts, and since 1980 these abstracts have contained approximately 350 words. Nearly all accredited institutions in North America that award doctoral degrees submit their dissertations to ProQuest Information and Learning for listing in DAI. Copies of dissertations may be ordered through this commercial vendor at the following Web address: www.ProQuest.com.

Masters Abstracts International. *Masters Abstracts International* (MAI) is published every other month. It contains author-written 150-word abstracts of master's theses. More than 12,000 new abstracts are published each year. Because master's abstracts are submitted on a voluntary basis, only a small percentage of U.S. master's theses appear in MAI. These abstracts also may be obtained from ProQuest Information and Learning.

ELECTRONIC SOURCES

As previously mentioned, electronic sources have become the preferred format for accessing the literature. According to Sparks (1999), electronic communication is changing how information is retrieved and disseminated and is also impacting the conduct and communication of research results. Electronic sources include online catalogs, CD-ROMs, and online databases.

ONLINE CATALOGS

In most libraries, that wonderful old piece of furniture called the "card catalog" has disappeared. It has been replaced with computer terminals. Users are able to determine the holdings of their particular library (as well as other libraries) through this medium. The online catalog will contain an alphabetical listing of books under several different categories such as (a) title, (b) author, (c) subject heading, and (d) keyword. A keyword search finds the word(s) anywhere in the item record; it is a much broader search than is a subject heading search. The records in a keyword search are usually arranged by relevance rather than being in alphabetical order.

Book titles are filed according to the first word of the title unless the first word is an article (a, an, the), and then the second word of the title is used to file the book in the catalog. Authors are filed in alphabetical order according to surnames. Subject headings are filed according to broad categories, such as nursing, and then subcategories are filed under the broad categories.

Each book is assigned a call number that specifies the physical location of the item in a particular library. These call numbers may contain numbers only or a combination of letters and numbers, according to the filing system used by that library.

For some time, libraries have been aware that they cannot function as independent units and still provide optimum service to their clientele. No one library can afford all of the holdings that might be desired. Library networks help librarians to determine whether to purchase certain books and also allow them to inform library users of the location of reference materials.

A listing of books held by libraries throughout the world may be obtained through the Online Computer Library Center, Inc. (OCLC) in Dublin, Ohio. The database that contains books is titled WorldCat. This database contains material from more than 24,000 member libraries, including academic, public, federal, medical, and corporate libraries. This database is updated continuously.

OCLC is a nonprofit, membership computer library service and research organization that was founded in 1967 by university presidents for the purpose of sharing library resources, and, thereby, reducing costs. An online-shared cataloging system has been available since 1971. The OCLC Interlibrary Loan service allows libraries to borrow and lend through an online network of almost 7000 libraries. The services of OCLC are not available directly to individuals. These services must be accessed through libraries.

The newest innovation in accessing books is called "eBooks." Some libraries now have books available electronically through a system labeled "netLibrary." After locating an eBook in a library's resources, the visitor receives the option of viewing the book or checking it out online. The user will then have exclusive online access to the book during the check-out period. What will they think of next?

CD-ROMs

Many databases have been made available on **CD-ROMs** (Compact Disk-Read Only Memory). One of these disks can store the equivalent of 275,000 pages of text. These databases provide user-friendly assistance that allows the viewer to conduct searches without the assistance of a librarian. This type of resource was popular in the late 1980s and the 1990s. Library users were able to pick up a disk and search a database using a computer in the library. One of the disadvantages of CD-ROMs compared to an online database is that the CD-ROM database is usually split over a series of disks and is outdated as soon as it is released. Most of the databases that are available on CD-ROM are also available in print form and online versions. Therefore, the various databases that are available for this type of resource are not discussed here.

ONLINE BIBLIOGRAPHIC DATABASES

For those who own personal computers, it is possible to access databases without using the library resources. If you are a student, you will probably be able to use a microcomputer and modem at home to tie in with the online services at your university. Some universities allow students to have free accounts that will provide access to the World Wide Web. You might also purchase online services yourself through a commercial vendor.

The Web is a massive collection of files. These files are called pages. A "browser" is needed to read and print these pages. Popular browsers are Internet Explorer and Netscape. If you are unsure of the source you wish to access, you will need to use a "search engine," such as Lycos, WebCrawler, AltaVista, Hotbot, Excite, Northern Light, or Google to search the Web for you. You may want to use more than one search engine because no engine indexes more than about 16% of the material on the web (Lawrence & Giles, 1999). Recently, megasearch engines, such as Dogpile and Ask Jeeves, have been developed; both combine results from many search engines.

If you know exactly where you wish to go on the Web, you will need to enter the URL (Uniform Resource Locator) of the source. These usually begin with http (Hyper-Text Transfer Protocol). It is generally not necessary to type the http part of the URL. The browser automatically assumes that the URL begins with http. Some URLs are case-sensitive, so you must be aware of the need for capital letters for some addresses. One part of the URL indicates the domain name. Three initials are used to designate the various domains. For example, "com" is used for commercial organizations, "edu" is used for educational institutions, "gov" denotes government institutions, and "org" is used for such agencies as professional societies and charities. Because of the huge amount of material on the Web, new domains have recently been developed. Two of these new domains are "biz" and "name." "Biz" has been designated for general use by businesses, and "name" has been designated for general use by individuals for personal Web sites.

Before beginning a computer search, the researcher must define and narrow the topic. A manual search of the indexes may help to determine key words and concepts to use in the search. A computer-assisted search should always be augmented with the traditional search methods, and consultation with experts in the field may help you locate information on appropriate studies.

Computer-assisted searches have revolutionized the review of the literature process. These searches, however, for a variety of reasons may not provide the desired references. Finding information on the Web may be time-consuming and unpredictable, according to Schloman (1999), because there are so many sites and Web pages. In a report released in October 2000, researchers at OCLC (Online Computer Library Center, Inc.) estimated that there were approximately 7.1 million unique Web sites in 2000, which was about a 50% increase from the 4.7 million sites in 1999 (OCLC Researchers Measure The World Wide Web, October 16, 2000). Currently, there is no official gatekeeper for the Web. Therefore, care must be exercised when accessing information from this medium.

There are many reliable and accurate online databases. Some of those considered to be most useful to nurses are discussed next. In contrast to the print versions of these databases, the online versions contain abstracts for some of the entries.

CINAHL®.   The online CINAHL database corresponds to the *Cumulative Index to Nursing & Allied Health Literature.* Access is provided to more than 1200 journals in nursing and 17 other allied health disciplines. This database provides records from journals as well as books, book chapters, pamphlets, audiovisuals and educational software, nursing dissertations, some conference proceedings, and standards of professional practice.

There are more than 10,000 subject headings. Approximately 70% of these headings appear in MEDLINE. The CINAHL database contains more than 200 terms that were designed specifically for nursing and allied health. Subjects may be searched via the CINAHL Subject Heading List.

Of the 1200 journals covered, abstracts are included for more than 800 of them. Articles from 280 of these journals are available in full text format. With permission of the journal's publisher, cited references are listed for articles published from 1994 to the present.

The CINAHL database is available from commercial vendors such as *SilverPlatter Information* (www.silverplatter.com), *OVID Technologies* (www.ovid.com), *OCLC* (www.oclc.org), EBSCO Publishing (www.epnet.com), and *PaperChase,* (www.paperchase.com). Since 1994, the CINAHL database has been available directly through CINAHL Information Services. This service is titled CINAHL®*direct* and is available at www.cinahl.com. Selected articles that are stored as pdf (portable document format) files may be downloaded from this site for a fee. At the present time, the cost is $12 for each article. Journal articles also may be ordered by fax or mail.

RNdex.   RNdex is a bibliographic database that was established in 1992 by SilverPlatter, Inc. In 1997, Information Resources Group, Inc. took over the development and production of this database (www.rndex.com). RNdex offers citations and abstracts from more than 150 leading nursing and case management journals. Selected references are provided from related health care and critical care medicine journals. The database is available in versions designed for institutions, professionals, and students. The RNdex Student Edition is available on CD-ROM. This version contains references to over 100 nursing journals. It is published at the beginning of each academic year and is available from campus bookstores and directly from Delmar Publishers.

MEDLINE.   MEDLINE is the online counterpart of *Index Medicus.* The material in MEDLINE constitutes the main component of the National Library of Medicine's (NLM) MEDLARS® system. The six initials stand for Medical Literature, Analysis, and Retrieval System. This system was established in 1966 to provide access to journals in the life sciences, with a concentration on biomedicine. It also includes information from nursing, dentistry, veterinary medicine, and pharmacy. The online version, MEDLINE (MEDLARS On-Line), was initiated in 1971. About 4300 titles are included in MEDLINE, with more than 11 million references contained in the database. More than 85% of the journals are published in English. About 76% of the article citations are accompanied by abstracts written by the authors of the articles. New references are added each Saturday. More than 400,000 references are added each year. MEDLINE is available through the NLM home page at www.nlm.nih.gov and can be searched for free. After you enter the home page, you may proceed to one of two web-based services—PubMed® or Internet Grateful Med. You also may access Internet Grateful Med directly at igm.nlm.nih.gov. Each of these search mechanisms has advantages. Internet Grateful Med provides access to other NLN databases on topics such as AIDS, bioethics, toxicology, and health services research, while PubMed offers links to molecular biology databases. Hutchinson (1999) has contended that PubMed is easier for the novice to use. However, Stephenson (1999) disagreed with Hutchinson and asserted that the pull-down menus for age groups, languages, and publication types make Internet Grateful Med easier for the new searcher who may also be a novice computer user. She also pointed out the value of the 14 other databases that are available through Internet Grateful Med.

A search of MEDLINE may be done using the MeSH® (Medical Subject Headings) controlled vocabulary or by author name, title word, text word, journal name, phrase, or any combination of these. The search will provide a citation that includes authors, title, and source. Often, an abstract is included. Both PubMed and Internet Grateful Med search MEDLINE daily for in-process citations.

One of the features of both PubMed and Internet Grateful Med is that full-text copies of articles may be ordered through a service called Loansome Doc®. A copy of the article will be delivered to a local medical library. Registration is required, and the local library may charge a fee.

MEDLINE is also available from many online vendors. The advantage of using one of these vendors is that they provide superior search capabilities and offer special features (Polit & Hungler, 1999).

HealthSTAR.   HealthSTAR corresponds to the *Hospital and Health Administration Index*. This database, produced by NLM, provides access to the published literature from 1975 to the present on health services technology, administration, and research. From 1979 until 1999, this database and its predecessors were produced through a cooperative arrangement between the American Hospital Association (AHA) and the NLM. Health-STAR is now one of the many databases of MEDLARS. It became available in 1996 and is divided into two files: (a) current file covering 1992 to present and (b) backfile covering 1975 to 1991. The current file is updated weekly. Citations and abstracts are provided for journal articles, monographs, technical reports, meeting abstracts, book chapters, and government documents. HealthSTAR can be accessed 24 hours a day through Internet Grateful Med at igm.nlm.gov.

ERIC.   The ERIC database is the world's largest source of education information. It contains nearly 1 million abstracts of documents and journal articles on education research and practice. It corresponds to two print sources: *Current Index to Journals in Education* (CIJE) and *Resources in Education* (RIE). This database is at the heart of the ERIC (Educational Resources Information Center) system. This national information system is supported by the U.S. Department of Education's Office of Educational Research and Improvement and is administered by the National Library of Education (NLE). The ERIC database covers material from 1966 to the present. Many libraries throughout the country have complete collections of ERIC documents. Information for the ERIC database is supplied by a group of educational clearinghouses throughout the United States. Each clearinghouse disseminates information on a certain special area in education. The ERIC database is updated monthly. Free public access to this database is available at www.accesseric.org.

PsycINFO.   The PsycINFO database corresponds to the print *Psychological Abstracts*. The American Psychological Association prepares this database. It covers psychological literature from 1887 to the present. Materials are selected from more than 1500 journals written in more than 25 languages. More than 55,000 references are added annually. The database is updated online in February, May, August, and November. As was mentioned under the section on the print version, several nursing journals are covered by this database. At the present time, individuals may purchase a 24-hour search for $9.95. This service is available through PsycINFO Direct at www.psycinfo.com.

DISSERTATION ABSTRACTS ONLINE. DISSERTATION ABSTRACTS ONLINE (DA Online) offers libraries electronic access to the entire *Dissertation* Abstracts database. It is produced by ProQuest Information and Learning. DA Online includes American dissertations accepted since 1861 at accredited institutions. Selected master's theses have been included since 1962. Abstracts are included for doctoral dissertations from July 1980 and for master's theses from 1988. More than 50,000 new dissertations and 7000 new theses are added to the database each year. The database is updated monthly and is searchable in a number of ways, including key words in the title and the abstract. The database is available online at www.ProQuest.com and through commercial vendors such as Ovid Online, Dialog, and EPIC/First Search.

Nursing Research Index. In Spring 1999, Sigma Theta Tau International introduced the Nursing Research index. This online database covers all nursing journals in which 50% or more of the articles are considered research articles. The index covers articles from 1996 until the present. It is a user-friendly database. This database may be found at www.stti.iupui.edu/lit_indexes/journals.html. The following steps are used. Click on the letter of the concept of interest. A list of all concepts beginning with that letter appears. Then click on the concept. A list of all terms linked with that concept will appear. For example, if you had been interested in "postpartum depression" you could click on either postpartum or depression and finally get to the point in the search where the two terms are combined. Then search the list of journal articles relating to postpartum depression (there were 19 when I did my search). Click on the article of interest. If the article is indexed in MEDLINE or International Nursing Index, a PubMed abstract number will appear at the bottom of the citation. You are then able to go directly to that abstract.

Other Online Databases. Many other online databases may be searched for free by nurses. Some of them are listed here along with their Internet addresses:

AIDSLINE	igm.nlm.nih.gov
BIOETHICSLINE	igm.nlm.nih.gov
CANCERLIT	cnetdb.nci.nih.gov
CHID (Combined Health Information Database)	chid.nih.gov
TOXLINE	igm.nlm.nih.gov

ONLINE JOURNALS

An increasing number of journals are now available both in print and online. Online journals are frequently called **ejournals.** Online magazines are called **ezines.** Ejournals are becoming a necessary means of meeting the demands for knowledge dissemination, according to Jones and Cook (2000). These authors describe an ejournal as a digital periodical that is published on the Internet or World Wide Web. The process of preparation and review of manuscripts is essentially the same as with print journals; it is the means of submission and dissemination that is different. A fee is usually charged for online access to full-text articles.

Knowing that many "starving students" are reading this textbook, information about free online sources is presented. Table 5–1 presents free online journals. Table 5–2 presents journals that have an online version and allow readers to view their table of contents and some abstracts of articles. Some journals offer viewers other options. For example *The Online Journal of Knowledge Synthesis for Nursing* presents one sample article and some editorials that may be read online without a fee. The *Journal of Neonatal Nursing* (published in the United Kingdom) allows viewers to read one free article each month. Military nurses are allowed free access to *Military RN Online*. Some journals allow access to articles that are set up for CE credit. These include *American Journal of Critical Care, AAOHN Journal* (American Association of Occupational Health Nurses), *and RN.*

OBTAINING INFORMATION FROM LITERATURE SOURCES

After literature sources are located, pertinent material must be extracted from these sources. This can be a formidable task. Some people try to avoid this task as long as possible by photocopying every article on a certain topic. They then gather up mounds of printed material and head for home, with the belief that the task will be easier or more pleasant at home. Whether in the library or at home, the researcher must finally read the literature sources and decide what material is appropriate for the study under consideration.

Before recording bibliographic material such as the author's name or title of the report, determine the requirement for reference citations in your particular school or class.

TABLE 5–1. Free Online Journals/Magazines	
Journal/Magazine	**URL Address**
Imprint (magazine for nursing students)	www.nsna.org
Internet Journal of Advanced Nursing Practice	www.ispub.com/journals/ijanp.htm
Journal of Undergraduate Nursing Scholarship	juns.nursing.arizona.edu
Online Journal of Issues in Nursing	www.nursingworld.org/ojin
On-Line Journal of Nursing Informatics	milkman.cac.psu.edu/~dxm12/OJNI.html
NurseWeek	www.nurseweek.com

TABLE 5–2. Journals with Free Online Table of Contents and Abstracts	
Journal	**URL Address**
American Journal of Nursing	www.nursingcenter.com
Computers in Nursing	www.nursingcenter.com
*Evidence-Based Nursing**	www.evidencebasednursing.com
Geriatric Nursing	www.mosby.com
Heart & Lung: The Journal of Acute and Critical Care	www.mosby.com
*Journal of Advanced Nursing**	www.blackwell-science.com/online
Journal of Nursing Administration	www.nursingcenter.com
Journal of Pediatric Oncology Nursing	www.jopon.org
MCN: The American Journal of Maternal/Child Nursing	www.nursingcenter.com
Nursing Research	www.nursingcenter.com
Research in Nursing & Health	www3.interscience.wiley.com

*Table of Contents only.

The American Psychological Association (1994) format has become quite popular in the nursing literature, and many nursing education programs are using this style of references.

A great deal of psychological pain will be avoided if complete reference material is recorded for each literature source. It is frustrating to have to return to the library or go back on the Web to search for missing items (such as volume numbers). You may discover that some part of the reference citation is missing as you are hurrying to type your paper at 2 AM, the morning before the paper is due. The motto is "Record References Accurately (RRA)." If direct quotations will be used, copy this material very carefully, word for word. Use quotation marks to indicate the quoted material. Be careful to write down the page number for the quotation (or another trip to the library or the Web site will be necessary!). For references obtained from the Web, provide the date when the page was viewed as well as its location on the Web.

In taking notes, be as brief as possible, but do not omit important information. It is better to have too much information from a source than not enough. For relevant research articles, you will probably want to record information on the problem of the study, hypotheses, methodology, type of sample, findings, and conclusions.

Bibliographic material and important information from sources may be recorded on index cards, in spiral notebooks, or on loose-leaf paper. The advantage of index cards and loose-leaf paper is that references can be arranged and rearranged at will according to any classification system that is devised by the researcher. The advantage of the spiral notebook is that your references are all in one place and will not get misplaced as easily as individual cards or scraps of paper. Use the method that is most appealing to you.

CRITIQUING THE LITERATURE REVIEW

It is difficult to critique a literature review section of a research article if you are not familiar with the literature on the study topic. For example, you will not be able to determine if the researcher has included classic sources and the most recent sources. However, there are many aspects of the literature review that you will be able to evaluate, even if you are not an expert in the content area.

Although you may not be able to determine if the most recent references have been included, if all sources appear to be older than 5 years, you might wonder if some recent references may have been omitted. Also, if the topic is one that you know has been studied for many years, such as preoperative teaching, you would expect to see older studies cited as well as recent ones.

The literature review should contain mostly paraphrases, rather than direct quotes. Sources should be critically appraised, and the relevance of the sources should be clear. The review should be concise and to the point.

It will be important to determine if the researcher has presented both supporting and opposing literature. Are there studies in which support for the theory was not demonstrated? If this is the case, the researcher should present this information in the literature review section. Sometimes the discerning reader will find opposing studies included in the discussion section of the article, and it may appear to the reader that the researcher went back to the library to find new sources to support nonsignificant findings!

It is important to determine if the researcher is citing primary sources or secondary sources when reporting results of studies conducted in the past. Although it may not always be possible to determine if a source is a primary one, an examination of the reference list at the end of the article will provide some clues. If most of the references are from research journals, you will have more confidence that the sources are primary ones. If the reference list contains book chapters and literature reviews on a certain topic, it is likely that some secondary sources are being cited. Guidelines for critiquing the literature review section of a research article are presented in Box 5–1.

Box 5–1. Guidelines for Critiquing the Literature Review

1. Is the literature review comprehensive?
2. Is the literature review concise?
3. Does the review flow logically from the purpose(s) of the study?
4. Are all sources relevant to the study topic?
5. Are sources critically appraised?
6. Are both classic and current sources included?
7. Are paraphrases or direct quotes used most often?
8. Are both supporting and opposing theory and research presented?
9. Are most of the references primary sources?

SUMMARY

The most important reason for reviewing the literature before conducting a research study is to determine what is already known about the study topic. Previous studies are located and a theoretical or conceptual basis for the study is sought in the literature.

Literature sources may be classified as primary or secondary. A **primary source** in the research literature is a description of a study that was written by the original researcher(s). A **secondary source** provides a summary or description of a research study written by someone other than the study investigator(s).

Literature sources can be located through print sources and electronic sources. Print sources include **Indexes** and **abstracts. Indexes** are used to obtain references to periodical articles. **Abstracts** contain brief summaries of articles and contain the purpose, methods, and major findings of studies. Electronic sources include online catalogs, **CD-ROMs,** and online bibliographic databases. Online journals and magazines, or **ejournals** and **ezines,** are becoming popular.

Accuracy in recording bibliographic material is essential. Direct quotations must be recorded word for word and the page number indicated. Bibliographic material and important information from literature sources may be recorded on index cards, in spiral notebooks, or on loose-leaf paper.

 ## NURSING RESEARCH ON THE WEB

For additional online resources, research activities, and exercises, go to www.prenhall.com/nieswiadomy. Select Chapter 5 from the drop down menu.

✕ GET INVOLVED ACTIVITIES

1. Choose a topic to use in a computer search (such as cancer, teenage pregnancy, or social support). Using your own computer or one in your library, conduct a computer search. Determine the number of references on that topic. Then consult the thesaurus for the database that you used and determine if the term that you entered in your search is a valid descriptor. If not, conduct another search using the valid descriptor that you have located in the thesaurus. Did you obtain more references using the new term?

2. Examine the reference lists of two research articles. Are you able to determine the number of references that appear to be primary sources and the number of references that appear to be secondary sources?

3. Examine these same reference lists again and try to determine if the researcher has used classical sources and current sources.

4. Divide into pairs. Have one person in each pair conduct a search of the printed indexes and one person in each pair conduct a computer search. Each pair will be given the same term to search. See which person in each pair is able to locate a reference first. How many of the people using the index were able to locate a reference faster than the people using the computer search?

✷ SELF-TEST

Circle the letter before the *best* answer.

1. Which of the following is the *most* important reason for conducting a review of the literature before conducting a research study?

   A. The research design can be copied from a previous study.
   B. A determination will be made about the existing knowledge in the identified problem area.
   C. An instrument may be uncovered that will be appropriate for the proposed study.
   D. The feasibility of the study can be determined.

2. A primary source for a nursing research study is:

   A. the retrieval mechanism that is first used in locating the research study.
   B. an index that directs the reader to the research study.
   C. a description of the study written by the researcher who conducted the study.
   D. a summary of research on the study topic.

3. Most research articles that appear in the journal *Research in Nursing and Health* are examples of:

   A. primary sources.
   B. secondary sources.
   C. both primary and secondary sources.
   D. neither primary nor secondary sources.

4. What is one of the advantages of conducting a computerized literature search rather than using the printed indexes?

   A. Primary sources are easier to locate.
   B. The entire articles may always be printed at the end of the search.
   C. No libraries have printed indexes available.
   D. Search terms can be combined.

5. Which of the following databases are appropriate for nurses to use?

   A. CINAHL
   B. MEDLINE
   C. HealthSTAR
   D. All of the above
   E. None of the above

6. Which of the following sources would provide the most current information on literature sources?

   A. printed indexes
   B. CD-ROMs
   C. online databases

7. Which of these printed indexes DOES NOT have an online version?

   A. Cumulative Index to Nursing & Allied Health Literature
   B. Index Medicus

    C. Health and Hospital Administration

    D. Nursing Studies Index

8. Which of the following sources should be used to obtain a 1962 reference in the *American Journal of Nursing*?

    A. *International Nursing Index*

    B. *Cumulative Index to Nursing Literature*

    C. *Index Medicus*

    D. *Cumulative Index to Nursing and Allied Health Literature*

9. In conducting a literature review, the reader is *least* interested in which of the following information about a research study?

    A. research study results

    B. opinions about the research study

    C. how the research variables were operationally defined

    D. research study methodology

10. Which of the following statements is true about online databases?

    A. No online databases are available to the general public.

    B. Some online databases are available to the general public.

    C. Many online databases are available to the general public.

✖ REFERENCES

Dougherty, M. C. (1999). Electronic research dissemination. *Nursing Research, 48,* 239.

Hill, D. R., & Stickell, H. N. (2000). Brandon/Hill selected list of print nursing books and journals. *Nursing Outlook, 48,* 10–21.

Hutchinson, D. (1999). *MEDLINE for health professionals: How to search PubMed on the Internet.* Sacramento, CA: New Wind Publishing.

Jones, S. L., & Cook, C. B. (2000, January 31). Electronic journals: Are they a paradigm shift? *Online Journal of Issues in Nursing.* Retrieved November 25, 2000 from the World Wide Web: www.ana.org/ojin/topic11/tpc11_1.htm.

Lawrence, S., & Giles, L. (1999). Accessibility and distribution of information on the Web. Retrieved November 21, 2000 from the World Wide Web: www.wwwmetrics.com.

OCLC Researchers Measure the World Wide Web (2000, October 16). Retrieved November 24, 2000 from the World Wide Web: www.oclc.org/oclc/press/20001016a.htm.

Polit, D. F., & Hungler, B. P. (1999). *Nursing research: Principles and Methods* (6th ed.). Philadelphia: Lippincott.

Pravikoff, D. (2000). On the information highway, or sitting on the curb? *Journal of Nursing Education, 39,* 99–100.

Schloman, B. F. (1999, August 19). Needle in a haystack? Finding health information on the Web. *Online Journal of Issues in Nursing.* Retrieved November 15, 2000 from the World Wide Web: www.ana.org/ojin/infocol/info_2.htm.

Sparks, S. M. (1999). Electronic publishing and nursing research. *Nursing Research, 48,* 50–54.

Stephenson, P. L. (1999). MEDLINE for health professionals: How to search PubMed on the Internet (book review). *Computers in Nursing, 17,* 149, 152–154.

CHAPTER 6

Theory and Nursing Research

✖ OUTLINE

✖ OBJECTIVES

On completion of this chapter, you will be prepared to:

1. Define theory, concept, construct, proposition, empirical generalization, model, and conceptual models
2. Discuss four nursing conceptual models
3. Distinguish between theoretical and conceptual frameworks
4. Describe deductive and inductive reasoning processes in theory generation and development
5. Identify theories used in nursing
6. Identify the steps used in testing a theory
7. Critique the study framework section of research reports

✖ NEW TERMS DEFINED IN THIS CHAPTER

concept
conceptual framework
conceptual model
construct
deductive reasoning
empirical generalization
grand theories

inductive reasoning
middle-range theories
model
proposition
theoretical framework
theory

It is Christmas Eve and you are trying to find a particular toy for your nephew. You congratulate yourself as you finally locate one. Then you notice the price! The toy is twice as expensive as you had thought. Knowing that members of the media have been discussing the popularity of this particular toy (in 2000 it was PlayStation 2, a game console/DVD player), you wonder if the theory of "supply and demand" is a plausible explanation for the outrageous cost of this toy. You pay for the toy, get back in your car, and head for home. As you drive down the freeway in the busy afternoon traffic, you notice the discourtesy of the drivers and the continual honking of horns. Many drivers appear tense and impatient. You think about the problems these people may have encountered during the day as well as the added inconvenience of the traffic congestion. Without a conscious awareness, you may be considering a stress theory as the explanation for the behaviors that you have observed.

Theories are used by people to explain happenings in their lives and in their environments. Theories also are used by nurses to explain happenings of significance to nursing. Nursing research and nursing practice should be theory based. When research is guided by a theoretical framework, the theory guides the research process from the beginning to the end—that is, from the identification of the research problem to the formulation of the study conclusions. You may ask, where does a researcher "get" a theory for a study or determine which theory would be most appropriate? This chapter will help answer these questions and, it is hoped, help you to recognize the value of theory-based nursing research.

THEORY TERMINOLOGY

Confusion is experienced by many nurses when confronted with the terms in this chapter. There is no absolute or "correct" definition for many of these terms. The lack of agreement in terminology sometimes leaves you wondering which definition to use. It is more important for you to gain a basic understanding of the terminology than to memorize definitions. You will be in a better position to recognize the terms when you encounter them in the research literature. Rather than memorizing one "correct" definition of the word "theory," for example, try to gain an understanding of what a theory is and how it is useful in nursing.

To help you understand the content of this chapter, some definitions and explanations of theory terminology are presented first. These definitions and explanations were generated after reviewing the most recent literature on the use of theory in nursing.

THEORY

One of the most commonly quoted definitions of a theory was formulated by Kerlinger (1973): "A theory is a set of interrelated constructs (concepts), definitions, and propositions that present a systematic view of phenomena by specifying relations among variables, with the purpose of explaining and predicting the phenomena" (p. 9). A more easily understood (although not as comprehensive) definition that will be used in this book is the following: A **theory** is a set of related statements that describes or explains phenomena in a systematic way. Theories explain why one event is associated with another event or what causes an event to occur. Theories are composed of concepts and the relationships between these concepts. Relationships between concepts are presented in theoretical statements, which are frequently called propositional statements. These propositions are connected in a logical system of thought.

Theory development is the basic aim of science (Kerlinger, 1986). Theories makes scientific findings meaningful and generalizable. The facts that are derived from many separate and isolated investigations take on meaning when placed within a theoretical context.

Theory comes from the Greek word "theoria," which means a beholding, spectacle, or speculation. "Speculation" is an appropriate word to use when discussing theories. Theories are always speculative in nature and are never considered to be true or proven. They provide description and explanation of the occurrence of phenomena and are always subject to further development or revision or may even be discarded if not supported by empirical evidence.

CONCEPT

Concepts are the building blocks of theory. A **concept** is a word picture or mental idea of a phenomenon. Concepts are words or terms that symbolize some aspect of reality. The meaning of a concept is conveyed by the use of a definition and examples of instances of the concept. A concept may be very concrete, such as the human heart, or may be very abstract, such as love. Concrete concepts may be specified and defined more easily than abstract concepts.

CONSTRUCT

A highly abstract, complex phenomenon (concept) is denoted by a "made up" or constructed term. **Construct** is the term used to indicate a phenomenon that cannot be directly observed but must be inferred by certain concrete or less abstract indicators of the phenomenon. Examples of constructs are wellness, mental health, self-esteem, and assertiveness. Each of these constructs can be identified only through the presence of certain measurable concepts. Wellness might be inferred through laboratory data or clinical observation. The laboratory data would be a very objective indicator of wellness, whereas the clinical observation would be a less objective indicator of wellness.

PROPOSITION

A **proposition** is a statement or assertion of the relationship between concepts. Propositional statements are derived from theories or from generalizations based on empirical data. A propositional statement may indicate the relationship between concepts in several ways. A propositional statement may assert simply that two events or phenomena tend to vary together. For example, "There is a relationship between pulse rates and respiration rates." Propositional statements may also assert that one variable causes another variable; for example, "Bacteria cause disease."

EMPIRICAL GENERALIZATION

When a similar pattern of events is found in the empirical data of a number of different studies, the pattern is called an **empirical generalization** (Reynolds, 1971). Empirical generalizations summarize the results of several empirical studies. Jacox (1974) proposed an example of a nurse who observes 40 or 50 preoperative patients and finds that each is anxious. The nurse thus makes an empirical generalization that all preoperative patients are anxious. Many studies have shown that women attend church more often than men. The empirical generalization can be made, therefore, that women are more frequent church attendees than men.

HYPOTHESIS

The term hypothesis was defined in Chapter 2. A hypothesis predicts the relationship between two or more variables. Hypotheses present the researcher's expectations about the outcome of a study. Through hypotheses, theoretical propositions are tested in the real world. The investigator can then advance scientific knowledge by supporting or failing to support the tested theory.

MODEL

The more complex the issues, the greater is the need to "create order out of chaos" by constructing models (Blackwell, 1985, p. 169). A **model** is a symbolic representation of some phenomenon or phenomena. Bush (1979) wrote that a model "represents some aspect of reality, concrete or abstract, by means of a likeness which may be structural, pictorial, diagrammatic, or mathematical" (p. 16). Probably the most common usage of the term model is when discussing structural types of models, such as model trains, model airplanes, and models of the human heart. The types of models that nurses are interested in when conducting nursing research are generally of the structural or diagrammatic form. A diagram or a picture can portray a theory in a fashion that clearly demonstrates the structure and parts of the theory. Whereas a theory focuses on statements or explanations of the relationships between phenomena, a model focuses on the structure or composition of the phenomena.

CONCEPTUAL MODELS

Conceptual models are made up of concepts and propositions that state the relationship between the concepts. These concepts are generally very abstract and are not readily observable in the empirical world. Conceptual models in nursing present broad general concepts of interest to nursing. Common concepts identified in nearly all of the nursing models are person, environment, health, and nursing (Fawcett, 1995; Fitzpatrick & Whall, 1996; George, 1995). Each nursing model addresses these elements in a unique fashion.

NURSING CONCEPTUAL MODELS

Several nurse theorists have developed conceptual models concerned with the phenomena of importance to nursing. These nurses include Dorothea Orem, Martha Rogers, Callista Roy, and Betty Neuman. A brief overview of the models introduced by these four nurse theorists will be presented.

OREM'S SELF-CARE MODEL

Dorothea Orem has been developing her ideas about self-care since the early 1950s. Concepts in her model are self-care, self-care agency, self-care demand, self-care deficit, nursing agency, and nursing system. Three theories have been derived from Orem's self-care model: theory of nursing systems, theory of self-care deficit, and theory of self-care. Recent modifications of her ideas are found in the fifth edition of her text *Nursing: Concepts of Practice,* which was published in 1995.

Orem's model is particularly appropriate today with the general public's increased interest in self-care. An article published in *Nursing Science Quarterly* in April 2000 (Taylor, Geden, Isaramalai, & Wongvatunyu, 2000) identified 66 published research studies that had used components of Orem's theories.

> McCaleb and Cull (2000) used Orem's theory of self-care to examine self-care practices of middle adolescents and to determine the influence of sociocultural characteristics, including socioeconomics and church attendance, on these self-care practices. Responses from 425 adolescents (ages 15 and 16) revealed that they engage in self-care practices only 58% of the time. The researchers pointed out that parents and health care providers should be concerned about this finding. The lowest self-care practice score was in the area of nutrition, with safety self-care practices receiving the highest score. In regard to sociocultural factors, as the father's education level increased and as the adolescent's church attendance increased, so did the self-care practices of these adolescents.

ROGERS' MODEL OF UNITARY HUMAN BEINGS

One of the most unusual conceptual models in nursing is that proposed by Martha Rogers. She presented her ideas in her 1970 book *An Introduction to the Theoretical Basis of Nursing.* By the time that she died in 1994, her ideas had made a great impact on nursing and probably will continue to do so for many years to come. Much of Rogers' work is contained in the book *Martha E. Rogers: Her Life and Her Work* by Malinski and Barrett (1994). The book was released shortly after Rogers' death.

Rogers continually refined her model, and when she spoke to groups of nurses (including myself), she frequently asked that they discuss her most current ideas rather than those presented in her 1970 book (which she called "the purple book"). Just as she viewed humans as continually evolving, her ideas were continually evolving. She originally used the term "man" in her writings. After 1983, she used the term "unitary human beings."

Humans and their environment are viewed as two energy fields that are always open to each other. Each human field is unique, and change is always toward increasing complexity and diversity. Aging is viewed as a "creative process directed toward growing diversity of field pattern and organization" (Rogers, 1980, p. 336).

Rogers' model is unique in that the person is viewed as a unified whole. No parts or subsystems are separated out. Although other models propose to present a holistic view of people, this view is often contradicted by the models' examination of the parts or subsystems of people.

> Rogers' conceptual model was used as the framework for Wall's (2000) study of changes in hope and power in lung cancer patients who exercise. The 104 participants were randomly assigned to an exercise or no-exercise group. The exercise group's power increased while the no-exercise groups' power decreased. No differences were found between the two groups in regard to hope. Positive correlations were found between hope and power. Using terms congruent with Rogers' model, Wall wrote, "Findings suggest that exercise is a form of knowing participation in change and illustrate a relation between one's ability to envision a better future and one's potential to actualize options through choice" (p. 234).

ROY'S ADAPTATION MODEL

Roy first published her ideas about adaptation as a framework for nursing in a 1970 article in *Nursing Outlook*. She has continued to publish extensively on her model. A thorough presentation of her ideas is found in the second edition of her text *Introduction to Nursing: An Adaptation Model,* which was published in 1984. Recent refinements of her model are found in the second edition of *The Roy Adaptation Model* by Roy and Andrews (1999).

Roy has pointed out that nursing focuses on the person as a total being, whereas medicine focuses on the patient's disease process. Humans are considered to be biopsychosocial beings in constant interaction with the changing environment. People are viewed as adaptive systems with cognator and regulator coping mechanisms that act to maintain adaptation in four response modes: physiological, self-concept, role function, and interdependence. In a 1988 publication, Roy described a cognitive information processing model that she had developed, which is based on her understanding of the cognator and regulator processors of adaptation.

> Cognitive adaptation and self-consistency in hearing-impaired older persons was studied by Zhan (2000), using Roy's adaptation model, with a specific focus on the cognator subsystem aspect of the model. The researcher found that three cognitive processes (clear focus and methods, knowing awareness, and self-perception) made significant contributions to the maintenance of self-consistency. Zhan concluded that understanding these cognitive processes would help nurses to promote effective adaptation in older persons.

NEUMAN'S SYSTEMS MODEL

The Neuman model first appeared in a 1972 article in *Nursing Research.* It was also presented in Riehl and Roy's *Conceptual Models for Nursing Practice* (both in the 1974 and the 1980 editions). Neuman presented refinements of the model in the 1982, 1989, and 1995 editions of her book *The Neuman Systems Model.*

Neuman has proposed a model that focuses on the total person. The person or client system (individual, group, community) is subject to environmental stressors that are intrapersonal, interpersonal, and extrapersonal in nature. The client system is composed of physiological, psychological, sociocultural, developmental, and spiritual variables. The client is protected from stressors by a flexible line of defense that is dynamic. The next barrier to stressors is the person's normal line of defense that has been built over time. When this defense is penetrated, the internal lines of resistance are activated to stabilize the client system.

Nursing interventions may occur at the primary, secondary, or tertiary levels of prevention. Primary prevention is appropriate before reaction to a stressor has occurred. Secondary prevention is used when reaction to a stressor has already occurred. Tertiary prevention is used to foster rehabilitation and a return to wellness. The nursing process is divided into three steps: nursing diagnosis, nursing goals, and nursing outcomes.

Neuman's model was used to examine mood and blood pressure responses in Black female caregivers and noncaregivers (Picot, Zauszniewski, Debanne, & Holston, 1999). The researchers' study model described how the flexible line of defense, the normal line of defense, and the lines of resistance should protect the basic structure from moods that disrupt the system's state of wellness. It was hypothesized that caregivers would report greater anger, anxiety, and sadness than noncaregivers and would, therefore, have higher blood pressures. Caregivers did not present with higher moods and blood pressures than noncaregivers. Surprisingly, lowered anger in the caregivers was associated with increased diastolic blood pressure. The authors suggested that the caregivers' lower anger scores might indicate denial or suppression of their anger.

THEORETICAL AND CONCEPTUAL FRAMEWORKS

A framework for a research study helps to organize the study and provides a context for the interpretation of the study findings. Either a theoretical or a conceptual framework should be used in all quantitative studies. Theoretical and conceptual frameworks are often used interchangeably in the literature. The two frameworks are similar in that both provide a background or foundation for a study. However, there are differences in these two types of frameworks.

A **theoretical framework** presents a broad, general explanation of the relationships between the concepts of interest in a research study; it is based on one existing theory. When using a theoretical framework, each main study concept is related back to a concept from an existing theory. A proposition from the selected theory is tested in any study based on that particular theory.

Suppose a teacher wanted to know if contracting for grades would motivate students to earn higher grades. After exploring different theories, she might decide to test a proposition from Carl Rogers (1969) theory of learning. One of Rogers' propositions is that learning is facilitated when the student participates responsibly in the learning process. The two theory concepts are "learning" and "participates responsibly in the learning process." The two study concepts that can be matched up with these two theory concepts are "earn higher grades" (which would match up with "learning") and "contracting for grades" (which would match up with "participates responsibly in the learning process"). Thus, based on the stated proposition from Rogers' theory, the researcher would be able to predict that students who contract for grades would earn higher grades than students who do not contract for grades.

If there is no existing theory that will fit the concepts to be studied, the researcher may construct a conceptual framework to be used in the proposed research study. A **conceptual framework** helps to explain the relationship between concepts, but rather than being based on one theory, this type of framework links concepts selected from several theories, from previous research results, or from the researcher's own experiences. The researcher relates the concepts in a logical manner. A conceptual framework is a less well-developed structure than a theoretical framework but may serve as the impetus for the formulation of a theory.

A friend of mine decided to study nurses' job satisfaction levels and their levels of empathy in their interactions with patients. After searching the literature, she was able to find an empathy theory and a job satisfaction theory. However, she could locate no theory that combined these two concepts. Therefore, she constructed a conceptual framework using these two theories. Based on the empathy theory, she reasoned that being empathetic requires being satisfied with self. She further reasoned that if people are happy in their jobs, they will be satisfied with themselves. Therefore, she proposed that job satisfaction and empathy are positively related.

The findings of a study should be related back to the study framework. Otherwise, numerous isolated findings would exist for each study. The concrete findings are linked to the abstract ideas of the theory or to the propositions proposed by the researcher in the conceptual framework. Thus, an explanation for the study findings is presented, and the body of knowledge on the study topic is increased.

THEORY GENERATION AND DEVELOPMENT

Researchers are concerned with both theory generation and the development of theories. The two activities go hand in hand. The processes of theory generation and the development of theories through testing are shown in Figure 6–1. As can be seen, theory generation and development involve both inductive and deductive reasoning processes. **Deductive reasoning** proceeds from the general (theory) to the specific (empirical data). **Inductive reasoning,** on the other hand, proceeds from the specific (empirical data) to the general (theory).

The deductive process moves from a general abstract explanation to a specific event in the real world. A hypothesis is deduced from a theory, and the hypothesis is empirically tested in a real-life situation. The researcher asks the question, If this theory is valid, what kind of behavior or event would I expect to find in my study? For example, you might test a propositional statement from Maslow's (1970) theory of motivation that states: If a person's safety needs are not met, safety needs will take precedence over self-esteem needs. If this statement is valid, you would expect to find that people are more concerned about receiving the correct medications than they are about being told that they are "good" patients.

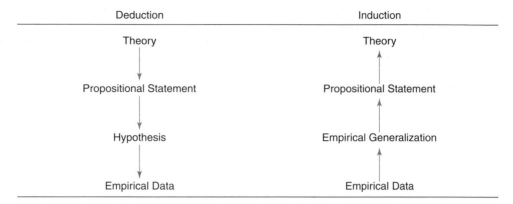

Figure 6–1. Deductive and inductive processes in theory generation and development.

When an inductive process is used, data are gathered from a real-life situation and the researcher tries to derive a general explanation of this behavior or event. The question is asked, How can I explain what I have been observing? For example, you might observe that patients who are occupied in some activity, such as watching television, seem to be less anxious than patients who are not involved in any activity. You continue to observe many patients and find that this pattern seems to hold true for most of the patients on the unit where you work. Your explanation for this phenomenon would involve an inductive reasoning process. An existing anxiety theory might provide an explanation for the phenomenon that was just discussed. If no existing theory can be located that explains this phenomenon, the researcher may start the process of generating a new theory. After empirical data are gathered on a number of occasions, empirical generalizations are made. The next step is to develop propositional statements. Finally, the propositional statements are logically related to form a theory.

TYPES OF THEORIES

Theories can be described according to the range of phenomena they describe and explain. Two types of theories are grand theories and middle-range theories. There is lack of consensus among nursing experts about the definition and scope of these two types of theories. Generally, **grand theories** are considered to address a broad range of phenomena in the environment or in the experiences of humans. **Middle-range theories** are considered to have a much more narrow focus; they are concerned with only a small area of the environment or of human experiences and incorporate a small number of concepts.

Grand theories are important in every discipline. According to Fitzpatrick and Whall (1996) a grand theory "serves as a guiding light, as a historical holder of disciplinary beliefs, and as a provider of visions of the future" (p. 2). Although grand theories are revered by many nurses, middle-range theories have been found to be more valuable to nursing research than have grand theories. The works of many of the nurse theorists have been identified as conceptual models at the grand theory level. Some nurses have contended that these models do not drive research (Tripp-Reimer, Woodworth, McCloskey, & Bulechek, 1996).

As you may recall, the nurse theorists have broadly discussed health, environment, person, and nursing. It is difficult to isolate a propositional statement from these broad concepts that can then be tested in a research study. For example, if a nurse wanted to find out if backrubs promote sleep in hospitalized patients, a middle-range theory, probably one that focuses on a proposition from a relaxation theory, would be needed to guide the study.

One of the shortcomings of the use of middle-range theories appears to be that most of them are from other disciplines. Examples of these theories include social support, coping, anxiety, adult learning, body image, stress, and helplessness. Although knowledge does not belong to any one discipline, each discipline looks at phenomena from a different perspective. Few disciplines are concerned with people who are ill. For example, learning theories that may be useful with well people may not be appropriate for sick people who not only are ill but are under a great deal of stress. An individual whose normal preferred learning mode is auditory may need a totally different approach when hospitalized. This person may now need visual as well as auditory learning signals, and the signals may need to be repeated several times. So, one cannot assume that a theory used in one discipline should be transferred directly over for use in another discipline. Modifications may be needed or the theory may be deemed to be inappropriate for use in nursing.

SOURCES OF THEORIES FOR NURSING RESEARCH

Nurses have available to them a wealth of theories on which to base their research. These theories have been developed in nursing and in many other disciplines. At the present time, nurses continue to use many theories from other disciplines.

THEORIES FROM NURSING

Although there are a number of nursing conceptual models, only a few theories have been derived from these models. Additionally, there have been few studies in which these theories have been tested. Abdellah and Levine (1994) wrote that one of the gaps in nursing research is the lack of tested nursing theories.

Some nurses have questioned the usefulness of nursing theories. Others, such as Rosemarie Parse, have made strong pleas for the use of nursing theories in nursing research. In an editorial in *Nursing Science Quarterly,* Parse (2000) strongly argued that a nursing research study must use a nursing framework or theory. Fawcett (2000) wrote a similar editorial in *Western Journal of Nursing Research.* The following month Brink (2000) published an editorial in the same journal and disagreed with Fawcett's position. She asserted that any research that has a direct bearing on nursing practice is considered to be nursing research. She further asserted that nursing is an applied discipline and draws knowledge from many sources. She asserted that if we were to ignore factual data simply because it came from another discipline, we would have to redo a lot of previous research or admit to "culpable ignorance."

Although nurse researchers have generally used theories that were not developed by nurses, there are many examples in the literature of studies that relied on the theoretical work of nurses. Examples of studies that used the models of Orem, Rogers, Roy, and Neuman were presented earlier in this chapter. Additional theories developed by nurses may be identified in published studies. Some of these include Cox's (1982) interaction model of client health behavior (IMCHB), Mishel's (1981) uncertainty in illness theory, King's (1981) theory of goal attainment, Pender's (1996) health promotion model, and Peplau's interpersonal theory (1988). An example of a study that used Mishel's theory and one that used Pender's model of health promotion is presented.

> Mishel's model of uncertainty was the framework for the study by Wunderlich, Perry, Lavin, and Kathz's (1999) of 19 patients' perceptions of uncertainty and stress during weaning from mechanical ventilation. The researchers found that critical care nurses can help minimize patients' stress and uncertainty during weaning trials by providing information. Patients were questioned within 3 months after being weaned from mechanical ventilation. Although most patients reported that they had high levels of uncertainty and stress, they revealed a positive attitude toward the information provided by critical care nurses.

> Pender's health promotion model was used by Lucas, Orshan, and Cook (2000) to study determinants of health-promoting behavior among women 65 years of age and older who were living in the community. Lucas et al. found that age, marital status, race, education, self-esteem, and the two health-related factors of perceived health and health self-determinism made significant contributions to the health-promoting behaviors of physical activity, nutrition, spiritual growth, and interpersonal relations.

THEORIES FROM OTHER DISCIPLINES

Nursing is referred to as a practice discipline. It has often been said that nursing, as a practice discipline, has "borrowed" knowledge from other disciplines, such as chemistry, biology, sociology, psychology, and anthropology. Levine (1995) has opposed the use of the term *borrowed*. She said it indicates that something needs to later be "returned." Levine wrote, "The fruits of knowledge are not the private domain of one discipline, to be returned like a borrowed cup of sugar to a neighbor" (p. 12).

The use of knowledge from other disciplines is necessary, but frequently this knowledge is not suitable to the needs of the nursing profession. Nurses must find ways to adapt the numerous theories from other disciplines. Once these theories have been adapted, they should be considered as shared knowledge rather than as borrowed theories (Stevens, 1979). Table 6–1 presents theories from other disciplines that have been used to explain phenomena in nursing. These theories concern concepts such as social learning, adult learning, role socialization, stress, helplessness, cognitive dissonance, human development, motivation, crisis, relaxation, pain, anxiety, body image, job satisfaction, family interactions, communication, coping, moral reasoning, health behaviors, and change. Many nursing studies have used theories from other disciplines.

Carson (1996) used Benson's theoretical work on relaxation to study the impact of a relaxation technique on the lipid profiles of 60 males with known hyperlipidemia. Lacko, Bryan, Dellasega, and Salerno (1999) used changed theory to involve nurses in a research study on delirium. The theory of stress and coping developed by Lazarus was used by Bouvé, Rozmus, and Giordono (1999) to study a nursing intervention designed to diminish the anxiety level of parents of children being transferred from a pediatric intensive care unit to a general pediatric floor. Moon and Becker (2000) used Bandura's self-efficacy theory to examine the relationships among self-efficacy, outcome expectancy,

TABLE 6–1.   Theories from Other Disciplines

1. Social learning theory: Bandura (1986); Rotter (1954)
2. Adult learning theory: Knowles (1990)
3. Role theory: Mead (1934)
4. Stress: Selye (1976)
5. Helplessness: Seligman (1975)
6. Cognitive dissonance: Festinger (1957)
7. Developmental theory: Piaget (1926); Freud (1938); Erikson (1950) Havighurst (1952)
8. Motivation: Maslow (1970)
9. Crisis: Caplan (1964)
10. Relaxation: Benson (1975)
11. Pain: Melzack and Wall (1983)
12. Anxiety: Spielberger (1972)
13. Body image: Schilder (1952)
14. Job satisfaction: Herzberg (1966)
15. Family theory: Minuchin (1974); Duvall (1977)
16. Family communication theory: Satir (1967)
17. Coping: Lazarus (1966)
18. Moral reasoning: Kohlberg (1978)
19. Health behaviors: Becker (1985)
20. Change theory: Lewin (1951)

and postoperative behaviors in patients who had experienced a total joint replacement. Kolberg's model on stages of moral development was used by Riesch, von Sadovszky, Norton, and Pridham (2000) to examine moral reasoning used by graduate nursing students. The gate control theory of pain by Melzack and Wall served as the framework for Kotzer's (2000) study of factors that would predict postoperative pain in children and adolescents following spine fusion.

Many published studies have reported the use of more than one theory. Three theories (Lazarus's stress theory, Izard's differential emotions theory, and Spielberger's personality trait theory) were compared in a study by Yarcheski, Mahon, and Yarcheski (1999) that examined state anger in early adolescents. The researchers found that all three theories provided sound and relevant explanations of state anger in early adolescents. However, the trait theory provided the most powerful explanation.

COMBINING THEORIES FROM NURSING AND OTHER DISCIPLINES

In some studies, nurse researchers have determined that a combination of theories from nursing and other disciplines would guide their research more appropriately than a theory from only one discipline. Two examples will be provided.

In the previous section on "Theories from Nursing" an example was given of Wunderlich et al.'s (1999) study that used Mishel's Uncertainty Model to study patients' perceptions of uncertainty and stress during weaning from mechanical ventilation. These researchers also used Lazarus's theory of stress and coping to describe the relationship between patients' needs to cope effectively and the uncertainty and stress that they felt while being weaned from a ventilator.

Kosco and Warren (2000) combined Martha Rogers' Theory of Unitary Human Beings with Maslow's Hierarchy of Needs theory and crisis theory in their study of critical care nurses' perceptions of family needs as being met compared with the family members' perceptions of these needs as being met. The population consisted of 45 family members in a large county hospital designated as a Level 3 trauma center. The top 10 needs were reported in order of importance and whether or not these needs had been met. There was agreement in many areas of needs. However, the family members found it more important than the nurses to have a specific person to call at the hospital when they were unable to visit and to have someone be concerned with the relative's own health.

THEORY TESTING IN NURSING RESEARCH

In the early stages of a research project, the researcher should consider the theoretical or conceptual framework for the study. The framework for the study is usually determined after a thorough review of the literature. If nursing is to build a scientific knowledge base, nursing studies should be based on a theoretical or conceptual framework so that the findings may be placed within the existing knowledge base for the profession. The most efficient way to obtain a body of knowledge for nursing is to build on the work of other researchers who have used the same theoretical base. Even a small research project becomes quite important when the findings of the study can be added to those of others who have used the same theoretical frame of reference.

Many studies are conducted in which a researcher wishes to study a particular problem but has no theory in mind that will be tested. In such cases, an attempt should be made to select a theory that will be useful in guiding the study. Sometimes more than one theory might be appropriate, but the researcher should choose the one that seems to describe and explain the relationship between the study variables better than other available theories. Choosing a theory for a study may be a difficult task, especially for the beginning researcher. To choose an appropriate theory, familiarity with various theories will be necessary. Descriptions of theories may be obtained through many sources. Various books and articles contain information about theories.

Once a theory has been selected, it is wise to consult the original or primary source of the theory. For example, if information is sought on Maslow's theory of motivation, Maslow's (1970) book should be read. By using a primary source, the researcher will gain the most accurate description of the theory as presented by the theorist.

The chosen theory should be considered throughout the research process. A step-by-step use of the chosen theory requires that the researcher:

1. Review various theories that may be appropriate to examine the identified problem.

2. Select a theory to be tested in the study.

3. Review the literature on this theory.

4. Develop study hypothesis(es) or research questions based on a propositional statement or statements from the theory.

5. Define study variables using the selected theory as the basis of the theoretical definitions.

6. Choose study instruments that are congruent with the theory.

7. Describe study findings in light of the explanations provided by the theory.

8. Relate study conclusions to the theory.

9. Determine support for the theory based on study findings.

10. Determine implications for nursing based on the explanatory power of the theory.

11. Make recommendations for future research concerning the designated theory.

Theory generation and building through research are essential to the development of scientific knowledge. Because the nursing profession is very concerned at present with the need for nursing knowledge, it can be seen that an understanding and use of theory are critical for all nurses. Theory is of little benefit to the profession if it is deemed to be unimportant by the rank-and-file members. It is hoped you will become convinced of the value of theory that has been tested through research. You can help spread the message to your nursing colleagues.

CRITIQUING THE STUDY FRAMEWORK

Many nursing studies that are published today contain a clearly identified theoretical or conceptual framework for the study. Others do not. Therefore, the first determination to make is whether the researcher identified a framework for the study. Sometimes, the research report will contain a heading for this section of the study. Other times, the discussion of the theoretical or conceptual framework will be included in the introductory section or the review of literature section. The important point is to determine if the researcher clearly identifies a framework.

If a theoretical or conceptual framework has been clearly identified in the report, the next evaluation step concerns the basis for the framework. Is it based on a nursing theory or a theory from another discipline? At the present time, many nursing studies are based on concepts and theories from other disciplines.

The reader then evaluates the appropriateness of the framework for the study. The entire research report must be read before the evaluation of the framework is made. Then the reader might ask the question: Would another theory have been more appropriate to guide the study? Several theories might be used in any given study. Imagine that, after reading the research report, it appears to you that the researcher was interested in helping subjects alter an unhealthy behavior—smoking. The researcher used a learning theory and taught subjects about the dangers of cigarette smoking. Considering the great amount of publicity about the dangers of cigarette smoking, you might wonder if another theory might have been more useful in helping to predict a change in an unhealthy behavior. It is possible that the subjects had knowledge of the dangers of cigarette smoking but did not perceive themselves as vulnerable. "Cancer won't happen to me." A theory, such as the health belief model, might have been used. The researcher might focus on the concepts of perceived susceptibility or perceived seriousness of the disease when presenting material about the dangers of smoking to the subjects.

You may be thinking, "I don't know that many theories. How can I evaluate this part of a study and decide whether the most appropriate theory was used?" This is a difficult task, but my guess is that you know more theories than you think you do. You may not know the name of the theorist, but you are familiar with the ideas in the theory. If you have some nagging doubt when you read the framework section of an article, ask other nurses what they think about the framework.

If you think that the framework seems appropriate for the study, determine if there is a thorough explanation of the concepts and their relationship to each other.

An entire theory is rarely tested in one study. Thus, is a specific proposition from the theory identified that will guide the hypothesis(es) or research question(s)? Are operational definitions provided for the concepts that will be measured in the study? Guidelines for critiquing the theoretical/conceptual framework of a study are presented in Box 6–1.

SUMMARY

An understanding of theory in nursing and the use of theory in research requires familiarity with terms such as theory, concept, construct, proposition, empirical generalization, model, conceptual models, theoretical frameworks, and conceptual frameworks.

A **theory** is a set of statements that describes or explains phenomena in a systematic way. Theories are composed of concepts and the relationship between these concepts. These relationships are presented in propositional statements that are connected in a logical way.

Concepts are the building blocks of theory. A **concept** is a word picture or mental idea of a phenomenon. Concepts may be concrete or abstract.

Box 6–1.   Guidelines for Critiquing the Study Framework

1. Is the framework clearly identified?
2. Is the framework based on a nursing theory or a theory from another discipline?
3. Does the framework appear to be appropriate for the study?
4. Are the concepts clearly defined?
5. Are the relationships among the concepts clearly presented?
6. Is (are) the propositional statement(s) identified that will guide the research question(s) or hypothesis(es)?
7. Are operational definitions provided for the theoretical concepts that will be tested?

A **construct** is a phenomenon (concept) that cannot be directly observed but must be inferred by certain concrete or less abstract indicators of the phenomenon. Examples of constructs are wellness and mental health.

Propositions are statements of the relationship between concepts. All theories contain propositional statements.

An **empirical generalization** is a summary statement of the findings of a number of different studies concerning the same phenomenon.

A **model** is a symbolic representation of phenomena. A model can be structural, pictorial, diagrammatic, or mathematical. Models focus on the structure of phenomena rather than on the relationships between phenomena, as is the case with theories.

Conceptual models are made up of concepts and propositions. The concepts are usually abstract. Conceptual models in nursing identify concepts of interest to nursing such as person, environment, health, and nursing.

Theoretical frameworks differ from conceptual frameworks in that they are based on propositional statements from a theory or theories. **Conceptual frameworks** link concepts from several theories, from previous research results, or from the researcher's own experience. In developing a conceptual framework, the researcher relates concepts in a logical manner to form propositional statements.

Researchers are concerned with the generation and development of theories through testing. Both inductive and deductive reasoning processes are used in theory generation and development. **Deductive reasoning** proceeds from the general (theory) to the specific (empirical data). **Inductive reasoning** flows from the specific (empirical data) to the general (theory).

Two types of theories are grand theories and middle-range theories. **Grand theories** are concerned with a broad range of phenomena in the environment or in the experiences of humans; **middle-range theories** are concerned with only a small area of the environment or of human experiences.

Nurses have used theories from nursing and from other disciplines when conducting nursing research. These theories from other disciplines concern concepts such as social learning, adult learning, role socialization, stress, helplessness, cognitive dissonance, human development, motivation, crisis, relaxation, pain, anxiety, body image, job satisfaction, family interactions, communication, coping, moral reasoning, change, and health behaviors.

A theoretical or conceptual framework should be used in all quantitative research. The framework will guide the steps in the research process and is the mechanism through which a generalizable body of knowledge is developed.

NURSING RESEARCH ON THE WEB

For additional online resources, research activities, and exercises, go to www.prenhall. com/nieswiadomy. Select Chapter 6 from the drop down menu.

✖ GET INVOLVED ACTIVITIES

1. Write the name of a theory on the blackboard. No duplicates will be allowed, so it is to your advantage to write your theory on the board as soon as you can get there!

2. Bring a research article to class that contains a theory. See how many different theories the class has identified in published studies.

3. Using the same articles from activity 2, try to identify other theories that might have been used as the frameworks for these studies.

4. Identify some specific area where you think additional theories are needed to guide nursing practice.

5. Divide into teams. Each team will choose a nurse theorist. Debate which of these theorists have made the most valuable contributions to nursing research.

✖ SELF-TEST

Match the description of terms in Column B with terms in Column A.

Column A	Column B
1. theory	A. word picture or mental idea of a phenomenon
2. concept	B. contains prepositional statements
3. construct	C. a statement that asserts the relationship between concepts
4. proposition	D. highly abstract phenomenon that cannot be directly observed
5. model	E. symbolic representation of some phenomenon or phenomena

Circle the letter before the *best* answer.

6. Nursing research has used which of the following reasoning processes?
   A. inductive
   B. deductive
   C. both inductive and deductive
   D. neither inductive nor deductive

7. Deriving a propositional statement from a theory involves the logical reasoning process called:
   A. deduction.
   B. conceptualization.
   C. induction.
   D. critical analysis.

8. Which of the following statements regarding theory is *false*?
   A. proves the relationship between variables
   B. describes the relationship between variables
   C. explains the relationship between variables
   D. contains propositional statements

9. Which of the following is *not* one of the common concepts that are included in nearly all of the nursing conceptual models?
   A. person
   B. environment

    C. death

    D. health

    E. nursing

10. Nursing has used theories from:

    A. sociology.

    B. psychology.

    C. anthropology.

    D. all of the above.

✖ REFERENCES

Abdellah, F. G., & Levine, E. (1994). *Preparing nursing research for the 21st century.* New York: Springer.

Bandura, A. (1986). *Social foundations of thought and action: A social cognitive theory.* Englewood Cliffs, NJ: Prentice-Hall.

Becker, M. H. (1985). Patient adherence to prescribed therapies. *Medical Care, 23,* 539–555.

Benson, H. (1975). *The relaxation response.* New York: Morrow.

Blackwell, B. (1985). Models: Their virtues and vices. *Journal of Cardiac Rehabilitation, 5,* 169–171.

Bouvé, L. R., Rozmus, C. L., & Giordono, P. (1999). Preparing parents for their child's transfer from the PICU to the pediatric floor. *Applied Nursing Research, 12,* 114–120.

Brink, P. J. (2000). A response to Fawcett. *Western Journal of Nursing Research, 22,* 653–655.

Bush, H. (1979). Models for nursing. *Advances in Nursing Science, 1*(2), 13–21.

Caplan, G. (1964). *Principles of preventive psychiatry.* New York: Basic Books.

Carson, M. A. (1996). The impact of a relaxation technique on the lipid profile. *Nursing Research, 45,* 271–276.

Cox, C. (1982). An interaction model of client health behavior: Theoretical prescription for nursing. *Advances in Nursing Science, 5*(1), 41–56.

Duvall, E. (1977). *Marriage and family development* (5th ed.). Philadelphia: Lippincott.

Erikson, E. (1950). *Childhood and society.* New York: W. W. Norton & Co.

Fawcett, J. (1995). *Analysis and evaluation of conceptual models of nursing* (3rd ed.). Philadelphia: F. A. Davis.

Fawcett, J. (2000). But is it *nursing* research? *Western Journal of Nursing Research, 22,* 524–525.

Festinger, L. (1957). *A theory of cognitive dissonance.* Stanford, CA: Stanford University Press.

Fitzpatrick, J. J., & Whall, A. L. (1996). *Conceptual models of nursing: Analysis and application* (3rd ed.). Stamford, CT: Appleton & Lange.

Freud, S. (1938). *The basic writings of Sigmund Freud.* New York: Random House.

George, J. B. (1995). *Nursing theories: The base for professional nursing practice* (4th ed.). Norwalk, CT: Appleton & Lange.

Havighurst, R. (1952). *Developmental tasks and education.* New York: Longmans, Green.

Herzberg, F. (1966). *Work and the nature of man.* Cleveland: World Publishing.

Jacox, A. (1974). Theory construction in nursing. *Nursing Research, 23,* 4–13.

Kerlinger, F. (1973). *Foundations of behavioral research* (2nd ed.). New York: Holt, Rinehart & Winston.

Kerlinger, F. (1986). *Foundations of behavioral research* (3rd ed.). New York: Holt, Rinehart & Winston.

King, I. M. (1981). *A theory for nursing: Systems, concepts, process.* New York: John Wiley & Sons.

Knowles, M. (1990). *The adult learner: A neglected species* (4th ed.). Houston: Gulf Press.

Kohlberg, L. (1978). The cognitive developmental approach to moral education. In P. Scharf (Ed.), *Readings in moral education* (pp. 36–51). Minneapolis: Winston Press.

Kosco, M., & Warren, N. A. (2000). Critical care nurses' perceptions of family needs as met. *Critical Care Nursing Quarterly, 23,* 60–72.

Kotzer, A. M. (2000). Factors predicting postoperative pain in children and adolescents following spine fusion. *Issues in Comprehensive Pediatric Nursing, 23,* 83–102.

Lacko, L., Bryan, Y., Dellasega, C., & Salerno, F. (1999). Changing clinical practice through research: The case of delirium. *Clinical Nursing Research, 8,* 235–250.

Lazarus, R. (1966). *Psychological stress and the coping process.* New York: McGraw-Hill.

Levine, M. Y. (1995). The rhetoric of nursing theory. *Image: Journal of Nursing Scholarship, 27,* 11–14.

Lewin, K. (1951). *Field theory in social science.* Westport, CT: Greenwood.

Lucas, J. A., Orshan, S. A., & Cook, F. (2000). Determinants of health-promoting behavior among women ages 65 and above living in the community. *Scholarly Inquiry for Nursing Practice: An International Journal, 14,* 77–99.

Malinski, V. M., & Barrett, E. A. M. (Eds.) (1994). *Martha E. Rogers: Her life and her work.* Philadelphia: F. A. Davis.

Maslow, A. (1970). *Motivation and personality* (2nd ed.). New York: Harper & Row.

McCaleb, A., & Cull, V. V. (2000). Sociocultural influences and self-care practices of middle adolescents. *Journal of Pediatric Nursing, 15,* 30–35.

Mead, G. (1934). *Mind, self and society.* Chicago: University of Chicago Press.

Melzack, R., & Wall, P. (1983). *The challenge of pain* (rev. ed.). New York: Basic Books.

Minuchin, S. (1974). *Families and family therapy.* Cambridge, MA: Harvard University Press.

Mishel, M. H. (1981). The measurement of uncertainty in illness. *Nursing Research, 30,* 258–263.

Moon, L. B., & Becker, J. (2000). Relationships among self-efficacy, outcome expectancy, and postoperative behaviors in total joint replacement patients. *Orthopaedic Nursing, 19,* 77–85.

Neuman, B. (1982). *The Neuman systems model.* Norwalk, CT: Appleton-Century-Crofts.

Neuman, B. (1989). *The Neuman systems model* (2nd ed.). Norwalk, CT: Appleton & Lange.

Neuman, B. (1995). *The Neuman systems model* (3rd ed.). Norwalk, CT: Appleton & Lange.

Orem, D. (1995). *Nursing: Concepts of practice* (5th ed.). St. Louis, MO: Mosby Year Book.

Parse, R. R. (2000). Obfuscating: The persistent practice of misnaming. *Nursing Science Quarterly, 13,* 91.

Pender, N. J. (1996). *Health promotion in nursing practice* (3rd ed.). Norwalk, CT: Appleton & Lange.

Peplau, H. E. (1988). *Interpersonal relations in nursing.* London: Macmillan Education, Ltd.

Piaget, J. (1926). *The language and thought of the child.* New York: Harcourt, Brace, and World.

Picot, S. J. F., Zauszniewski, J. A., Debanne, S. M., & Holston, E. C. (1999). Mood and blood pressure responses in Black female caregivers and noncaregivers. *Nursing Research 48,* 150–161.

Reynolds, P. (1971). *A primer in theory construction.* Indianapolis: Bobbs-Merrill.

Riehl, J., & Roy, C. (Eds.). (1974). *Conceptual models for nursing practice.* Norwalk, CT: Appleton-Century-Crofts.

Riehl, J., & Roy, C. (Eds.). (1980). *Conceptual models for nursing practice* (2nd ed.). Norwalk, CT: Appleton-Century-Crofts.

Riesch, S. K., von Sadovszky, V., Norton, S., & Pridham, K. F. (2000). Moral reasoning among graduate students in nursing. *Nursing Outlook, 48,* 73-80.

Rogers, C. (1969). *Freedom to learn.* Columbus, OH: Charles E. Merrill.

Rogers, M. (1970). *An introduction to the theoretical basis of nursing.* Philadelphia: F. A. Davis.

Rogers, M. (1980). Nursing: A science of unitary man. In J. P. Riehl and C. Roy (Eds.), *Conceptual models for nursing practice* (2nd ed.) (pp. 329–337). New York: Appleton-Century-Crofts.

Rotter, J. (1954). *Social learning and clinical psychology.* Englewood Cliffs, NJ: Prentice-Hall.

Roy, C. (1970). Adaptation: A conceptual framework for nursing. *Nursing Outlook, 18,* 42–45.

Roy, C. (1984). *Introduction to nursing: An adaptation model* (2nd ed.). Englewood Cliffs, NJ: Prentice-Hall.

Roy, C. (1988). Human information processing. In J. J. Fitzpatrick, R. L. Taunton, & J. Q. Benoliel (Eds.). *Annual review of nursing research* (pp. 237–261). New York: Springer.

Roy, C., & Andrews, H. A. (1999). *The Roy adaptation model* (2nd ed.). Stamford, CT: Appleton & Lange.

Satir, V. (1967). *Conjoint family therapy* (rev. ed.). Palo Alto, CA: Science & Behavior Books.

Schilder, P. (1952). *The image and appearance of the human body.* New York: International University Press.

Seligman, M. (1975). *Helplessness: On depression, development, and death.* San Francisco: W. H. Freeman.

Selye, H. (1976). *The stress of life* (rev. ed.). New York: McGraw-Hill.

Spielberger, C. (1972). Anxiety as an emotional state. In C. D. Spielberger (Ed.), *Anxiety: Current trends in theory and research* (Vol. 1) (pp. 3–47). New York: Academic Press.

Stevens, B. (1979). *Nursing theory.* Boston: Little, Brown.

Taylor, S. G., Geden, E., Isaramalai, S., & Wongvatunyu, S. (2000). *Nursing Science Quarterly, 13,* 104–110.

Tripp-Reimer, T., Woodworth, G., McCloskey, J. C., & Bulechek, G. (1996). The dimensional structure of nursing interventions. *Nursing Research, 45,* 10–17.

Wall, L. M. (2000). Changes in hope and power in lung cancer patients who exercise. *Nursing Science Quarterly, 13,* 234–242.

Wunderlich, R. J., Perry, A., Lavin, M. A., & Katz, B. (1999). Patients' perceptions of uncertainty and stress during weaning from mechanical ventilation. *Dimensions of Critical Care Nursing, 18,* 2–8.

Yarcheski, A., Mahon, N. E., & Yarcheski, T. J. (1999). An empirical test of alternate theories of anger in early adolescents. *Nursing Research, 48,* 317–323.

Zhan, L. (2000). Cognitive adaptation and self-consistency in hearing-impaired older persons: Testing Roy's adaptation model. *Nursing Science Quarterly, 13,* 158–165.

CHAPTER 7

Hypotheses and Research Questions

OUTLINE

Purposes of Hypotheses
Sources or Rationale for Hypotheses
Classifications of Hypotheses
- Simple and Complex Hypotheses
- Null and Research Hypotheses
- Nondirectional and Directional Research Hypotheses

Hypothesis Criteria
- Is Written in a Declarative Sentence
- Is Written in the Present Tense
- Contains the Population
- Contains the Variables
- Reflects the Problem Statement
- Is Empirically Testable

Hypothesis Format
Hypotheses and Theory Testing
Research Questions
Critiquing Hypotheses and Research Questions
Summary
Nursing Research on the Web
Get Involved Activities
Self-test

OBJECTIVES

On completion of this chapter, you will be prepared to:

1. Determine the purposes of hypotheses in research studies
2. Identify sources or rationale for study hypotheses
3. Describe classifications of hypotheses
4. Distinguish between simple and complex hypotheses
5. Compare null hypotheses and research hypotheses
6. Differentiate nondirectional and directional research hypotheses
7. List the criteria to be considered when formulating a hypothesis
8. Discuss the format for writing hypotheses
9. Recognize the use of hypotheses in the testing of theories
10. Determine the types of studies for which hypotheses are not needed
11. Critique study hypotheses and research questions in research reports and articles

✕ NEW TERMS DEFINED IN THIS CHAPTER

complex hypothesis
directional research hypothesis
interaction effect
nondirectional research hypothesis

null hypothesis
research hypothesis
simple hypothesis

You check on your cake that has been in the oven for 30 minutes and see that it is not rising. You start thinking of possible reasons. The oven may not have been turned on. After placing a hand on the oven and feeling its warmth, you discard this hunch. Maybe the temperature was not set correctly. You check and see that the oven is set on 350°F, which is the desired setting. Next, you consider the possibility that some ingredient might have been left out of the batter. Suddenly, you spot the unopened can of baking soda. Ahha! The reason for the flat cake has become apparent. The hunches you had about the reasons for your flat cake could be considered hypotheses. After the facts were gathered, you find that your last hunch was correct. The missing baking soda is the cause of the flat cake.

In scientific research, hypotheses are intelligent guesses that assist the researcher in seeking the solution to a problem. Kerlinger (1986) has defined a hypothesis as a "conjectural statement of the relations between two or more variables" (p. 17). Polit and Hungler (1999) presented a similar definition by calling a hypothesis a "tentative prediction or explanation of the relationship between two or more variables" (p. 61). The following definition will be used in this book: A hypothesis is a statement of the predicted relationship between two or more variables. Research studies may have one or several hypotheses. There should be as many hypotheses as are needed to test all aspects of the research problem.

Whereas the problem statement presents the question that is to be asked in the study, the hypothesis presents the answer to the question. The hypothesis links the independent and the dependent variables. You will recall that an independent variable is the "cause," and the dependent variable is the "effect" in experimental studies. The researcher manipulates the independent variable. In nonexperimental studies, the words "cause" and "effect" are not appropriate because the researcher does not manipulate the independent variable. The researcher, however, may be able to make a determination of which variable might have an influence on the other variable. The direction of influence runs from the independent variable to the dependent variable. If a researcher were trying to examine the relationship between age and the amount of exercise that people perform, the independent variable would be age and the dependent variable would be exercise performance. It would not be appropriate to say that age is the "cause" of the amount of exercise that one performs, but the direction of influence logically flows from age to exercise performance. It would make no sense to say that exercise performance influences the age of a person.

Hypotheses should always be written before the study and should not be changed after the study results are examined. This is like changing your choice of who will win a race after you have already watched the finish of the race.

PURPOSES OF HYPOTHESES

Hypotheses serve several purposes in research studies. They lend objectivity to scientific investigations by pinpointing a specific part of a theory to be tested. Through hypotheses, theoretical propositions can be tested in the real world. The investigator can then advance scientific knowledge by supporting or failing to support the tested theory. Even when the research hypothesis is not supported, scientific knowledge is gained. Negative findings are sometimes as important as positive ones. Hypotheses also guide the research design and dictate the type of statistical analysis to be used with the data. Finally, hypotheses provide the reader with an understanding of the researcher's expectations about the study before data collection begins.

SOURCES OR RATIONALE FOR STUDY HYPOTHESES

Hypotheses are not wild guesses or shots in the dark. The researcher should be able to state the source or rationale for each hypothesis. This source or rationale for the hypothesis may come from personal experience, previous research studies, or theoretical propositions.

A nurse may have a hunch that comes from personal experiences or observations. For example, you may have noticed that psychiatric patients seem to become more anxious as the time for their discharge approaches. Observations continue to be made. Patients' charts are examined to determine behaviors reported by other staff members. The behaviors recorded on the charts seem to agree with your observations. An empirical generalization induced from these observations might be the following: As the time for discharge draws near, the anxiety levels of psychiatric patients increase. The following hypothesis might then be tested: The anxiety levels of psychiatric patients are higher immediately before discharge than they are 3 days before discharge. Recall the difference between induction and deduction. This hypothesis was derived through induction. It was based on an empirical generalization derived from your observations as a nurse.

Even when a study is based on empirical generalizations from the researcher's own experiences, a review of the literature should be conducted in the study area to determine what is already known on the topic. Then an attempt should be made to find a theoretical explanation for the observed phenomenon.

Hypotheses for nursing research studies can also be derived from the literature or from the findings of other studies. The researcher may test the assumptions of another study or test a hypothesis based on the findings of another study.

Finally, the most important source of a hypothesis is the theoretical or conceptual framework developed for the study. This process of hypothesis derivation involves deductive reasoning. A propositional statement is isolated from the study framework and empirically tested. For example, using Maslow's theory of human needs (see Chapter 6), you might decide to test the proposition that safety needs take precedence over self-esteem needs. This proposition could then be transferred into a hypothesis to be tested in a research study. You might ask a group of patients to rate a list of nursing actions and then you could determine if they rated actions that concern patient safety higher than actions that concern meeting the self-esteem needs of patients.

CLASSIFICATIONS OF HYPOTHESES

Hypotheses may be categorized as simple and complex. They may also be classified as research hypotheses or null hypotheses. Research hypotheses may be further divided into nondirectional and directional hypotheses.

SIMPLE AND COMPLEX HYPOTHESES

A **simple hypothesis** concerns the relationship between one independent and one dependent variable. Independent and dependent variables were discussed in Chapter 2. If you recall, in experimental studies the independent variable may be considered as the "cause," or reason that a phenomenon occurs, and the dependent variable may be considered as the "effect," or the occurrence of the phenomenon. Independent and dependent variables may also be identified in many nonexperimental studies by examining the direction of the influence of one variable on the other or by determining which variable occurred before the other one. The independent variable occurs first in chronological time (but not necessarily first in the hypothesis statement itself).

A **complex hypothesis** concerns a relationship where two or more independent variables, two or more dependent variables, or both, are being examined in the same study. A simple hypothesis might be called bivariate and a complex hypothesis might be considered as multivariate. Remember, hypotheses are not required if only one variable is being examined.

Simple hypotheses contain one independent variable and one dependent variable; complex hypotheses may contain several independent and dependent variables. As long as there is more than one independent variable, more than one dependent variable, or both, the hypothesis is considered to be complex. Table 7–1 lists examples of simple and complex hypotheses.

Caution should be exercised when using complex hypotheses. It may be better to divide a complex hypothesis into two or more simple hypotheses. Although you may read about "partial support" for a hypothesis, this is inaccurate. If only part of the hypothesis is supported, the researcher is in the "partial support" crisis. In actuality, a hypothesis is either supported totally, or it is not supported. For example, consider this hypothesis: There is a positive relationship between patients' perception of pain control and (a) complaints of pain and (b) requests for pain medications. Statistically, two hypotheses will be tested: (a) the relationship between perception of pain control and complaints of pain and (b) the relationship between perception of pain control and requests for pain medications. What if a significant relationship is found between perception of pain control and complaints of pain but not between perception of pain control and requests for pain medication? The "partial support" crisis has occurred. The researcher cannot decide to divide the original hypothesis at this time but must admit that the research hypothesis has not been supported. This problem could have been solved by writing two simple hypotheses rather than one complex hypothesis.

There are times when complex hypotheses are necessary. Whenever the researcher wants to examine an interaction effect, a complex hypothesis is called for. An **interaction effect** concerns the action of two variables in conjunction with each other. Consider hypothesis 3 in Table 7–1. The researcher believes that the combination of diet and exercise is necessary for weight loss.

NULL AND RESEARCH HYPOTHESES

Those of you who have had a course in statistics will recall that a **null hypothesis** (H_o) predicts that no relationship exists between variables, and it is the null hypothesis that is subjected to statistical analysis. For those of you who have repressed statistics into your

TABLE 7–1.   Simple and Complex Hypotheses

Population	Independent Variable	Dependent Variable	Type of Hypothesis	Hypotheses
1. Infants	Level of alcohol use of mothers	Birth weight	Simple	1. Birth weight is lower among infants of alcoholic mothers than among infants of nonalcoholic mothers.
2. Intensive care unit patients	Sleep deprivation	Anxiety	Simple	2. The greater the degree of sleep deprivation, the higher the anxiety level of intensive care unit patients.
3. Adults	a. Type of diet b. Exercise	Weight	Complex	3. Daily weight loss is greater for adults who follow a reduced calorie diet and exercise daily than for those who do not follow a reduced calorie diet and do not exercise daily.
4. Nurse practitioners	Type of nurse practitioner	Job mobility	Simple	4. The level of job mobility is different for psychiatric nurse practitioners than for medical-surgical nurse practitioners.
5. Women	Method of delivery	a. Postpartum depression b. Feelings of inadequacy	Complex	5. More postpartum depression and feelings of inadequacy are reported by women who give birth by cesarean delivery than by those who deliver vaginally.
6. Myocardial infarction patients	Denial	Anxiety	Simple	6. There is a negative relationship between denial and reports of anxiety among postmyocardial infarction patients.

unconscious and for those who have not yet taken a statistics course, the null hypothesis is tested even when the research hypothesis is stated in the study. A **research hypothesis** or alternative hypothesis (H_1) states the expected relationship between variables. Other names for the research hypothesis are *scientific, substantive,* and *theoretical.* With this type of hypothesis, the reader of a research report can determine exactly what the researcher expects to find after analyzing the data.

Statistical logic requires that a testable hypothesis must state the expectation of no correlation between the variables or no difference between groups on the variable that is being measured. If the research hypothesis states that a difference exists between two groups, the null hypothesis states that no difference exists. If the research hypothesis proposes that a correlation exists between two variables, the null hypothesis states that no correlation exists. Although some research studies express hypotheses in the null form, it is more desirable to state the researcher's expectations (Batey, 1977; Kerlinger, 1986; Polit & Hungler, 1999). A review of the current nursing research journals shows that the research hypothesis has replaced the statistical null hypothesis as the preferred way of expressing the predictions for studies. The use of theoretical frameworks in nursing research has brought about this change. Study predictions should be based on the study framework.

The level of significance for rejecting the statistical null hypothesis should always be stated before data are collected. In nursing, as in many other disciplines, the level of significance is usually set at .05. A significance level of .05 means that the researcher is willing to risk being wrong 5% of the time, or 5 times out of 100, when rejecting the null hypothesis (see Chapter 14). Generally, the aim of the researcher is to reject the null hypothesis because this provides support for the research hypothesis. Sir Ronald Fisher (1951) stated, "Every experiment may be said to exist only in order to give the facts a chance of disproving the null hypothesis" (p. 16).

Occasionally, the null hypothesis and the research hypothesis are the same. The researcher actually expects no correlation between variables or no difference between groups being compared on a certain variable. For example, an in-service educator at a hospital might believe that a certain inexpensive teaching program is as effective as an expensive teaching program for patients with diabetes. The educator might predict that there would be no difference in patients' learning of the subject matter when the two different teaching programs are used. Usually, the researcher does expect to find a difference or a correlation; otherwise, the study would not have been conducted.

> A null hypothesis was used by Pridham, Kosorok, Greer, Carey, Kayata, and Sondel (1999) in their study of the effects of prescribed versus ad libitum feedings and formula caloric density on premature infant dietary intake and weight gain. Their null hypothesis stated that dietary intake and weight change would not differ for infants fed on a prescribed or on an ad libitum feeding regimen.

NONDIRECTIONAL AND DIRECTIONAL RESEARCH HYPOTHESES

Research hypotheses may be described as being nondirectional or directional. In a **nondirectional research hypothesis,** the researcher merely predicts that a relationship exists. The direction of the relationship is not presented.

The use of distraction to reduce reported pain, fear, and behavioral distress in children and adolescents was studied by Carlson, Broome, and Vessey (2000). They used two nondirectional hypotheses. The first one stated: There will be a significant difference in observed behavioral distress, self-reported pain, and children's fear between children/adolescents using a kaleidoscope for distraction during venipuncture and IV insertion and those who do not.

In the **directional research hypothesis,** the researcher further predicts the type of relationship. Directional hypotheses have several advantages. They make clear the researcher's expectation, allow more precise testing of theoretical propositions, and allow the use of one-tailed statistical tests. As you may remember, statistical significance is more easily achieved when one-tailed tests are used.

Hypotheses that are derived from theory will nearly always be directional. Theories attempt to explain phenomena; therefore, propositional statements from theories present the rationale for predictive hypotheses.

A directional hypothesis was used in a study by Kelly, Doughty, Hasselbeck, and Vacchiano (2000). They hypothesized that patients receiving warmed irrigation solution (40° C) during arthroscopic knee surgery would maintain a higher core body temperature than those whose irrigation solution was at room temperature.

When a study is not theory-based or the findings of related studies are contradictory, the investigator may decide to use a nondirectional hypothesis. Examine the hypotheses in Table 7–1. Try to determine the directional and nondirectional hypotheses. Only one of them is a nondirectional hypothesis.

HYPOTHESIS CRITERIA

The important criteria for a hypothesis require that the hypothesis:

1. Is written in a declarative sentence
2. Is written in the present tense
3. Contains the population
4. Contains the variables
5. Reflects the problem statement
6. Is empirically testable

Is WRITTEN IN A DECLARATIVE SENTENCE

Problem statements are written in interrogatory sentences; hypotheses are written in declarative sentences. This is one of the major differences between the problem statement and the hypothesis for a study. The problem statement asks a question about some phenomenon or phenomena, and the hypothesis presents an answer or tentative solution to the problem. Hypotheses should be written in the present tense.

It is possible to transpose only two words in some problem statements and change them into nondirectional research hypotheses. Examine the two examples below.

- *Problem Statement:* Is there a change in the anxiety levels of preoperative patients after listening to a relaxation tape?
- *Hypothesis:* There is a change in the anxiety levels of preoperative patients after listening to a relaxation tape.
- *Problem Statement:* Is there a correlation between the number of sources of stress reported by nurses in a thoracic intensive care unit and the nurses' desire to leave employment in that setting?
- *Hypothesis:* There is a correlation between the number of sources of stress reported by nurses in a thoracic intensive care unit and the nurses' desire to leave employment in that setting.

Generally, it is not quite so easy to compose the hypothesis. As previously stated, directional hypotheses, rather than the nondirectional type presented in the two examples, are the preferred type. These will require more deliberation and consideration of the framework for the hypothesis. A theoretical proposition or an empirical generalization will need to be isolated and then developed into a testable hypothesis that predicts the relationship the researcher expects to find. For example, the first hypothesis might be changed to a directional hypothesis in the following way: The anxiety levels of preoperative patients are lower after listening to a relaxation tape. This hypothesis is based on the theoretical proposition that anxiety is reduced if relaxation can be achieved.

Is Written in the Present Tense

Hypotheses found in the literature are frequently written in future tense. However, hypotheses are tested in the present and should be written in present tense.

- *Future Tense:* There *will* be a positive relationship between the number of times children have been hospitalized and their fear of hospitalization.
- *Present Tense:* There *is* a positive relationship between the number of times children have been hospitalized and their fear of hospitalization.

Contains the Population

The population needs to be specifically identified in the hypothesis, just as it is in the problem statement. Usually, the population will be described or stated exactly as it was in the problem statement. If the problem statement identifies the population as "middle-aged females who are about to undergo a hysterectomy," these same terms should be contained in the hypothesis. It would not be correct to identify the population in the hypothesis only as "hysterectomy patients."

Contains the Variables

If you are observant, and I'm sure that you are, you noticed that the word variable is written as a plural noun in the heading above. In the problem statement section of Chapter 4, this same heading was written as variable(s). In the problem statement you might have only one variable. Remember, a univariate research problem statement is acceptable. A scientific hypothesis, however, contains at least two variables. The hypothesis links two or more variables together.

The variables in the hypothesis are the same as those in the corresponding problem statement. These variables may be expanded on or made clearer in the hypothesis. Frequently, the hypothesis will contain the instrument or tool that will be used to measure the dependent variable. This instrument links the hypothesis more closely to the actual data-gathering procedure and helps to operationalize the dependent variable. Here is an example of two ways to write the same hypothesis:

- Anxiety levels are lower for preoperative hysterectomy patients who have practiced relaxation exercises than for preoperative hysterectomy patients who have not practiced relaxation exercises.
- Anxiety levels, as measured by the State Anxiety Scale of Spielberger's State-Trait Anxiety Inventory, are lower for preoperative hysterectomy patients who have practiced relaxation exercises than for preoperative hysterectomy patients who have not practiced relaxation exercises.

As you can see, the second example contains the instrument that will be used to measure the dependent variable. The hypothesis will still need further clarification, however, before it is ready to be tested. For example, relaxation exercises would have to be operationally defined before the study could actually be conducted.

Reflects the Problem Statement

To reemphasize the point, the hypothesis should contain essentially the same material as the problem statement. Occasionally you read a research report in which it appears that one person wrote the problem statement and another person wrote the hypothesis without ever reading the problem statement. For example, the problem statement might identify "depression" as the dependent variable, and the hypothesis lists "anxiety" as the dependent variable. Congruency is a must!

Is Empirically Testable

The ability to obtain empirical data should have been determined as the research problem was formalized. If there is no possibility of obtaining empirical data, it will not be possible to conduct a quantitative study. A hypothesis that cannot be empirically tested has no scientific merit. Ethical and value issues are two areas that are inappropriate for hypothesis testing because data cannot be obtained that can be empirically verified.

HYPOTHESIS FORMAT

As discussed in the problem statement format section in Chapter 4, research problems that examine more than one variable are usually written in the form of a correlational statement or a comparative statement. The same holds true for hypotheses. The issue of correlations and comparisons becomes important when the data are submitted for statistical analysis, because statistical tests are basically designed to examine correlations between variables or comparisons among sets of data. A study might compare the average pulse rates of two different groups, for example, or the correlation between pulse rates and respirations in one group of subjects.

A directional research hypothesis should contain a predictive term such as *more than, greater than, decrease in,* or *positive correlation.* Let's take the problem statement examples in Chapter 4 and examine corresponding hypotheses.

- *Problem Statement:* Is there a correlation between anxiety and midterm examination scores of baccalaureate nursing students?

- *Hypothesis:* There is a negative correlation between anxiety and midterm examination scores of baccalaureate nursing students.

- *Problem Statement:* Is there a difference in readiness to learn about preoperative teaching between preoperative patients who have high anxiety levels compared with preoperative patients who do not have high anxiety levels?

- *Hypothesis:* Readiness to learn about preoperative teaching is less among preoperative patients who have high anxiety levels compared with preoperative patients who do not have high anxiety levels.

HYPOTHESES AND THEORY TESTING

The statistical testing of a hypothesis is discussed in Chapter 14. It seems important at this point, however, to mention hypothesis testing and its relation to theory.

Hypotheses are never proved or disproved. Novice researchers can be spotted easily if they discuss trying to "prove" their hypotheses. Remember, neither theories nor hypotheses are "proved." In my research classes, a student has to bring cookies to the next class if he or she says the word "prove" out loud in a class discussion.

If the null hypothesis is rejected, the research hypothesis is supported. If the research hypothesis is supported, the theory from which the hypothesis was derived will also be supported. Likewise, if the research hypothesis is not supported, the theory is also not supported. When the data fail to support the theory, a critical reexamination of the theory is needed. Beginning researchers frequently have difficulty in explaining their findings when these findings fail to support the tested theory. In some cases, the researcher will point out all the limitations of the study and intimate that the theory is probably valid and that the study results failed to support the theory because of design or methodology problems that are the fault of the researcher. Study limitations may, in fact, have influenced the results of the study, but it is also possible that the theory is not valid.

RESEARCH QUESTIONS

As has been previously mentioned, some studies do not call for hypotheses. Unless a study is examining the relationship between variables, hypotheses are not required. Qualitative research studies (Chapter 9) generally do not test hypotheses. Other types of studies that frequently do not test hypotheses are single-variable descriptive studies and methodological studies, which are concerned with the development of research instruments and research methodology.

When hypotheses are not tested in a research study, research questions are posed. Research questions are more precise and specific than the broad question that is found in the problem statement. Consider the following problem statement: What are the sources of stress identified by parents of chronically ill children? Specific research questions might be: How many different sources of stress are identified by parents of chronically ill children? What sources of stress are identified by fathers of chronically ill children? What sources of stress are identified by mothers of chronically ill children?

In some studies where hypotheses are tested, research questions are also posed. These questions do not relate to the hypotheses but are additional areas of interest concerning the study topic. For example, suppose a researcher is testing a new intervention for weight loss. The hypothesis might be: People who are overweight and are allowed to eat a candy bar each day as part of their diet lose more weight over a 6-week period than those who are not allowed to eat a candy bar (This is my kind of diet!). The researcher might also ask such questions as: Which type of candy bars do people choose? How many calories are in the candy bars that are chosen? What percentage of their daily calories are consumed in the candy bars?

CRITIQUING HYPOTHESES AND RESEARCH QUESTIONS

First, the evaluator of a research report determines if the report contains a hypothesis or hypotheses. Generally, there is a section heading that clearly labels the hypotheses. If the study contains no hypotheses, a determination should be made as to whether the study is appropriate for hypothesis testing.

If the study report contains a hypothesis or hypotheses, there are a number of factors to be considered. Criteria for evaluating study hypotheses are presented in Box 7–1.

Hypotheses should be clear and concise declarative sentences and should be written in the present tense. Hypotheses should reflect the problem statement and be derived from the study framework, if there is a clearly identified study framework. If there is no identified study framework, the source or rationale for each hypothesis should be apparent to the critiquer of the research report. For example, a hypothesis might be based on previous research findings. The preferred type of hypothesis is a directional research hypothesis. It is easy to determine that the hypothesis is directional when there is a word or phrase such as "greater than," "increase in," or "negative correlation." The hypothesis should contain the population and the study variables. Each hypothesis should be empirically testable and contain only one prediction. The hypothesis may contain the name of the specific research instrument or instruments that will be used to measure the study variables. If not, the research report should contain an operational definition of each of the study variables.

Box 7–1. Guidelines for Critiquing Hypotheses and Research Questions

1. Does the study contain a hypothesis or hypotheses?
2. Is each hypothesis clearly worded and concise?
3. Is the hypothesis written in a declarative sentence?
4. Is each hypothesis directly tied to the study problem?
5. If there is a clearly identified study framework, is each hypothesis derived from this framework?
6. Does each hypothesis contain the population and at least two variables?
7. Is each hypothesis stated as a directional research hypothesis? If not, is the rationale given for the type of hypothesis that is stated?
8. Is it apparent that each hypothesis can be empirically tested?
9. Does each hypothesis contain only one prediction?
10. If the study contains research questions, are the questions precise and specific?
11. Do the research questions further delineate the problem area of the study?

It is not uncommon for a study to test many more hypotheses than are stated. This fact may be discovered when examining the statistical results. For every statistical test result and accompanying probability value, the researcher has tested a hypothesis, whether or not the hypothesis was actually stated. Frequently, after eyeballing the data, the researcher may decide to make some additional statistical analyses. For example, suppose a determination was being made about the effectiveness of preoperative relaxation exercises in controlling postoperative anxiety. The study results indicate that the postoperative anxiety levels of subjects are not significantly different between those who practiced relaxation and those who did not practice relaxation exercises preoperatively. However, when the researcher looked at the data, it appeared that the relaxation exercises might have been effective for women, but not for men. An additional statistical comparison might be made between the women who practiced relaxation and those who did not practice relaxation. This type of statistical analysis is labeled a post hoc (after the fact) comparison.

If the study report contains research questions rather than hypotheses, the reader should evaluate the appropriateness of the research questions. Do they further specify the problem area of the study?

SUMMARY

A hypothesis is a statement of the predicted relationship between two or more variables. Hypotheses allow theoretical propositions to be tested in the real world, guide the research design, dictate the type of statistical analysis for the data, and provide the reader with an understanding of the researcher's expectations about the study before data collection begins.

The rationale or sources of hypotheses can come from the researcher's own personal experiences, from previous research studies, or from theoretical propositions. Nursing research involves both inductive and deductive means of formulating hypotheses.

Hypotheses may be categorized as simple or complex. **Simple hypotheses** contain one independent and one dependent variable; **complex hypotheses** contain two or more independent variables, two or more dependent variables, or both. An **interaction effect** concerns the action of two variables in conjunction with each other.

Hypotheses may also be classified as statistical null hypotheses or research hypotheses. The **null hypothesis** states that no difference exists between groups or that there is no correlation between variables. The **research hypothesis** states that a difference or correlation does exist. Research hypotheses can be divided into nondirectional and directional hypotheses. The **nondirectional research hypothesis** indicates that a difference or correlation exists but does not predict the type. The **directional research hypothesis** states the type of correlation or difference that the researcher expects to find. The directional research hypothesis is the preferred type for nursing research studies, unless the study is not based on theory or if previous studies in the area have demonstrated contradictory findings.

Criteria for an acceptable hypothesis require that the hypothesis (a) is written in a declarative sentence, (b) is written in the present tense, (c) includes the population, (d) includes the variables, (e) reflects the problem statement, and (f) is empirically testable.

The results of statistical analysis will either support or fail to support the hypothesis. Hypotheses are never "proved" or "disproved." If the null hypothesis is rejected, the research hypothesis is supported. Thus, if a theoretical proposition is being tested and support is found for the research hypothesis, the theory is also supported.

In studies where hypotheses are not necessary, research questions are posed. These questions are more specific than the broad question that is found in the problem statement.

NURSING RESEARCH ON THE WEB

For additional online resources, research activities, and exercises, go to www.prenhall. com/nieswiadomy. Select Chapter 7 from the drop down menu.

✖ GET INVOLVED ACTIVITIES

1. Each student will bring a research article to class that contains a hypothesis. Share the hypotheses with classmates. Critique as many of the hypotheses as time allows.

2. Rewrite one of these hypotheses found in the literature that does not meet the criteria for an acceptable hypothesis.

3. Divide into groups and practice writing hypotheses. Each group will write two hypotheses. In the first one, use the word "headache" as an independent variable, and in the second one, use "headache" as the dependent variable.

4. Propose two study examples in which hypotheses would not be needed.

❉ SELF-TEST

Identify the independent variable(s) and dependent variable(s) in the following hypotheses.

1. Male appendectomy patients request more pain medication on the first postoperative day than do female appendectomy patients.
2. There is an inverse relationship between the number of prenatal classes attended by pregnant women and their degree of fear concerning labor and delivery.
3. The body image of unmarried pregnant teenagers is less positive than is the body image of married pregnant teenagers.
4. There is an inverse relationship between postoperative hysterectomy patients' anxiety levels and their requests for pain medication.
5. There is a higher incidence of marijuana usage among high school freshmen than among high school seniors.
6. Older adults demonstrate a lower self-image after retirement than before retirement.
7. The job turnover rate and job dissatisfaction levels of graduate nurses who have worked less than 2 years is higher than for those graduate nurses who have worked more than 2 years.

Evaluate the following hypotheses using the criteria presented in this chapter; identify any errors that exist in the hypotheses.

8. Baccalaureate-prepared nurses provide for more of the psychosocial needs of clients.
9. Is there a difference in the anxiety levels of cardiac patients who are taught guided imagery techniques compared with cardiac patients who are not taught guided imagery techniques?
10. Depression levels decrease as the amount of interpersonal involvement increases.
11. Nurses provide better health teaching instructions to clients than do doctors.
12. There is a positive relationship between nurses' job autonomy levels and their reported job satisfaction levels.

❉ REFERENCES

Batey, M. (1977). Conceptualization: Knowledge and logic guiding empirical research. *Nursing Research, 26,* 324–329.

Carlson, K. L. , Broome, M., & Vessey, J. A. (2000). Using distraction to reduce reported pain, fear, and behavioral distress in children and adolescents: A multisite study. *Journal of the Society of Pediatric Nurses, 5,* 75–85.

Fisher, R. (1951). *The design of experiments* (6th ed.). New York: Hafner.

Kerlinger, F. (1986). *Foundations of behavioral research* (3rd ed.). New York: Holt, Rinehart & Winston.

Kelly, J. A., Doughty, J. K., Hasselbeck, A. N., & Vacchiano, C. A. (2000). *Journal of PeriAnesthesia Nursing, 15,* 245–252.

Polit, D. F., & Hungler, B. P. (1999). *Nursing research: Principles and methods* (6th ed.). Philadelphia: Lippincott.

Pridham, K., Kosorok, M. R., Greer, F., Carey, P., Kayata, S., & Sondel, S. (1999). The effects of prescribed versus ad libitum feedings and formula caloric density on premature infant dietary intake and weight gain. *Nursing Research, 48,* 86–93.

PART III

Research Designs

Quantitative Research Designs

✖ OBJECTIVES

On completion of this chapter, you will be prepared to:

1. Define experimental research
2. Discuss internal and external validity of experimental designs
3. Identify six threats to internal validity
4. Identify three threats to external validity
5. Distinguish between true experimental, quasiexperimental, and preexperimental designs
6. Discuss three true experimental designs
7. Discuss two quasiexperimental designs
8. Discuss two preexperimental designs

9. Discuss four types of nonexperimental research designs
10. Describe two types of settings in which research is conducted
11. Critique the design section of quantitative studies

✖ NEW TERMS DEFINED IN THIS CHAPTER

comparative studies
comparison group
control group
correlation
correlation coefficient
correlational studies
descriptive studies
experimenter effect
explanatory studies
exploratory studies
ex post facto studies
external validity
extraneous variable
field studies
Hawthorne effect
history
instrumentation change
internal validity
laboratory studies
manipulation
maturation
methodological studies

mortality
negative relationship
nonequivalent control group design
one-group pretest-posttest design
one-shot case study
positive relationship
posttest-only control group design
preexperimental designs
pretest-posttest control group design
prospective studies
quasiexperimental designs
random assignment
reactive effects of the pretest
retrospective studies
Rosenthal effect
selection bias
simulation studies
Solomon four-group design
survey studies
testing
time-series design
true experimental designs

Do you sew? Do you cook? If so, you probably use patterns and recipes. These patterns and recipes provide guidelines that help you construct a beautiful piece of clothing or cook a delicious meal. This chapter introduces the concept of research design, which is the "pattern" or "recipe" for a research study. The choice of a research design concerns the overall plan for the study. It is concerned with the type of data that will be collected and the means used to obtain the needed data. The researcher must decide if the study will try to determine causative factors, explore relationships, or examine historical data, for example. The design is not concerned with the specific data-collection methods, such as questionnaires or interviews, but with the overall plan for gathering data. The design must be appropriate to test the study hypothesis(es) or answer the research question(s).

EXPLORATORY, DESCRIPTIVE, AND EXPLANATORY STUDIES

The amount of existing knowledge about the variable(s) can be used as the criterion for classifying research as exploratory, descriptive, or explanatory. Although there can be overlap between the first two categories, it is helpful to examine them separately.

Exploratory studies are conducted when little is known about the phenomenon of interest. For instance, you might decide to examine the needs of family members of a patient who will be receiving antibiotics at home by IV push method. In an article in the October 2000 issue of *RN,* Skokal discussed how patients and their caregivers are being taught to give medications via IV push. Shortened hospital stays and cost-cutting measures have brought about this change. To determine what questions need to be asked, you would conduct a review of the literature. It is likely that you would find little written on this topic. An exploratory research study would therefore be appropriate.

A flexible approach rather than a structured approach to data collection would be used. In exploratory studies, there is a greater interest in examining the qualitative aspects of the data rather than the quantitative aspects. Hypotheses are generally not appropriate for these types of studies.

In **descriptive studies,** phenomena are described or the relationship between variables is examined. A descriptive study is similar to an exploratory study. However, the two categories can be distinguished by considering the amount of information that is available about the variable(s) under investigation. As previously stated, exploratory studies are appropriate when little is known about the area of interest. When enough information exists to examine relationships between variables, descriptive studies may be conducted in which hypotheses are tested.

By the time you read this material, IV antibiotic push therapy at home will probably be commonplace. Therefore, enough information might be available to conduct a descriptive study on this topic. You might try to determine which of the new antibiotics causes the most venous spasm during IV push therapy at home.

Explanatory studies search for causal explanations and are much more rigorous than exploratory or descriptive studies. This type of research is usually experimental. There is enough knowledge about the variables of interest to allow the investigator to exercise some degree of control over the research conditions and manipulate one or more of the variables. This will become clearer as you read more in this chapter about experimental research.

In returning to the home IV antibiotic example, you may now have enough information to design an explanatory study. You might design an intervention to help patients and their caregivers reduce the incidence of venous spasm.

In summary, exploratory and descriptive studies describe phenomena and examine relationships among phenomena, whereas explanatory studies help provide explanations for the relationships among phenomena. Many nursing studies have been descriptive or exploratory in nature. Many explanatory studies have also been reported in the nursing literature.

RESEARCH DESIGNS

Although the terms *exploratory, descriptive,* and *explanatory research* can be used to indicate the type of study that is being conducted, these terms do not clearly indicate the study plan or specific design. There are several ways to classify research designs. This text presents designs under the two broad categories of quantitative and qualitative designs. As mentioned earlier, some studies combine aspects of quantitative and qualitative research in the same study.

TABLE 8–1. Quantitative Research Designs

Experimental Designs	Nonexperimental Designs
True experimental designs	Action studies
Pretest-posttest control group	Comparative studies
Posttest-only control group	Correlational studies
Solomon four-group	Developmental studies
Quasiexperimental designs	Evaluation studies
Nonequivalent control group	Meta-analysis studies
Time-series	Methodological studies
Preexperimental designs	Needs-assessment studies
One-shot case study	Secondary analysis studies
One-group pretest-posttest	Survey studies

Quantitative designs are discussed in this chapter, and qualitative designs are presented in the next chapter. Quantitative designs are divided into experimental and nonexperimental designs. Some of the various experimental and nonexperimental designs are presented in Table 8–1.

EXPERIMENTAL RESEARCH

Experimental research is concerned with cause-and-effect relationships. All experimental studies involve manipulation or control of the independent variable (cause) and measurement of the dependent variable (effect). Although experimental research designs are highly respected in the scientific world, causal relations are difficult to establish, and researchers should avoid using the word *prove* when discussing research results. Controls are difficult to apply when experimental research is conducted with human beings. This is one reason that many nursing studies have used nonexperimental designs.

VALIDITY OF EXPERIMENTAL DESIGNS

In experimental studies, as well as in other types of research, the researcher is interested in controlling extraneous variables that may influence study results. **Extraneous variables** are those variables that the researcher is not able to control, or does not choose to control, and that may influence the results of a study. Other names for extraneous variables are *confounding* and *intervening*. These variables are also called study limitations. The researcher acknowledges these study limitations in the discussion section of a research report. The extraneous variables, or competing explanations for the results, in experimental studies are labeled threats to internal and external validity (Campbell & Stanley, 1963).

In experimental studies, the researcher is trying to establish a cause-and-effect relationship. The **internal validity** of an experimental design concerns the degree to which changes in the dependent variable (effect) can be attributed to the independent variable (cause). Threats to internal validity are factors other than the independent variable that influence the dependent variable. These factors constitute rival explanations or competing hypotheses that might explain the study results.

External validity concerns the degree to which study results can be generalized to other people and other settings. Questions to be answered about external validity are these: With what degree of confidence can the study findings be transferred from the sample to the entire population? Will these study findings hold true with other groups in other times and places?

Internal and external validity are related in that as the researcher attempts to control for internal validity, external validity is usually decreased. Conversely, when the researcher is concerned with external validity or the generalizability of the findings to other settings and other people, the strict control that is necessary for high internal validity may be affected. Therefore, the researcher must decide how to balance internal and external validity.

Threats to internal and external validity are addressed before the discussion of the types of experimental designs so that you can better determine the strengths and weaknesses of the various designs as you read about them in this chapter.

THREATS TO INTERNAL VALIDITY

Campbell and Stanley (1963) and Cook and Campbell (1979) have identified threats to the internal validity of a study. Six of these threats will be discussed: selection bias, history, maturation, testing, instrumentation change, and mortality.

Selection Bias.   The **selection bias** threat occurs when study results are attributed to the experimental treatment or the researcher's manipulation of the independent variable when, in fact, the results are due to subject differences before the independent variable was manipulated. This selection threat should be considered in experimental studies when subjects are not randomly assigned to experimental and comparison groups. For example, suppose the researcher decides to offer a seminar to help people stop cigarette smoking. Fifteen volunteers are obtained who indicate they would like to stop smoking. This group is designated as the experimental group. Fifteen other people are recruited who have not shown a desire to stop smoking. This group will become the control group. The 15 subjects in the experimental group may have been more motivated to stop smoking before the treatment than the 15 subjects in the control group. The selection process for the groups, therefore, may have biased the eventual results of the study.

History.   The threat of **history** occurs when some event other than the experimental treatment occurs during the course of a study, and this event influences the dependent variable. A researcher might be interested in determining the incidence of breast self-examination (BSE) among women after attending a 3-week teaching program on BSE. During the time that the study is being conducted, an article is published in the newspaper concerning the rise in the number of women with breast cancer. This "history" event could result in an increase in the incidence of BSE behaviors. At the conclusion of the study, the researcher would not be able to determine if the teaching program (independent variable) was the reason for the increase in the incidence of BSE (dependent variable) or if the newspaper article was the impetus for an increase in BSE among the study subjects.

History is controlled by the use of at least one simultaneous comparison group. Additionally, random assignment of subjects to groups will help control the threat of history. Environmental events (history) would therefore be as likely to occur for subjects in one group as in another. If a difference is found between the groups at the conclusion of the study, the researcher is much more confident that the manipulation of the independent variable is the cause of this difference.

Maturation. **Maturation** becomes a threat when changes that occur within the subjects during an experimental study influence the study results. People may become older, taller, or sleepier from the time of the pretest to the posttest. If a school nurse was interested in the weight gain of children who receive a hot breakfast at school each day, she would have to keep in mind that changes may occur in these children during the course of the study that are not related to the experimental treatment. The children will probably gain some weight regardless of whether they eat a hot breakfast at school. Again, a comparison group helps control for this threat. Maturation processes are then as likely to occur in one group as in another.

Testing. The testing threat may occur in studies where a pretest is given or where subjects have knowledge of baseline data. **Testing** refers to the influence of the pretest or knowledge of baseline data on the posttest scores. Subjects may remember the answers they put on the pretest and put the same answers on the posttest. Also, subjects' scores may be altered on the posttest as a result of their knowledge of baseline data. For example, if subjects were weighed and told their weight before an experimental weight reduction program, these subjects might make some effort on their own to lose weight because they have discovered that they are overweight. This knowledge of baseline data could be considered as a pretest.

Instrumentation Change. When mechanical instruments or judges are used in the pretest and posttest phases of a study, the threat of instrumentation must be considered. **Instrumentation change** involves the difference between the pretest and posttest measurement caused by a change in the accuracy of the instrument or the judges' ratings, rather than as a result of the experimental treatment. Judges may become more adept at the ratings or, on the other hand, may become tired and may make less exact observations. Training sessions for judges and trial runs to check for fatigue factors may help to control for instrumentation changes. Also, if mechanical instruments are used, such as sphygmomanometers, these instruments should be checked for their accuracy throughout the study.

Mortality. The **mortality** threat occurs when the subject dropout rate is different between the experimental and comparison groups. The observed effects may occur because subjects who dropped out of a particular group differ from those who remained in the study. For example, if a large number of experimental group subjects who scored very high on an anxiety pretest dropped out of the study, the average anxiety scores on the posttest for the experimental group might be deceivingly low. The researcher might falsely conclude that the treatment really worked well! There is no research design that will control for mortality because participants can never be forced to remain in a study.

The longer a study lasts, the more likely that subject dropout will occur. Fogg and Gross (2000) pointed out that if subjects dropped out of a study at random, the problem might not be so bad, However, the reasons that people drop out could make the resultant two groups quite different than they were at the beginning of the study. For example, if the dependent variable were depression, it is possible that people with the highest or lowest levels of depression would be the ones to drop out of the study.

Subject mortality is a problem that plagues nurse researchers in nearly all clinical studies. To control for this threat, the researcher should try to establish a relationship with the study participants and help them recognize the importance or their continued participation in a particular study.

THREATS TO EXTERNAL VALIDITY

Campbell and Stanley (1963) have identified four threats to external validity, and Bracht and Glass (1968) delineated ten threats to the external validity of a study. Three threats are discussed here: the Hawthorne effect, the experimenter effect, and the reactive effects of the pretest.

Hawthorne Effect.   The **Hawthorne effect** occurs when study participants respond in a certain manner because they are aware that they are being observed. This term came about as the result of the studies on worker productivity at the Hawthorne plant of the Western Electric Company. Working conditions were varied, such as changing the length of the working day. Worker productivity was found to increase no matter what changes were made. The increase in productivity was finally determined to be the result of the subjects' knowledge that they were involved in a research study. The Hawthorne effect may also be considered a threat to internal validity.

Experimenter Effect.   The **experimenter effect** is a threat to study results that occurs when researcher characteristics or behaviors influence subject behaviors. Examples of researcher characteristics or behaviors that may be influential are facial expressions, clothing, age, gender, and body build. Although the term experimenter effect is appropriate to use only when discussing experimental research, a term with a similar meaning is used in nonexperimental research. The **Rosenthal effect,** named after the person who identified this phenomenon, is used to indicate the influence of an interviewer on respondents' answers. It has been shown that researcher characteristics such as gender, dress, and type of jewelry may influence study participants' answers to questions.

Reactive Effects of the Pretest.   When a pretest and a posttest are used in an experimental study, the researcher must be aware not only of the internal validity threat that may occur but also of the external validity threat that may exist. The **reactive effects of the pretest,** which is sometimes called the measurement effect (Polit & Hungler, 1999), occurs when subjects have been sensitized to the treatment through taking the pretest. This sensitization may affect the posttest results. People might not respond to the treatment in the same manner if they had not received a pretest. In other words, a researcher could not say that the experimental treatment would bring about the same results with another group of people unless he or she said that the new group would also be given the pretest before the treatment. The pretest does not have to be a paper-and-pencil test. As mentioned previously, if study participants were told their weight before a weight reduction study, this knowledge of baseline data would be considered a pretest.

You might say, "I still don't see how this threat is different from the internal validity threat of 'testing.'" The internal validity threat occurs if the pretest or knowledge of baseline data is the *cause* of the results on the posttest, rather than the independent variable being the cause of the results on the posttest. An external validity threat occurs if the pretest acts as a *catalyst* in bringing about the results on the posttest. In this situation, the pretest is not the direct cause of the change in the posttest measurements. It is the indirect cause.

Are you ever going to know for sure if the pretest threat has occurred? Probably not. The important thing is to remember that there is a possibility that this threat may occur if a pretest is given in a study or if subjects have knowledge of their baseline data (such as their cholesterol levels) that will then be compared to posttest results (their decrease or increase in cholesterol levels). You may want to read this section several times. This material gives my students a headache!

SYMBOLIC PRESENTATION OF RESEARCH DESIGNS

Research designs are often easier to understand when seen in a symbolic form. The symbols used to depict the designs in this chapter are based on the notation scheme of Campbell and Stanley (1963).

R = random assignment of subjects to groups
O = observation or measurement of dependent variable
X = experimental treatment or intervention

The Xs and Os on one line apply to a specific group. The time sequence of events is read from left to right. If an X appears first and then an O, this means the intervention occurred first and then an observation was made. If a subscript appears after an X or O (X_1; X_2; O_1; O_2), the numbers indicate the first treatment, second treatment, first observation, second observation, and so forth.

$R \; O_1 \; X \; O_2$ (Experimental group)
$R \; O_1 \quad O_2$ (Comparison group)

In this example, there are two groups, both of which were formed through random assignment of subjects to groups. **Random assignment** is a procedure that ensures that each subject has an equal chance of being assigned or placed in any of the groups in an experimental study. Both groups in the example were measured or given a pretest (dependent variable). The experimental group was exposed to an experimental treatment (independent variable), but the comparison group was not exposed to this treatment. Then both groups were again measured or given the posttest (dependent variable).

TYPES OF EXPERIMENTAL DESIGNS

There are three broad categories of experimental research designs: true experimental, quasi-experimental, and preexperimental. The distinction between these designs is determined by the amount of control the researcher is able to exercise over the research conditions.

TRUE EXPERIMENTAL DESIGNS

The **true experimental designs** are those in which the researcher has a great deal of control over the research situation. Threats to the internal validity of the study are minimized. Only with the use of true experimental designs may causality be inferred with any degree of confidence. With these types of designs, the researcher has some confidence that the independent variable was the cause of the change in the dependent variable. There are three criteria for a true experimental design:

1. The researcher manipulates the experimental variable(s).
2. At least one experimental and one comparison group are included in the study.
3. Subjects are randomly assigned to either the experimental or the comparison group.

Sometimes there is misunderstanding of the term *manipulation* as it is used in experimental studies. The concept of manipulation might bring to mind the picture of puppets on a string; however, the term **manipulation** means that the independent, or experimental, variable is controlled by the researcher. The researcher has control over the type of experimental treatment that is administered and who will receive the treatment. Of course, human subjects always have the option of agreeing or not agreeing to participate in a research study.

The experimental treatment in nursing research usually concerns some type of nursing intervention. The researcher manipulates the independent variable, or nursing intervention, by administering it to some subjects and withholding it from others. The dependent variable, or the effects of the nursing intervention, will then be observed. For example, a nurse researcher might implement a new, structured, preoperative teaching program with a group of preoperative patients and use the routine teaching program with another group of preoperative patients. The anxiety levels of both groups of patients would be the dependent variable.

The second criterion for a true experimental design is the use of a comparison or control group. The term *control* group is seen more frequently in the literature than the term *comparison* group. A **control group** usually indicates a group in an experimental study that does not receive the experimental treatment. In nursing research, the withholding of a treatment may be unethical, however. In the previous example concerning preoperative patients, the withholding of preoperative teaching would not be considered ethical. In many nursing studies, therefore, a comparison group is used rather than a control group that receives no intervention. The comparison group usually receives the "normal" or routine intervention. The term **comparison group** is used in this text to indicate any group in an experimental study that either receives no treatment or a treatment that is not thought to be as effective as the experimental treatment.

Finally, the third criterion for true experimental studies is the random assignment of subjects to groups. As previously mentioned, random assignment ensures that each subject has an equal chance of being placed into any of the groups in an experimental study. Keep in mind that random sampling and random assignment are two entirely different concepts. These concepts are discussed further in Chapter 10. At this point, be aware that random assignment concerns the equality of groups in experimental studies. The random assignment of subjects to groups eliminates selection bias as a threat to the internal validity of the study.

Three types of true experimental designs are discussed. These designs are the pretest-posttest control group design, the posttest-only control group design, and the Solomon four-group design.

Pretest-Posttest Control Group Design.

The **pretest-posttest control group design** is probably the most frequently used experimental design (Campbell & Stanley, 1963). In this design, (a) the subjects are randomly assigned to groups, (b) a pretest is given to both groups, (c) the experimental group receives the experimental treatment and the comparison group receives the routine treatment or no treatment, and (d) a posttest is given to both groups.

$$R\ O_1\ X\ O_2\ \text{(Experimental group)}$$
$$R\ O_1\quad O_2\ \text{(Comparison group)}$$

The researcher is able to determine if the groups were equal before the treatment was administered. If the groups were not equivalent, the posttest scores may be statistically adjusted to control for the initial differences between the two groups that were reflected in the pretest scores.

A nurse researcher might be interested in the usefulness of a diabetic teaching film. A group of clients with diabetes are randomly assigned to the experimental or the comparison group. Both groups are then pretested on their knowledge of diabetes. The experimental group watches the diabetic teaching film. The comparison group is asked to read printed material that is similar to the information covered in the teaching film. Both groups are then posttested on their knowledge of diabetes. Finally, the differences between the posttest scores of the two groups are compared.

The pretest-posttest control group design controls for all threats to internal validity. The disadvantage of this design concerns the external threat of the reactive effects of the pretest. The results of the study can be generalized only to situations in which a pretest would be administered before the treatment.

A two-group pretest-posttest design was used by Bouvé, Rozmus, and Giordano (1999) to examine a nursing intervention designed to decrease the anxiety level of parents of children being transferred from a pediatric intensive care unit to a general pediatric floor. Parents in the experimental group were given a transfer-preparation letter along with a verbal explanation.

The control group parents were merely told, immediately before transfer, that their child was being transferred; this was the usual procedure that was in place at the time of the study. After statistically controlling for the parents' usual anxiety levels, measured by a pretest, results showed significantly lower anxiety levels 1 to 2 hours before transfer among the parents in the experimental group.

Posttest-Only Control Group Design. In the **posttest-only control group design,** (a) subjects are randomly assigned to groups, (b) the experimental group receives the experimental treatment, and the comparison group receives the routine treatment or no treatment, and (c) a posttest is given to both groups.

$$R \; X \; O_1 \text{ (Experimental group)}$$
$$R \quad O_1 \text{ (Comparison group)}$$

The posttest-only control group design is easier to carry out and superior to the pretest-posttest design. The researcher does not have to be concerned with the reactive effects of the pretest on the posttest. The generalizability of the results would be more extensive. A study similar to the example described under the pretest-posttest control group design could be developed. The only difference would be that the two groups would not receive a pretest on their knowledge of diabetes.

Random assignment of subjects into groups in the posttest-only control group design ensures equality of the groups. The use of a large sample size will increase the effectiveness of random assignment. Although random assignment should ensure equality of groups, researchers seem to be fearful that the groups may not, in fact, be similar. They, therefore, sometimes choose to administer a pretest.

Hayes (1998) reported the use of a two-group, experimental, posttest-only design in her study of a geragogy-based medication instruction program for elderly patients who were being discharged from an emergency department. Geragogy concerns the design of programs of instruction for elderly learners. Hayes asserted that a posttest-only design recognized that the information given about medications would be new information for these learners. Therefore, no pretest was given. Subjects in the intervention group demonstrated significantly more knowledge of medications 48 to 72 hours after discharge than did subjects in the group that received the usual discharge teaching method.

Solomon Four-Group Design. In the **Solomon four-group design,** (a) subjects are randomly assigned to one of the four groups; (b) two of the groups, experimental group 1 and comparison group 1, are pretested; (c) two of the groups, experimental group 1 and experimental group 2, receive the experimental treatment, whereas two of the groups, comparison group 1 and comparison group 2, receive the routine treatment or no treatment; and (d) a posttest is given to all four groups.

$$R \; O_1 \; X \; O_2 \text{ (Experimental group 1)}$$
$$R \; O_1 \quad O_2 \text{ (Comparison group 1)}$$
$$R \quad X \; O_2 \text{ (Experimental group 2)}$$
$$R \quad O_2 \text{ (Comparison group 2)}$$

The Solomon four-group design is considered to be the most prestigious experimental design because it minimizes threats to internal and external validity (Campbell & Stanley, 1963). This design not only controls for all of the threats to internal validity but also controls for the reactive effects of the pretest. Any differences between the experimental and the comparison groups can be more confidently associated with the experimental treatment. Unfortunately, this design requires a large sample, and statistical analysis of the data is complicated.

A Solomon four-group design was used by Swanson (1999) to study the effects of counseling with women who miscarry. All four groups were measured on three dependent variables: self-esteem, mood states, and the impact of miscarriage. One group received early counseling (at 6 weeks, 4 months, and 1 year). Another group received delayed counseling at 4 months and 1 year. One of the control groups received an early administration of tools for the dependent variables (6 weeks, 4 months and 1 year). The other control group received delayed administration of these tools (4 months and 1 year). Results showed that the caring received in the counseling sessions had significant effects on the women's integration of loss and on their well-being in the first year after a miscarriage.

QUASIEXPERIMENTAL DESIGNS

Sometimes researchers are not able to randomly assign subjects to groups, or for various reasons no comparison group is available for an experimental study. **Quasiexperimental designs** are those in which there is either no comparison group or subjects are not randomly assigned to groups. Generally, the researcher uses existing or intact groups for the experimental and comparison groups. Although the researcher does not have as much control in a quasiexperimental study as in a true experiment, there are some advantages to the use of quasiexperimental designs. By conducting experiments with naturally occurring groups, the real world is more closely approximated than when subjects are randomly assigned to groups.

Many different designs fall into the category of quasiexperimental designs. Two are discussed here: nonequivalent control group design and time-series design.

Nonequivalent Control Group Design. The **nonequivalent control group design** is similar to the pretest-posttest control group design except that there is no random assignment of subjects to the experimental and comparison groups.

$$O_1 \ X \ O_2 \ \text{(Experimental group)}$$
$$O_1 \quad O_2 \ \text{(Comparison group)}$$

A researcher might choose a group of patients with diabetes on one hospital floor for the experimental group and a group of patients with diabetes on another floor for the comparison group. The experimental treatment would be administered to the experimental group, and the comparison group would receive no treatment or some alternative treatment.

Threats to internal validity controlled by the nonequivalent control group design are history, testing, maturation, and instrumentation change. The biggest threat to internal validity is selection bias. The two groups may not have been similar at the beginning of the study. It is possible, however, to test statistically for differences in the groups. For example, it could be determined if the ages and educational backgrounds of the subjects in both groups were similar. If the groups were similar, more confidence could be placed in a cause-and-effect relationship between variables.

> MacDonald (1999) mentioned in the abstract of her study that she used a quasiexperimental nonequivalent control group pretest-posttest design. She examined the impact of the Cardiovascular Health Education Program (CHEP) on the cardiovascular health knowledge of eighth-grade adolescents. There were 88 students in the experimental group and 58 in the control group. They were enrolled in both rural and urban schools. Students were not randomly assigned to groups but, rather, were in naturally assembled classroom settings. The CHEP did have a significant positive impact on the cardiovascular health knowledge of rural adolescents, but it did not have a similar impact on urban adolescents.

Time-series Design. In a **time-series design,** the researcher periodically observes or measures the subjects. The experimental treatment is administered between two of the observations.

$$O_1 \; O_2 \; O_3 \; X \; O_4 \; O_5 \; O_6$$

A researcher might assess the pain levels of a group of clients with low back pain. After 3 weeks of pain assessment (O_1, O_2, O_3), subjects could be taught a special exercise to alleviate low back pain. During the next 3 weeks, pain levels would again be measured (O_4, O_5, O_6). The results of this study would help the researcher to determine if low back pain persists, if a specific exercise is effective in reducing low back pain, and if the effectiveness of the exercise persists.

The time-series design with its numerous observations or measurements of the dependent variable helps to strengthen the validity of the design. The greatest threats to validity are history and testing.

PREEXPERIMENTAL DESIGNS

Preexperimental designs is the name applied by Campbell and Stanley (1963) to experimental designs that are considered very weak and in which the researcher has little control over the research. Sometimes these types of designs are discussed to provide examples of how not to do research! The two preexperimental designs discussed here are the one-shot case study and the one-group pretest-posttest design.

One-shot Case Study. In a **one-shot case study,** a single group is exposed to an experimental treatment and observed after the treatment.

$$X \; O$$

A group of patients with diabetes might attend a diabetic class (X) and be tested on their knowledge of diabetes (O) after the class is completed. This design calls for no comparisons to be made. There is no way to determine if the level of knowledge about diabetes was the result of the class. The clients could have already possessed this knowledge before the class.

Threats to internal validity are history, maturation, and selection bias. The threats of testing and instrumentation change would not be applicable in this design. Selection bias would be a very serious threat in this particular design. The one-shot case study is the weakest of all the experimental designs because it controls for no threats to internal validity.

One-group Pretest-Posttest Design. The **one-group pretest-posttest design** provides a comparison between a group of subjects before and after the experimental treatment.

$$O_1 \ X \ O_2$$

A group of patients with diabetes could be given a pretest of their knowledge concerning diabetes (O_1). This group would then attend a diabetic class (X) and be posttested (O_2) at the end of the class.

Threats to internal validity would be history, maturation, testing, and instrumentation change. As you may have noticed, this design has two threats that were not applicable in the last design. Because of the existence of a pretest and posttest, testing and instrumentation change become threats to internal validity.

> A one-group pretest-posttest design was used in a study conducted by To and Chan (2000). In their article, the researchers reported that many mentally handicapped patients remain in mental hospitals in Hong Kong because of behavioral problems. The purpose of their study was to evaluate the effectiveness of progressive muscle relaxation in reducing the aggressive behaviors of 10 mentally handicapped patients. A 14.7% reduction in aggressive behaviors was found after the patients participated in muscle relaxation training.

NONEXPERIMENTAL RESEARCH

Nurse researchers have made great use of the nonexperimental research designs. Many times, experimental research cannot be conducted with human beings because of ethical reasons. At other times, nonexperimental research is the most proper type of research to obtain the needed data. In trying to determine clients' perceptions of pain, the only way to obtain this information would be to ask these clients about their pain. An experimental study would not be appropriate. All nonexperimental research is descriptive in nature because there is no manipulation or control of variables, and the researcher can only describe the phenomenon as it exists. Although the researcher cannot talk about a cause-and-effect relationship in nonexperimental research, it is important to obtain valid study results in this type of research. The researcher must attempt to control for extraneous variables through such means as careful selection of the study sample. Threats to internal validity and external validity are terms that are reserved for use in discussing experimental studies. However, in nonexperimental research, extraneous variables that threaten the validity of the study must also be considered.

TYPES OF NONEXPERIMENTAL DESIGNS

There are many types of nonexperimental research (Table 8–1). Four of the most common types are survey, correlational, comparative, and methodological.

SURVEY STUDIES

Survey studies are investigations in which self-report data are collected from samples with the purpose of describing populations on some variable or variables of interest. Surveys have probably been conducted as long as human beings have existed. Accounts of surveys are recorded in the Bible and in other historical books. People in our society today are very familiar with surveys. Probably everyone who is reading this material has been involved in some type of survey. Two of the more common public opinion surveys conducted in the United States are the Gallup and Harris polls. These national polls use scientific sampling techniques to obtain information from large groups of people through the sampling of a small percentage of the total groups.

The control exercised by the researcher in survey research lies in the sampling technique. The ability to generalize sample results to the population of interest depends on the sampling method. Probability sampling techniques and adequate sample sizes (see Chapter 10) are very important in survey research.

Many disciplines, especially the social sciences, have used survey research. Surveys generally ask subjects to report their attitudes, opinions, perceptions, or behaviors. A nurse researcher might use a survey to gather data on the health needs of clients, their sleep patterns, or their perceptions of the nursing care they have received.

Surveys may be conducted by phone, mail, or through personal contact with the subjects. The most common data collection methods used in survey research are questionnaires and interviews. In surveys, participants may be studied using a cross-sectional or a longitudinal approach (see Chapter 10). In a cross-sectional survey, subjects are studied at one point in time. Longitudinal surveys follow subjects over an extended period of time.

One of the chief virtues of survey research is its ability to provide accurate information on populations, using relatively small samples (Kerlinger, 1986). Another advantage of survey research concerns the large amount of data that can be obtained rather quickly and with minimal cost. Of course, one of the biggest disadvantages of the survey approach is the type of data that is obtained. Self-report responses may be unreliable because people may provide socially acceptable responses.

Emergency nurses' knowledge of pain management principles was examined in a survey study conducted by Tanabe and Buschmann (2000). Questionnaires were mailed to all 1000 members of the Illinois Emergency Nurses Association. Returns were received from 305 respondents. A 52-item questionnaire was used to measure knowledge of pain management principles and barriers to pain management. The researchers concluded that a deficit existed in the respondents' knowledge of the terms *addiction, tolerance,* and *dependence.* Additionally, there was a deficit in knowledge of various pharmacological analgesic principles. The two most common barriers to pain management were identified as (a) the inability to administer medication until a diagnosis was made (53%) and (b) inadequate assessment of pain and pain relief (48%).

CORRELATIONAL STUDIES

In **correlational studies,** the researcher examines the strength of relationships between variables by determining how changes in one variable are associated with changes in another variable. A **correlation** indicates the extent to which one variable (X) is related to another variable (Y). As X increases, does Y increase or decrease? In a simple correlational study, one group of subjects is measured on two variables (X and Y) to determine if there is a relationship between these variables. Other correlational studies may examine the relationship between more than two variables.

The magnitude and direction of the relationship between two variables are indicated by a **correlation coefficient.** Correlation coefficients may be positive (+) or negative (−) and range from −1.00 (perfect negative correlation) to 1.00 (perfect positive correlation). If the correlation coefficient has no sign in front of it (.80), a positive relationship is indicated. A negative correlation coefficient will be preceded by a negative sign (−.80). A correlation coefficient of .00 indicates no relationship between variables. Correlation coefficients will be reported through various statistics such as the Pearson's product-moment correlation (more commonly called the Pearson r) and the Spearman rho (see Chapter 13).

A **positive relationship,** or direct relationship, means that as the value of one variable increases, the value of the other variable increases. A **negative relationship,** or inverse relationship, means that as the value of one variable increases, the value of the other variable decreases. Suppose data are gathered on age and assertiveness levels of registered nurses. A correlation coefficient of .80 would indicate that there is a strong positive relationship between age and assertiveness levels of registered nurses. The older the nurse, the more assertive she or he is. On the other hand, a correlation coefficient of −.80 would indicate a strong negative relationship. The older the nurse, the less assertive she or he is.

The identification of an independent and a dependent variable may not be appropriate in some correlational studies. Generally, however, an independent and a dependent variable can be identified. In correlational research, the independent variable is that variable that comes first in chronological order and that influences the other variable. The researcher does not manipulate the independent variable. For example, if you were trying to determine if there is a correlation between age and assertiveness levels, the independent variable would be age, and the dependent variable would be assertiveness levels. The subject's age is a nonmanipulated, inherent variable that exists in time or chronological order before the variable of assertiveness. The researcher would be wrong in concluding that age causes assertiveness. There may, in fact, be some other variable or variables that bring about the assertiveness levels of people.

> The correlation between anger and blood pressure readings (BPR) in 230 third-grade children was studied by Hauber, Rice, Howell, and Carmon (1998). Study results revealed significant inverse relationships between anger suppression scores and diastolic BPR ($r = -.17$; $p = .02$) and between anger reflection/control scores and both systolic BPR and diastolic BPR ($r = -.18$; $p = .011$ and $r = -.14$; $p = .05$).

COMPARATIVE STUDIES

Comparative studies examine the differences between intact groups on some dependent variable of interest. This description may sound like the aim of many experimental studies. The difference between comparative studies and experimental studies lies in the researcher's ability to manipulate the independent variable. In comparative studies, there is no manipulation of the independent variable. Frequently, the independent variable is some inherent characteristic of the subjects, such as personality type, educational level, or medical condition.

There are many reasons for the choice of a comparative research design. One reason involves the ethics of research. When human subjects are studied, manipulation of the independent variable may not be possible. A researcher could not examine child abuse as an independent variable in an experimental study. It would not be ethical to select one group of children who would receive abusive treatment and another group of children who would not receive abusive treatment. A researcher, however, could use child abuse as an independent variable in a comparative study. The researcher would choose a group of children who had experienced abuse during their life and compare them with a group of children who had not been abused. The dependent variable might be self-esteem.

Comparative studies are frequently classified as retrospective or prospective. In **retrospective studies,** the dependent variable (effect) is identified in the present (a disease condition, for example), and an attempt is made to determine the independent variable (cause of the disease) that occurred in the past. In **prospective studies,** the independent variable or presumed cause (high cholesterol blood levels, for example) is identified at the present time, and then subjects are followed in the future to observe the dependent variable (incidence of coronary artery disease).

Retrospective studies are frequently called ex post facto. In **ex post facto studies,** data are collected "after the fact." Variations in the independent variable are studied after the variations have occurred, rather than at the time of the occurrence. For example, a researcher might be interested in the fear responses of children during physical examinations. A determination would be made of previous unpleasant experiences during physical examinations that might have influenced the children's present behaviors. These previous experiences might be considered the "cause" and the present fear responses might be considered the "effect."

> A comparative study was conducted to determine if fatigue was different among elders who were in caregiving roles compared with elders who were in noncaregiving roles (Teel & Press, 1999). Elders in the caregiving group (n = 92) were caring for spouses with Alzheimer's disease, Parkinson's disease, or cancer. The spouses of the noncaregiving group of elder respondents (n = 33) required no extra care. As was expected, caregiving spouses reported more fatigue, less energy, and more sleep difficulty that did the noncaregiving spouses.

Whereas a retrospective study starts by examining an "effect" and then looks back in time to determine the "cause," a prospective study starts with the determination of a "cause" and then looks forward in time to determine the "effect" on subjects. An example of prospective research is the well-publicized study concerning Agent Orange and Vietnam veterans. During the Vietnam war, many American servicemen were exposed to the chemical defoliant Agent Orange. After years of examining the effects of this chemical on veterans and their offspring, the Air Force finally issued a report in 1984 that revealed some of the problems linked with exposure to Agent Orange. Among the problems found in the veterans, or reported by them, were high rates of benign skin lesions, liver disorders, leg pulses that could be an indication of hardening of the arteries, and minor birth defects in their children ("Agent Orange," 1984). During the past decade, Americans have been concerned about symptoms of military personnel who served during the conflict in the Persian Gulf in 1991. The symptoms have been labeled the *Gulf War syndrome.* Much debate exists in the literature about this syndrome. Prospective research continues to be conducted.

Prospective studies may use an experimental approach, whereas retrospective studies would never use this type of design. In prospective studies, the researcher might manipulate the independent variable, or the "cause," and then observe subjects in the future for the dependent variable, or the "effect." Prospective studies are costly, and subject dropout may occur. These types of studies are less common than retrospective studies.

METHODOLOGICAL STUDIES

Nurse researchers must be concerned with the instruments they use in research projects because these instruments must be valid and reliable measures of the variables of interest. **Methodological studies** are concerned with the development, testing, and evaluation of research instruments and methods. There is a growing interest in methodological research.

Few instruments have been developed specifically to measure the phenomena of interest to nursing. Nurses frequently use tools developed by researchers in other disciplines. If these tools are appropriate for nursing research, they definitely should be used. But frequently, tools are used because of their availability rather than for their appropriateness to measure the variables of the study.

More methodological studies are now appearing in the nursing literature. It is hoped nurses will continue to focus interest on methodological studies. Nurses will thus develop a stockpile of research instruments to measure nursing phenomena. A cursory review of the issues of *Nursing Research* in the last few years revealed that at least one methodological study was included in each issue. As further evidence of the importance of measurement in nursing research, the *Journal of Nursing Measurement* began publication in 1993.

A postpartum depression screening scale was developed and tested by Beck and Gable (2000). The researchers contended that each year approximately 400,000 women in the United States experience postpartum depression but that only a small proportion of these women are identified as having this problem. The researchers pointed out the shortcomings of using existing depression tools to measure postpartum depression. After assessing the psychometric properties of the newly devised 35-item Postpartum Depression Screening Scale (PDSS), they were satisfied with the results of the validity and reliability analyses. They are continuing to determine the sensitivity, specificity, and positive predictive value of the PDSS.

SETTINGS FOR RESEARCH

Research may be classified as laboratory or field studies, according to the setting in which the study is conducted. In **laboratory studies,** subjects are studied in a special environment that has been created by the researcher. Although laboratory studies are not always highly standardized, the investigator usually attempts to control the research environment as much as possible. **Field studies** are conducted "in the field" or in a real-life situation.

Defloor and Grypdonck (2000) conducted a laboratory study to determine if pressure relief cushions actually relieve pressure. Interface pressures of 29 different types of cushions and a sheepskin were measured on 20 healthy volunteers in a laboratory setting. Participants were seated in an upright position with their back against the back of the chair, hands in their lap, knees bent at a 90° angle, and their feet resting on the floor. Only 13 of the cushions had any effect on reducing pressure. No pressure-relieving effect was found with either gel cushions or the sheepskin. The lowest interface pressures were found with three brands of air cushions and three brands of foam cushions. Some cushions reduced interface pressure by as much as 19% whereas others increased interface pressure by almost 40%.

Simulation studies are also considered to be laboratory studies. In a simulation study, the researcher might measure subjects' responses to descriptions of case studies that are intended to represent real-life situations. The control of the environment in this situation is through the researcher's descriptions of the case studies.

Problem-solving skills of senior nursing students were studied by Roberts (2000) using a videotape simulation exercise. The study was conducted to compare the problem-solving skills of senior nursing students (N = 235) enrolled in three types of nursing educational nursing programs in England. After viewing the videotape, participants were given 30 minutes in which to formulate a care plan. Roberts contended that the use of simulation in research allows for standardization and control of extraneous variables that is not possible when actual patients and real-life situations are used in the clinical setting.

A research study receives the classification of field study when it is conducted in a real-life setting. Phenomena are studied in the natural environments in which they occur. Most nursing research has been conducted in the field. The field approach is particularly appropriate for the nurse researcher because nursing is a practice discipline. Topf (1990) has called for studies that use both a laboratory and a field component. These two types of settings allow the researcher to better control for both internal and external validity of the study design.

CRITIQUING QUANTITATIVE RESEARCH DESIGNS

It may be very difficult for the reader to determine if an appropriate design has been used in a study. As has been said previously, critiquing is not easy! Advanced research knowledge may be necessary to make an accurate determination of the appropriateness of a study design. However, the beginning researcher or critiquer can make some overall evaluations of the design section of a research report. Criteria for evaluating quantitative research designs are presented in Box 8–1.

The entire research report must be read before a determination can be made as to whether the research design is appropriate for the study. The major consideration to be made when critiquing a study design concerns the ability of the study design to test the hypothesis(es) or answer the research question(s). Is the researcher trying to determine a cause-and-effect relationship or to merely describe a phenomenon from the point of view of the research subject?

> ### Box 8–1. Guidelines for Critiquing Quantitative Research Designs
>
> 1. Is the design clearly identified in the research report?
> 2. Is the design appropriate to test the study hypothesis(es) or answer the research question(s)?
> 3. If the study used an experimental design, was the most appropriate type of experimental design used?
> 4. If the study used an experimental design, what means were used to control for threats to internal validity? External validity?
> 5. Does the research design allow the researcher to draw a cause-and-effect relationship between the variables?
> 6. If the design was nonexperimental, would an experimental design have been more appropriate?
> 7. What means were used to control for extraneous variables, such as subject characteristics, if a nonexperimental design was used?

The research design determines how much control the researcher has over the research situation. In some studies, very tight controls are needed; in other studies tight controls would inhibit the collection of valid data. Therefore, the reader of a research report must determine the purpose of the study and what the researcher hoped to add to the body of knowledge on the selected phenomenon or phenomena.

SUMMARY

Exploratory, descriptive, and explanatory studies are classified according to the amount of knowledge about the variable(s) of interest. **Exploratory studies** are conducted when little is known about the topic of interest. In **descriptive studies,** the phenomenon of interest may have already been studied in the past, and there is enough information to ask questions about the relationship between variables. **Explanatory studies** search for causal explanations. The researcher exercises control over the research situation by manipulating one or more of the variables and examining the influence of this manipulation on another variable or variables.

Experimental research is concerned with cause-and-effect relationships. All experimental studies involve manipulation of the independent variable (cause) and measurement of the dependent variable (effect).

Extraneous variables are uncontrolled variables that may influence study results. In experimental studies, these extraneous variables are called threats to internal and external validity. **Internal validity** concerns the degree to which changes in the dependent variable (effect) can be attributed to the independent variable (cause). **External validity** concerns the degree to which study results can be generalized to other people and settings.

Six threats to internal validity are selection bias, history, maturation, testing, instrumentation change, and mortality. **Selection bias** occurs when study results are attributed to the experimental treatment when, in fact, the results occur because of subject differences before the treatment. **History** occurs when some event besides the experimental treatment occurs during the study, and this event influences the dependent variable. **Maturation** is a threat to internal validity when changes that occur within the subjects during an experimental study influence the study results. The **testing** threat involves the influence of the pretest on the posttest scores. **Instrumentation change** concerns the difference between the pretest and the posttest measurements that is due to a change in the accuracy of the instrument or the judges' ratings. The **mortality** threat occurs when the subject dropout rate is different between the experimental and comparison groups, and this difference in dropout rate influences the posttest results.

Three threats to external validity are the Hawthorne effect, the experimenter effect, and the reactive effects of the pretest. The **Hawthorne effect** occurs when study participants respond in a certain manner because they are aware that they are being observed. A researcher's behavior that influences subject behavior is called the **experimenter effect.** The **reactive effects of the pretest** threat occurs when subjects' responses to the experimental treatment are indirectly influenced by the pretest.

Random assignment is a procedure that ensures that each subject has an equal chance of being assigned or placed into any of the groups in an experimental study.

There are three broad categories of experimental research designs: true experimental, quasiexperimental, and preexperimental. **True experimental designs** are determined by three criteria: the researcher manipulates the experimental variable, at least one experimental and one **comparison** or **control group** are included in the study, and subjects are randomly assigned to either the experimental or the comparison group. **Manipulation** means that the independent variable is controlled by the researcher. Three types of true experimental designs are the **pretest-posttest control group design,** the **posttest-only control group design,** and the **Solomon four-group design.**

Quasiexperimental designs are those in which there is either no comparison group or no random assignment of subjects to groups. Two quasiexperimental designs are the **nonequivalent control group design** and the **time-series design.**

Preexperimental designs are those in which the researcher has little control over the research. Two types of preexperimental designs are the **one-shot case study** and the **one-group pretest-posttest design.**

Survey studies obtain data from samples on certain variables to determine the characteristics of populations on those same variables. **Correlational studies** examine the strength of relationships between variables. A **correlation** indicates the extent to which one variable (X) is related to another variable (Y). The magnitude and direction of the relationship between two variables are indicated by a **correlation coefficient.** These coefficients may be positive (+) or negative (−) and range from −1.00 (perfect negative correlation) to 1.00 (perfect positive correlation). A **positive relationship** (direct) means that as the value of one variable increases, the value of the other variable increases. A

negative relationship (inverse) means that as the value of one variable increases, the value of the other variable decreases.

Comparative studies examine the difference between intact groups on some dependent variable of interest. Many comparative studies are called **ex post facto studies** because the variation in the independent variable has already occurred, and the researcher, "after the fact," tries to determine if the variation that has occurred in the independent variable has any influence on the dependent variable that is being measured in the present. Ex post facto studies may also be called **retrospective studies. Prospective studies** are comparative studies in which the independent variable is identified in the present and the dependent variable is measured in the future.

Methodological studies are concerned with the development, testing, and evaluation of research instruments and methods. A paucity of instruments have been developed specifically to measure the phenomena of interest to nurses.

Research may be conducted in a laboratory or field setting. **Laboratory studies** are conducted in a special environment that has been created by the researcher. **Simulation studies** are considered to be laboratory studies. **Field studies** are conducted in real-life settings. Most experimental studies in nursing research have been field studies.

NURSING RESEARCH ON THE WEB

For additional online resources, research activities, and exercises, go to www.prenhall. com/nieswiadomy. Select Chapter 8 from the drop down menu.

✖ GET INVOLVED ACTIVITIES

1. Examine the first five research articles that you can locate in the library. Identify the number of studies that used a quantitative design.

2. Using the CINAHL computerized database, type in "experimental design" and see how many nursing studies in the last 10 years have used an experimental design.

3. Bring a research article to be discussed. Determine the design that was used. Share this information with your peers. Decide if the design appears to be the most rigorous one that could have been used for the study.

4. Divide into groups and develop an idea for a study that would require a quantitative design. Decide on the specific design that your group thinks is most appropriate. Then exchange your ideas among groups and see if other groups chose the same design as was chosen by your group. All groups should give the rationale for the design selected.

✖ SELF-TEST

Each item in Column A represents a statement by a subject in a research study. Match the statements on the left with the threats to internal and external validity that are listed in Column B.

Column A	Column B
1. "It's a good thing I'm in this new diet experiment. I couldn't believe it when that researcher told me that I was 10 pounds overweight."	A. Hawthorne effect
	B. selection bias
2. "Aren't we lucky to be part of this experiment?"	C. history
	D. experimenter effect
3. "That researcher scares me. I guess I'd better act like he wants me to act."	E. testing
4. "I volunteered to be in the experimental group."	
5. "I watched this show about lung cancer. It made me realize that I really should try to stop smoking while I'm in this study that is trying to help smokers quit."	

Circle the letter before the *best* answer.

6. Which of the following items distinguishes true experimental research from quasi-experimental research?

   A. size of sample
   B. the use of a nonprobability sample
   C. random assignment of subjects to groups
   D. the introduction of an experimental treatment

7. Which of the following designs would be most appropriate to use in trying to determine if clients' low back pain changes after they were taught an exercise to help correct back alignment?

   A. one-group pretest-posttest design
   B. posttest-only control group design
   C. one-shot case study
   D. pretest-posttest control group design

8. Which of the following designs controls for the sensitization of subjects to a pretest?

   A. pretest-posttest control group design
   B. Solomon four-group design
   C. one-shot case study
   D. time-series design

9. Which of the following is present in every experimental study?

   A. manipulation of the independent variable
   B. a control group
   C. random assignment of subjects to groups
   D. random selection of subjects from the population

10. Collecting data from a sample to determine the characteristics of a population is the purpose of what type of research?

    A. correlational
    B. survey
    C. methodological
    D. quasiexperimental

11. Ex post facto studies are also called:

    A. prospective.
    B. retrospective.
    C. longitudinal.
    D. descriptive.

✂ REFERENCES

Agent orange study finds health problems (1984, February 25). *Dallas Morning News,* p. 1A, 5A.

Beck, C. T., & Gable, R. K. (2000). Postpartum Depression Screening Scale: Development and psychometric testing. *Nursing Research, 49,* 272–282.

Bouvé, L. R., Rozmus, C. L., & Giordono, P. (1999). Preparing parents for their child's transfer from the PICU to the pediatric floor. *Applied Nursing Research, 12,* 114–120.

Bracht, G., & Glass, G. (1968). The external validity of experiments. *American Educational Research Journal, 5,* 437–474.

Campbell, C., & Stanley, J. (1963). *Experimental and quasi-experimental designs for research.* Chicago: Rand McNally.

Cook, C., & Campbell, D. (1979). *Quasi-experimentation: Design and analysis issues for field settings.* Chicago: Rand McNally.

Defloor, T., & Grypdonck, M. H. F. (2000). Do pressure relief cushions really relieve pressure? *Western Journal of Nursing Research, 22,* 335–350.

Fogg, L., & Gross, D. (2000). Threats to validity in randomized clinical trials. *Research in Nursing and Health, 23,* 79–87.

Hauber, R. P., Rice, M. H., Howell, C. C., & Carmon, M. (1998). Anger and blood pressure readings in children. *Applied Nursing Research, 11,* 2–11.

Hayes, K. S. (1998). Randomized trial of geragogy-based medication instruction in the emergency department. *Nursing Research, 47,* 211–218.

Kerlinger, F. (1986). *Foundations of behavioral research* (3rd ed.). New York: Holt, Rinehart & Winston.

MacDonald, S. A. (1999). The Cardiovascular Health Education Program: Assessing the impact on rural and urban adolescents' health knowledge. *Applied Nursing Research, 12,* 86–90.

Polit, D. F., & Hungler, B. P. (1999). *Nursing research: Principles and methods* (6th ed.) Philadelphia: Lippincott.

Roberts, J. D. (2000). Problem-solving skills of senior student nurses: An exploratory study using simulation. *International Journal of Nursing Studies, 37,* 135–143.

Skokal, W. A. (2000). IV push at home? *RN, 63,* 26–29.

Swanson, K. M. (1999) Effects of caring, measurement, and time on miscarriage impact and women's well-being. *Nursing Research, 48,* 288–298.

Tanabe, P., & Buschmann, M. (2000). Emergency nurses' knowledge of pain management principles. *Journal of Emergency Nursing, 26,* 299–305.

Teel, C. S., & Press, A. N. (1999). Fatigue among elders in caregiving and noncaregiving roles. *Western Journal of Nursing Research, 21,* 498–520.

To, M. Y. F., & Chan, S. (2000). Evaluating the effectiveness of progressive muscle relaxation in reducing the aggressive behaviors of mentally handicapped patients. *Archives of Psychiatric Nursing, 14,* 39–46.

Topf, J. (1990). Increasing the validity of research results with a blend of laboratory and clinical strategies. *Image: Journal of Nursing Scholarship, 22,* 121–123.

CHAPTER 9

Qualitative Research Designs

✳ OBJECTIVES

On completion of this chapter, you will be prepared to:

1. Define qualitative research
2. Compare qualitative and quantitative research
3. Describe five types of qualitative research designs
4. Identify two of the most common data collection methods used in qualitative research
5. Recognize reliability and validity issues in qualitative research
6. Discuss the complexity of analyzing qualitative data
7. Determine the benefits of combining quantitative and qualitative research methods
8. Critique qualitative research reports

✳ NEW TERMS DEFINED IN THIS CHAPTER

case studies
content analysis
ethnographic studies
external criticism
focus groups
grounded theory studies

historical studies
internal criticism
phenomenological studies
saturation
triangulation

Are you more interested in individuals and their subjective feelings than you are in objective data on groups of people? If your answer is "yes," you may like this chapter.

Nurse researchers have conducted quantitative research for many years and have demonstrated the usefulness of this methodology. However, in recent years, some nurses have begun to question the appropriateness of using this approach to examine some of the phenomena of interest to nursing. Nursing has traditionally focused on the individual and the holistic nature of the person. This value system is more consistent with qualitative research philosophy than with quantitative research philosophy. In qualitative research, the individual's perspective is very important, whereas in quantitative research, the focus is on the group or population rather than on the individual.

The interest in qualitative research is growing rapidly. DeSantis and Ugarriza (2000) wrote that during the 1990s "qualitative methodology surged to the forefront of nursing research" (p. 351).

Using the computerized database of the Cumulative Index to Nursing and Allied Health (CINAHL), a search was done in November 2000 of the term *qualitative nursing research*. A total of 3410 records were found! To determine the number of published books on qualitative nursing research, a search was done of the on-line book seller Amazon.com. This search revealed 31 matches. Some of these were duplicates because hardcover and paperback copies were listed separately. However, there were still more than 25 separate books listed on qualitative nursing research.

COMPARISON OF QUALITATIVE AND QUANTITATIVE RESEARCH

Quantitative research is based on the concepts of manipulation and control of phenomena and the verification of results, using empirical data gathered through the senses. Qualitative research focuses on gaining insight and understanding about an individual's perception of events. Verification of results through the senses is not called for. The individual's interpretation of events or circumstances is of importance, rather than the interpretation made by the researcher.

According to Porter (1989), "while the qualitative researcher attempts to obtain rich, real, deep and valid data, the quantitative researcher aims for hard, replicable and reliable data" (p. 98). Streubert and Carpenter (1999) asserted that the inability of researchers to quantitatively measure certain phenomena and the dissatisfaction with the results of measurement of other phenomena have led to the acceptance of qualitative research approaches to gain knowledge.

Qualitative research is concerned with in-depth descriptions of people or events, and data are collected through such methods as unstructured interviews and participant observation. Connelly and Yoder (2000) pointed out that nurses should be comfortable with these two methods of data collection because of their nursing educational preparation and clinical experiences.

In qualitative research, the researcher searches for patterns and themes in the data, rather than focusing on the testing of hypotheses. While quantitative research frequently uses a deductive or theory-testing approach, qualitative research uses an inductive approach. The qualitative researcher is not limited by existing theories, but rather must be open to new ideas and new theories.

At first glance, it might appear that qualitative research would be easier to conduct than quantitative research. The researcher does not have to be as concerned with numbers and complicated statistical analyses. However, qualitative research is not recommended for the beginning researcher. The guidelines for this type of research are not as clear-cut and easy to follow as are the guidelines for conducting quantitative research. The beginning qualitative researcher should seek a mentor.

TYPES OF QUALITATIVE RESEARCH

There are many different types of qualitative research (Table 9–1). Field and Morse (1985) identified eight approaches: ethnography, grounded theory, ethnology, ethology, ethnoscience, ethnomethodology, analytic sociology, and phenomenology. Leininger (1985) added the ethnonursing method. Wilson and Hutchinson (1996) listed ten types of qualitative research: grounded theory, ethnography, phenomenology, ethnoscience, hermeneutics, historical inquiry, ethical inquiry, feminist inquiry, critical social theory, and case study. Burns and Grove (1997) presented six approaches to qualitative research: phenomenological, grounded theory, ethnographic, historical, philosophical inquiry, and critical social theory. Polit and Hungler (1999) listed ten qualitative research traditions: ethnography, ethnoscience, phenomenology, hermeneutics, ethology, ecological psychology, grounded theory, ethnomethodology, symbolic interaction, and discourse analysis. Five common types of qualitative studies are described in this chapter: phenomenological, ethnographic, grounded theory, historical, and case study.

PHENOMENOLOGICAL STUDIES

Phenomenological studies examine human experiences through the descriptions that are provided by the people involved. These experiences are called "lived experiences." The goal of this type of research is to describe the meaning that experiences hold for each subject (Cohen, 1987; Streubert & Carpenter, 1999). This type of research includes the qualities of "humanness, such as individualism, self-determination, wholeness, uniqueness,

TABLE 9–1. Qualitative Research Process	
Case study	Ethnoscience
Critical social inquiry	Ethology
Discourse analysis	Feminist inquiry
Ecological psychology	Grounded theory
Ethical inquiry	Herrmeneutics
Ethnography	Historical
Ethnology	Phenomenology
Ethnomethodology	Philosophical inquiry
Ethnonursing	Symbolic interaction

and an open system" (Ramer, 1989, p. 7). Streubert and Carpenter (1999) asserted that phenomenological inquiry is appropriate for nursing research because nursing practice is enmeshed in the life experiences of people.

In phenomenological research, subjects are asked to describe their experiences as they perceive them. To understand the lived experience from the vantage point of the subject, the researcher must first identify what she or he expects to discover and then deliberately put aside this idea. This process is called "bracketing." Only when the researcher puts aside her or his own ideas about the phenomenon will it be possible to see the experience from the eyes of the person who has lived the experience.

Phenomenological research would ask such questions as, "What is it like for a mother to live with a teenage child who is dying of cancer?" The researcher might perceive that she, herself, would feel very hopeless and frightened. These feelings would need to be identified and then put aside in order to listen to what the mother is saying about how she is living through this experience. It is possible that this mother has discovered an important reason for living, where previously she had not felt needed anymore by her teenage child.

Parse, Coyne, and Smith (1985) wrote that the analysis of data from these types of studies requires that the researcher "dwell with the subjects' descriptions in quiet contemplation" (p. 5). The researcher then tries to uncover the meaning of the lived experience for each subject. Themes and patterns are sought in the data. Data collection and data analysis occur simultaneously.

Phenomenological research methods are very different from the methods used in quantitative research. Mariano (1990) asserted that phenomenology could be difficult to understand, particularly if a person has had a limited background in philosophy. Although phenomenological research has sometimes been viewed as "soft science," Streubert and Carpenter (1999) have contended that this research method is a "rigourous, critical, systematic method of investigation" (p. 43). They called for the beginning researcher to seek a mentor who has experience in phenomenological research.

A phenomenological study was conducted to examine the experiences of working Americans who are medically uninsured (Orne, Fishman, Manka, & Pagnozzi, 2000). A purposive sample of 12 individuals was asked, "What is it like to be working and without medical insurance?" Data were grouped into four theme clusters: "a marginalized life," "up against rocks and hard places," "making choices-chancing it," and "getting by-more or less." The researchers concluded that being a medically uninsured American worker is an experience of "living on the edge." When you do not have health insurance life is full of uncertainty, vulnerability, and fear.

ETHNOGRAPHIC STUDIES

Ethnographic studies involve the collection and analysis of data about cultural groups. Agar (1986) described ethnography as "encountering alien worlds and making sense of them" (p. 12). He further stated that ethnographers try to show how actions in one world make sense from the point of view of another world. Cameron (1990) wrote that ethnography means "learning from people" (p. 5). According to Leininger (1985), ethnography can be defined as "the systematic process of observing, detailing, describing, documenting, and analyzing the lifeways or particular patterns of a culture (or subculture) in order to grasp the lifeways or patterns of the people in their familiar environment" (p. 35).

In ethnographic research, the researcher frequently lives with the people and becomes a part of their culture. The researcher explores with the people their rituals and customs. An entire cultural group may be studied or a subgroup in the culture. The term *culture* may be used in the broad sense to mean an entire tribe of Indians, for example, or in a more narrow sense to mean one nursing care unit.

Ethnographers interview people who are most knowledgeable about the culture. These people are sometimes called *key informants.* Data are generally collected through participant observation and interviews. As was discussed under phenomenological studies, the researcher brackets, or makes explicit, her or his own personal biases and beliefs, sets them aside, and then tries to understand the daily lives of individuals as they live them. Data collection and analysis occur simultaneously. As understanding of the data occurs, new questions emerge. The end purpose of ethnography is the development of cultural theories.

Although ethnography is relatively new to nurse researchers, the method has been used in anthropological research for a long time. This method is the one used by Margaret Mead (1929) to study the Samoans. Ethnography has been the principal method used by anthropologists to study people all over the world. Ethnographers study how people live and how they communicate with each other.

The use of the ethnographic method in nursing research began in the 1960s. Ethnography is useful in nursing because nurse researchers can view nursing and health care in the context in which it occurs.

An ethnographic study was conducted by Schulte (2000) to describe the culture of public health nurses (PHNs) in a large, midwestern urban health department. The data were placed into categories, domains, and cultural themes. The main theme that emerged was that public health nurses try to create connections among three interacting communities: the local community, the community created by individuals and families, and the community of resources. Schulte suggested that the study accented the holistic focus of public health nursing and that PHNs require a variety and range of knowledge to facilitate client wholeness.

GROUNDED THEORY STUDIES

Grounded theory is a qualitative research approach developed by two sociologists, Glaser and Strauss (1967). **Grounded theory studies** are studies in which data are collected and analyzed and then a theory is developed that is *grounded* in the data. Some of the terms used by Glaser and Strauss are difficult for nurses to understand. Leininger (1985) wrote that in 1980 she began to translate their terms into what she called "standard English."

The grounded theory method uses both an inductive and a deductive approach to theory development. According to Field and Morse (1985), "constructs and concepts are grounded in the data and hypotheses are tested as they arise from the research" (p. 23). These authors argued that given the state of development of nursing theories, theory generation is more critical than theory testing for the development of nursing knowledge.

Rather than using probability sampling procedures, purposeful sampling is used (see Chapter 10). The researcher looks for certain subjects who will be able to shed new light on the phenomenon that is being studied. Diversity rather than similarity is sought in the people who are sampled.

Data are gathered in naturalistic settings (field settings). Data collection primarily consists of participant observation and interviews, and data are recorded through hand-written notes and tape recordings. Data collection and data analysis occur simultaneously. A process called *constant comparison* is used, in which data are constantly compared to data that have already been gathered. Pertinent concepts are identified and assigned codes. These codes are constantly reviewed as new interpretations are made of the data. The researcher keeps an open mind and uses an intuitive process in interpreting data. The codes that are developed frequently are gerunds (words ending in "ing") like soothing, placating, and asserting (note the "ing" words in the following study example by Draucker and Stern).

Once concepts have been identified and their relationships specified, the researcher consults the literature to determine if any similar associations have already been uncovered. Consulting the literature for the first time at this stage of a research project is quite different from quantitative methods where the literature is always consulted early in the research process. Leininger (1985) asserted that a prestudy literature search could lead to "premature closure." This means that the researcher would go into the research setting expecting to find what is reported in the literature. When an instance is found that is similar to that reported in the literature, the researcher would say, "Yes, that's it!" and go home and write the same thing.

Despite the great diversity of the data that are gathered, the grounded theory approach presumes that it is possible to discover fundamental patterns in all social life. These patterns are called basic social processes.

Grounded theory is more concerned with the generation rather than the testing of hypotheses. The theory that is generated is self-correcting, which means that as data are gathered, adjustments are made to the theory to allow for the interpretation of new data that are obtained.

Although the grounded theory approach was developed by two sociologists, Glaser and Strauss, to study questions in the discipline of sociology, the approach seems quite appropriate to nurse researchers. Nursing is very concerned with social interactions.

> Women's responses to sexual violence by a male intimate were studied by Draucker and Stern (2000) using a grounded theory approach. Data were gathered from the point of view of 23 women who had experienced sexual violence at some time during their adult lives by a man they knew (boyfriend, partner, spouse, relative, friend, date). The theoretical framework that emerged from the data focused on three variations of "forging ahead." These variations were "getting back on track," "starting over," and "surviving the long, hard road." Processes used by these women to forge ahead included "telling others," "making sense of the violence," and "creating a safer life."

HISTORICAL STUDIES

Nurses are increasingly interested in establishing a body of nursing knowledge and defining the role of professional nurses. One means of achieving these aims is to examine the roots of nursing through historical research. **Historical studies** concern the identification, location, evaluation, and synthesis of data from the past. Historical research seeks not only to discover the events of the past but to relate these past happenings to the present and to the future. Leininger (1985) wrote, "Without a past, there is no meaning to the present, nor can we develop a sense of ourselves as individuals and as members of groups" (p. 109).

Although there is a need for historical research in nursing, this research approach has been chosen by a limited number of nurse researchers. According to the noted nursing historian Teresa Christy (1975), nurses are action oriented and have preferred experimental research to historical research. She contended that many nurses think of historical research as more "search than research" (p. 189). But the process of historical research is basically the same as in many other types of scientific research. The problem area or area of interest is clearly identified and the literature is reviewed. Research questions are formulated. Finally, the data are collected and analyzed.

Historical research may be more difficult to conduct than some of the other types of research. Christy wrote that the historical researcher must develop the "curiosity, perseverance, tenacity and skepticism of the detective" (p. 192).

The data for historical research are usually found in documents or in relics and artifacts. Documents may include a wide range of printed material. Relics and artifacts are items of physical evidence. For example, you might examine the types of equipment used by nurses in another time period. Historical data can also be obtained through oral reports. The materials may be found in libraries, archives, or in personal collections. Much valuable material has probably been discarded because no one recognized its importance.

The sources of historical data are frequently referred to as primary and secondary sources. Primary sources are those that provide first-hand information or direct evidence. Secondary sources are second-hand information (or sometimes third-hand or fourth-hand). For example, a letter written by Florence Nightingale about nursing care during the Crimean War would be considered a primary source of data. If a friend summarized the information about nursing care during the Crimean War based on a letter she received from Florence Nightingale, this source of information would be considered a secondary source.

Primary sources should be used in historical research, when possible. There are many examples of primary sources: (a) oral histories, (b) written records, (c) diaries, (d) eyewitnesses, (e) pictorial sources, and (f) physical evidence. Suppose a nurse researcher wished to examine the practices of nurse midwives during the 1940s. An oral history might be obtained from an older member of the nursing profession who had practiced as a nurse midwife during that time. The researcher might also be able to obtain some of the field notes written by people who had practiced as nurse midwives during the 1940s. Some of the nurses may have kept diary accounts of the events that occurred during that period of their lives. It might also be possible to interview some women who had been cared for by nurse midwives during the 1940s. These women would be considered eyewitnesses. Some of the women or the nurse midwives might have photographs taken during the birthing events. Finally, it might be possible for the researcher to obtain some equipment used by nurse midwives during that period.

The data for historical research should be subjected to two types of evaluation. These evaluations are called external criticism and internal criticism. **External criticism** is concerned with the authenticity or genuineness of the data, and **internal criticism** examines the accuracy of the data. Whereas external criticism establishes the validity of the data, internal criticism establishes the reliability of the data.

External criticism would seek to determine if a letter was actually written by the person whose signature was contained on the letter. The writing paper might be examined to determine if that type of paper was in existence during the lifetime of the letter writer. False documents, such as a supposed copy of Adolf Hitler's diary, have been uncovered through the process of external criticism. Various methods, including carbon dating, can be used to determine the age of substances such as paper.

Internal criticism or evaluation of historical data is more difficult to conduct than external criticism. In the case of a written document, internal criticism would evaluate the material contained in the document. Motives and possible biases of the author must be considered in trying to determine if the material is accurate. It might be fairly easy to determine that a certain person was the writer of a letter that was being examined. It might not be so easy, however, to determine if the letter contained an accurate recording of events as they actually happened.

Although nurse researchers have conducted only a limited number of historical studies, there seems to be a growing interest in historical research, particularly among doctoral candidates who are writing dissertations. In 1993, the first issue of *Nursing History Review* was published. Members of the American Association for the History of Nursing (AAHN) receive the journal as a benefit of membership in the organization. The URL for the AAHN is http://www.aahn.org.

Many historical studies have focused on nursing leaders. There seem to have been few studies on the historical patterns of nursing practice (Burns & Grove, 1997). It is hoped that historical research will expand and that nursing will be provided with a recorded account of the significant events and developments of nursing practice as well as those of the nursing profession. As interest in historical nursing research increases, nursing archives, which are repositories of nursing memorabilia, are being established throughout the United States. Try to visit one of these storehouses of nursing history.

Kristman-Scott (2000) conducted a historical analysis of the concept of disclosure of terminal status to patients. She combined a manual and computerized search of popular, nursing, medical, sociological, psychological, and thanatological literature from 1930 to 1990 to discover books and articles that dealt with health care disclosure issues. The researcher discovered a long-standing tradition of nondisclosure of terminal status by health professionals. She concluded that this tradition of nondisclosure prohibits patients from being able to manage the end of their lives and make choices about how they will die. She asserted that nursing care is compromised when patients are uninformed.

CASE STUDIES

Case studies are in-depth examinations of people or groups of people. A case study could also examine an institution, such as hospice care for the dying. The case method has been used a great deal in anthropology, law, and medicine. In medicine, case studies have frequently been concerned with a particular disease.

A case study may be considered as quantitative or qualitative research depending on the purpose of the study and the design chosen by the researcher. As is true of other types of qualitative studies, for a case study to be considered as a qualitative study, the researcher must be interested in the meaning of experiences to the subjects themselves, rather than in generalizing results to other groups of people. Case studies are not used to test hypotheses, but hypotheses may be generated from case studies (Younger, 1985).

Patricia Benner is a qualitative researcher who has been interested in how a nurse moves from being a novice to an expert nurse. She has used the case study approach extensively. She contended that case studies help us to formalize experiential knowledge and thus promote quality nursing care (Benner, 1983).

Data may be collected in case studies through various means such as questionnaires, interviews, observations, or written accounts by the subjects. A nurse researcher might be interested in how people with diabetes respond to an insulin pump. One person or a group of people with diabetes could be studied for a time to determine their responses to the use of an insulin pump. Diaries might be used for the day-to-day recording of information. The nurse researcher would then analyze these diaries and try to interpret the written comments.

Content analysis is used in evaluating the data from case studies. **Content analysis** involves the examination of communication messages. The researcher searches for patterns and themes. After reading the diaries of the individuals who are using insulin pumps, the nurse researcher might come up with themes such as: "freedom from rigid schedule," "more normal life," and "release from self-inflicted pain."

When subjects are chosen for case studies, care must be taken in the selection process. In the previously discussed example, the researcher should avoid choosing only those clients who are expected to respond favorably or unfavorably to the insulin pump.

Case studies are time consuming and may be quite costly. Additionally, subject dropout may occur during this type of study. Whenever a study is carried out over an extended period, loss of subjects must be considered. A person may move from the locality or simply decide to discontinue participation in the study.

The case study approach was used by Sedlak (1997) to describe students' critical thinking abilities, from their perspectives, in making clinical decisions. Data were gathered from journal writings, interviews, and from the researcher's observations in the clinical laboratory. Four major themes emerged: development of the professional self-perspective, development of a perfectionist perspective, development of a caring perspective, and development of a self-directed learning perspective.

DATA COLLECTION IN QUALITATIVE STUDIES

Semistructured interviews and participant observation are probably two of the most common types of data-collection methods used in qualitative studies. These types of data collection allow for the flexibility that is needed in qualitative research. Other types of data-collection methods include open-ended questionnaires, life histories, diaries, personal collections of letters and photographs, and official documents (Field & Morse, 1985).

In qualitative research, the amount of time for data collection is generally not specified when a study begins. In some types of qualitative research, such as grounded theory methodology, data collection continues until the data are saturated (Thomas, 1990.) **Saturation** means that the researcher is hearing a repetition of themes or salient points as additional participants are interviewed. No new information is being obtained from participants. Data are becoming redundant. This may happen after interviewing 5 people or it may not happen until after 100 have been interviewed. Generally, the number of participants interviewed in qualitative research is quite small compared with the number of participants in quantitative research. Even considering the small number of participants, the amount of data is usually voluminous. Bernstein (2000) interviewed only eight subjects in her study of the experience of acupuncture for the treatment of substance dependence. She wrote, "sampling was terminated when no new information came forth from newly sampled units, which would indicate that redundancy was the primary criterion in sample selection" (p. 269).

The use of focus groups has increased in nursing studies. A **focus group** consists of a small group of individuals meeting together and being asked questions, by a moderator, about a certain topic or topics. The advantage of this approach is that it is a time-saver compared to individual interviews. However, there may not be equal participation by group members. Some people may be reluctant to express their views to others.

Many examples are found in the literature in which a focus group has been used. This approach has been found to be particularly effective with Hispanics (McQuiston & Gordon, 2000).

Views of Mexicans about condom use was studied by McQuiston and Gordon (2000). They used focus groups to examine (a) whether newly immigrated Mexican men and women in the Southeast United States discussed HIV/sexually transmitted disease prevention with each other, and (b) how condom use was discussed. Six focus groups were conducted at a Hispanic center. The groups were separated by gender. For the women, communication was equated with safe sex; for the men trust was the important element in safe sex. Women indicated the need to communicate with their partners before they could trust them; men indicated the need to trust their partners before they could communicate with them.

SAMPLE SIZE IN QUALITATIVE RESEARCH

One of the criticisms of qualitative studies is that sample sizes are generally smaller than in quantitative studies. However, there are no set rules about the necessary sample size for a qualitative study. Sandelowski's (1995b) article "Sample Size in Qualitative Research" is an excellent source on this topic. She claims that the quality of information obtained from each respondent is more important than is the amount of data obtained. She stated that samples may be "too small to support claims of having achieved either informational redundancy or theoretical saturation, or too large to permit the deep, case-oriented analysis that is the raison-d'etre of qualitative inquiry" (p. 179).

Frequently, sample sizes are quite small (10 to 12) in qualitative research. Saturation is a concept that is mentioned in regard to sampling in qualitative studies. As previously mentioned, saturation means that no new information is being obtained from participants. So rather than sampling a certain number of individuals, the researcher stops data collection when saturation of the data has occurred.

RELIABILITY AND VALIDITY OF QUALITATIVE DATA

The reliability and validity of research findings are of great importance in all studies. Although the methods may vary according to the type of study, both qualitative and quantitative researchers are interested in the credibility of their findings. Reliability in qualitative research may be defined as the "repeatability of scientific observations, and sources that could influence the stability and consistency of those observations" (Hinds, Scandrett-Hibden, & McAulay, 1990, p. 431). Validity means that the findings "reflect reality, and the meaning of the data is accurately interpreted" (Hinds et al., 1990, p. 431).

The rigor and objectivity of the methods and the desire for generalizability of findings of qualitative studies are not present to the same extent as in quantitative studies. Replication of a study is very desirable in quantitative research. However, qualitative studies are generally not replicated because knowledge of the findings of one study could bias the results of another study (Porter, 1989). Additionally, Leininger (1985) likened qualitative research to the detective studying for clues. Each situation is unique.

Rather than discussing the strict rigor and objectivity of their research, qualitative researchers often mention the relevance of their study findings. The subjects themselves are frequently considered as the persons most knowledgeable about the topic. Therefore, the researcher often returns to the subjects for their assessment of the accuracy of the researcher's interpretation of the data.

One of the ways that the rigor of a qualitative study is considered is through the long period of time spent collecting data. Data are generally collected until it becomes clear that no new information is being collected. Also, multiple sources of data are frequently used, which provides a check for both reliability and validity. Both the large amount of data collected and the length of time spent collecting data help to increase the reliability and validity of qualitative study findings.

ANALYSIS OF QUALITATIVE DATA

Thomas (1990) compared the analysis of quantitative and qualitative data. She likened quantitative analysis to grading multiple choice or true-false questions. Qualitative analysis is like grading essay questions. Essay questions may be easier to write, but they are much harder to grade.

Analysis of data in qualitative studies usually involves an examination of words rather than numbers, as is the case in quantitative studies. Frequently, a massive amount of data, in the form of words, is gathered in qualitative studies. The task of analyzing all of these data can be overwhelming. One large study might involve the analysis of several thousand pages of notes!

Data analysis is generally not a distinct step in qualitative studies as it is in quantitative studies. In many qualitative studies, the researcher begins interpreting data as data are collected. There are no universally accepted rules for analyzing qualitative data.

All qualitative studies involve content analysis procedures in one form or another (McLaughlin & Marascuilo, 1990). In general, content analysis involves creating categories of data and developing rules for coding data into these categories. The use of content analysis varies according to the type of qualitative study that is conducted. Grounded theory, ethnography, and phenomenological research are based on the specific techniques developed from the three disciplines that developed these methods: sociology, anthropology, and psychology, respectively. More information on specific content analysis methods can be found in other sources.

Data may be analyzed manually or through the aid of computer programs. With the advent of computer programs, data analysis has been greatly enhanced for qualitative researchers. Computer software programs can store data, edit data, retrieve segments of text, and assemble data according to themes or categories (Pilkington, 1996).

Ross' 1994 article in *Computers in Nursing* is a good source for understanding the use of computers in analyzing qualitative data. She discussed various software programs and indicated that existing word processing and flat-file databases can be used. *Ethnograph* was used by England (1996) in her analysis of data in a study of caregiver planning by adult offspring caregivers. This same software program was used to gain insights of nurses about assaults in hospital-based emergency departments (Levin, Hewitt, & Misner, 1998). The computer program *Nudist* (Nonnumerical Unstructured Data Indexing, Searching, and Theorizing) was used to examine mothers' responses to care given by male nursing students during and after birth (Morin, Patterson, Kurtz, & Brozowski, 1999). This program was also used by Forbes, Bern-Klug, and Gessert (2000) to study end-of-life decision making for nursing homes residents with dementia. Several other programs have been mentioned in the literature. Polit and Hungler (1999) identified *MARTIN, QUALPRO,* and *HyperQual2.* Streubert and Carpenter (1999) listed *Atlas/ti* and *Hyper Research for Windows.*

Sandelowski (1995a) issued a caution about the use of computer technology in the analysis of qualitative data. She wrote that this type of technology is changing the "look and feel" of qualitative research and that computer printouts of data give the information a "veneer" of objectivity. She jokingly wrote that even "soft" data can be considered as "hard" data when it is produced by "hardware." Sandelowski expressed a fear that the art of qualitative work will be adversely affected by this technology.

COMBINING QUALITATIVE AND QUANTITATIVE METHODS

Many nurse researchers have recommended the use of both qualitative and quantitative research methods in a single study. Ford-Gilboe, Campbell, and Berman (1995) called for nurse researchers to combine "numbers and stories." Combining both qualitative and quantitative methods increases the researcher's ability to rule out rival explanations for phenomena (Hinds, 1989). Field and Morse (1985) asserted that the strongest research findings are found in studies that use both research methods. These two authors described the sequential and simultaneous use of the two methods. In the sequential use of the methods, the qualitative method might be used initially, until hypotheses emerge. Then the hypotheses might be tested using a quantitative method. When qualitative and quantitative methods are used simultaneously, the technique is called **triangulation.**

Myers and Haase (1989) indicated that the integration of quantitative and qualitative approaches is inevitable and essential for nursing research. However, for the two approaches to be combined, the researcher must value both approaches. Haase and Myers

(1988) indicated that merely including open-ended questions in a study does not indicate a true combination of the two research approaches. Using a qualitative approach, the researcher must search for the underlying meanings in the data, rather than just identifying and counting the frequency of surface themes.

In two commentaries published four months apart in *Journal of Professional Nursing,* O'Connell (2000) and Cobb (2000) discussed their feelings about a study in which they combined two "world views" (qualitative and quantitative) in one study. These two researchers (who were personal friends) collaborated on a study of coping strategies used during smoking cessation. O'Connell (the quantitative researcher) wrote that there is a quantitative church and a qualitative church; they are not merely research methods. She asserted, "Although these two methods may appear to have similar goals, ie, the explication of new knowledge, they often disagree on everything else, even the definition of knowledge" (p. 74). Cobb (the qualitative researcher) asserted that "wrestling a bear would have been easier than struggling to wrest mutual understanding from two different world views, but, ultimately, the marriage worked relatively well, and we ended up happy with the outcome" (p. 188).

Frenn and Porter (1999) combined quantitative and qualitative methods in their study of exercise and nutrition among 15 adolescents. The researchers made the determination that combining these two methods would help them best understand adolescents' health promotion behaviors. The Health Habits and History Questionnaire (HHHQ) and the Child/Adolescent Activity Log (CAAL) were used to gather quantitative data. The qualitative data were collected through semistructured audio taped interviews and field observations. Although both qualitative and quantitative methods were used, the researchers identified their study as a qualitative study.

Many textbooks and articles discuss the issues involved in combining qualitative and quantitative research methods. Sandelowski (2000) has written a very good article on this topic. She discusses why there is still confusion about how to accomplish "mixed-method" studies. She places particular focus on sampling, data collection, and data analysis.

CRITIQUING QUALITATIVE RESEARCH DESIGNS

Qualitative studies should not be evaluated with the same set of criteria as quantitative studies. It is more difficult to evaluate qualitative studies using a standard set of criteria. Each qualitative method is unique. However, there are some general criteria by which qualitative research can be evaluated. Some of these criteria are presented in Box 9–1.

The beginning researcher may be very reluctant to critique qualitative studies. When unfamiliar with the study topic, the reviewer may believe that she or he lacks the expertise to critique the study. However, a determination can be made of how clearly the research report presents the process of data collection and analysis. The most important issue to consider is whether the data are provided to answer the research questions. Are the researcher's conceptualizations clearly based on the data? The reviewer should expect to

---

Box 9–1.   Guidelines for Critiquing Qualitative Designs
1. Does the phenomenon lend itself to study by qualitative methods, or would a quantitative approach have been more appropriate?
2. Does the study focus on the subjective nature of human experience?
3. Will the study findings have significance for nursing?
4. Does the researcher clearly describe how subjects were selected?
5. Is the data collection and recording process fully presented?
6. Is it clear how researcher bias in data collection was avoided?
7. Is the data analysis method consistent with the purpose of the study?
8. Have the research questions been answered?
9. Are recommendations made for future research?

---

see examples from the data and then make a judgment about how clearly the researcher has presented the interpretation of the data.

SUMMARY

Nurses are becoming more interested in qualitative research. Qualitative research focuses on gaining insight and understanding about an individual's perception of events and circumstances.

Five common types of qualitative research are phenomenological, ethnographic, grounded theory, historical, and case studies. **Phenomenological studies** examine human experiences through the descriptions that are provided by the people involved. **Ethnographic studies** collect data from groups, such as certain cultural groups. In **grounded theory studies,** a theory is developed that is *grounded* in the data. **Historical studies** concern the identification, location, evaluation, and synthesis of data from the past. Historical data should be subjected to both external and internal criticism. **External criticism** is concerned with the authenticity of the data, and **internal criticism** is concerned with the accuracy of the data. **Case studies** are in-depth examinations of people, groups of people, or institutions. **Content analysis** is the term used to indicate the examination of communication messages that are obtained in case studies, as well as in other types of qualitative studies.

The most commonly used methods of data collection in qualitative research are participant observation and semistructured interviews. **Saturation** means that the researcher is hearing a repetition of themes or salient points as additional participants are interviewed; data collection ceases at that time. Sample sizes may be quite small in qualitative research.

The reliability and validity of qualitative studies are determined differently than in quantitative studies. Qualitative studies are considered valid if the findings "reflect reality" from the point of view of the subject. Both the large amount of data collected and the length of time spent collecting data help to increase the reliability and validity of qualitative data.

Qualitative studies produce large amounts of data. The data generally consist of words, rather than numbers. Data analysis usually occurs all during the course of the study, rather than at the completion of the study. Data may be analyzed manually or through the aid of computer software programs.

Many nurse researchers have recommended the use of both qualitative and quantitative research methods in a study. When both methods are used simultaneously in a study, the term **triangulation** is used.

 ## NURSING RESEARCH ON THE WEB

For additional online resources, research activities, and exercises, go to www.prenhall. com/nieswiadomy. Select Chapter 9 from the drop down menu.

✖ GET INVOLVED ACTIVITIES

1. Each student will bring a published article that contains a report of a qualitative study. Using these qualitative research articles located in the literature, determine the specific type of qualitative design that was used. Determine the sample size obtained in each of these qualitative studies.

2. While searching the literature for a qualitative study, make a list of titles that indicate the study might be a qualitative study (for example, the title might contain a gerund, such as "becoming" or "transcending").

3. Divide into groups and develop an idea for a study in which the grounded theory method or the phenomenological method would be appropriate.

✖ SELF-TEST

Write T (True) or F (False) beside the following statements:

_____ 1. Qualitative research has been the type of research chosen by most nurse researchers in the past.

_____ 2. The researcher exerts tight controls over the research situation in qualitative research.

_____ 3. There has been an increase in the number of qualitative studies conducted in the past few years.

_____ 4. Many nurses are calling for a combination of both qualitative and quantitative methods in research.

_____ 5. Qualitative researchers are very concerned with the generalizability of their study findings.

_____ 6. The number of subjects is generally larger in qualitative research than in quantitative research.

Circle the letter before the *best* answer:

7. Which of the following types of studies is considered a qualitative study?

   A. correlational
   B. ethnographic
   C. comparative
   D. methodological

8. Which of the following statements is true when comparing qualitative research to quantitative research?

   A. Qualitative research is easier to conduct than quantitative research.
   B. The amount of data to be analyzed is usually greater in qualitative studies than in quantitative studies.
   C. The amount of time needed to conduct a qualitative study is usually less than in a quantitative study.
   D. Qualitative research most frequently uses a deductive approach, whereas quantitative research uses an inductive approach.

9. The most frequently used data-collection methods found in qualitative research are:

   A. closed-ended questions and nonparticipant observations.
   B. participant observations and semistructured interviews.
   C. structured interviews and physiological measures.
   D. closed-ended questions and structured interviews.

10. When both qualitative and quantitative research methods are used simultaneously in the same study, this procedure is called:

   A. triangulation.
   B. meta-analysis.
   C. multitrait/multimethod.
   D. methodological plurality.

✶ REFERENCES

Agar, M. H. (1986). *Speaking of ethnography.* Beverly Hills, CA: Sage Publications.

Benner, P. (1983). Uncovering the knowledge embedded in clinical practice. *Image: Journal of Nursing Scholarship, 19,* 36–41.

Bernstein, K. S. (2000). The experience of acupuncture for treatment of substance dependence. *Journal of Nursing Scholarship, 32,* 267–272.

Burns, N., & Grove, S. (1997). *The practice of nursing research: Conduct, critique and utilization* (3rd ed.). Philadelphia: W. B. Saunders.

Cameron, C. (1990). The ethnographic approach: Characteristics and uses in gerontological nursing. *Journal of Gerontological Nursing, 16*(9), 5–7.

Christy, T. (1975). The methodology of historical research. *Nursing Research, 24,* 189–192.

Cobb, A. K. (2000). Acculturation and accommodation in qualitative and quantitative research. *Journal of Professional Nursing, 16,* 188.

Cohen, M. Z. (1987). A historical overview of the phenomenological movement. *Image: Journal of Nursing Scholarship, 19,* 31–34.

Connelly, L. M., & Yoder, L. H., (2000). Improving qualitative proposals: Common problem areas. *Clinical Nurse Specialist, 14,* 69–74.

DeSantis, L., & Ugarriza, D. N. (2000). The concept of theme as used in qualitative nursing research. *Western Journal of Nursing Research, 22,* 351–372.

Draucker, C. B., & Stern, P. N. (2000). Women's responses to sexual violence by male intimates. *Western Journal of Nursing Research, 22,* 385–406.

England, M. (1996). Content domain for caregiver planning identified by adult offspring caregivers. *Image: Journal of Nursing Scholarship, 28,* 17–22.

Field, P. A., & Morse, J. M. (1985). *Nursing research: The application of qualitative approaches.* Rockville, MD: Aspen.

Forbes, S., Bern-Klug, M., & Gessert, C. (2000). End-of-life decision making for nursing home residents with dementia. *Journal of Nursing Scholarship, 32,* 251–258.

Ford-Gilboe, M., Campbell, J., & Berman, H. (1995). Stories and numbers: Coexistence without compromise. *Advances in Nursing Science, 18,* 14–26.

Frenn, M., & Porter, C. (1999). Exercise and nutrition: What adolescents think is important. *Applied Nursing Research, 12,* 179–184.

Glaser, B. G., & Strauss, A. C. (1967). *The discovery of grounded theory: Strategies for qualitative research.* New York: Aldine.

Haase, J. E., & Myers, S. T. (1988). Reconciling paradigm assumptions of qualitative and quantitative research. *Western Journal of Nursing Research, 10,* 128–136.

Hinds, P. S. (1989). Method triangulation to index change in clinical phenomena. *Western Journal of Nursing Research, 11,* 440–447.

Hinds, P. S., Scandrett-Hibden, S., & McAulay, L. S. (1990). Further assessment of a method to estimate reliability and validity of qualitative research findings. *Journal of Advanced Nursing, 15,* 430–435.

Krisman-Scott, M. A. (2000). An historical analysis of disclosure of terminal status. *Journal of Nursing Scholarship, 32,* 47–52.

Leininger, M. M. (Ed.) (1985). *Qualitative research methods in nursing.* Orlando, FL: Grune & Stratton.

Levin, P. F., Hewitt, J. B., & Misner, S. T. (1998). Insights of nurses about assault in hospital-based emergency departments. *Image: Journal of Nursing Scholarship, 30,* 249–254.

Mariano, C. (1990). Qualitative research: Instructional strategies and curricular considerations. *Nursing & Health Care, 11,* 354–359.

McLaughlin, F. E., & Marascuilo, L. A. (1990). *Advanced nursing and health care research: Quantification approaches.* Philadelphia: Saunders.

McQuiston, C., & Gordon, A. (2000). The timing is never right: Mexican views of condom use. *Health Care for Women International, 21,* 277–290.

Mead, M. (1929). *Coming of age in Samoa.* New York: New American Library.

Morin, K. H., Patterson, B. J., Kurtz, B., & Brzowski, B. (1999). Mothers' responses to care given by male nursing students during and after birth. *Image: Journal of Nursing Scholarship, 31,* 83–87.

Myers, S. T., & Haase, J. E. (1989). Guidelines for integration of quantitative and qualitative approaches. *Nursing Research, 38,* 299–301.

O'Connell, K. (2000). If you call me names, I'll call you numbers. *Journal of Professional Nursing, 16,* 74.

Orne, R. M., Fishman, S. J., Manka, M., & Pagnozzi, M. E. (2000). Living on the edge: A phenomenological study of medically uninsured working Americans. *Research in Nursing & Health, 23,* 204–212.

Parse, R. R., Coyne, A. B., & Smith, M. J. (1985). *Nursing research: Qualitative methods.* Bowie, MD: Brady.

Pilkington, F. B. (1996). The use of computers in qualitative research. *Nursing Science Quarterly, 9,* 5–7.

Polit, D. F., & Hungler, B. P. (1999). *Nursing research: Principles and methods* (6th ed.). Philadelphia: Lippincott.

Porter, E. J. (1989). The qualitative-quantitative dualism. *Image: Journal of Nursing Scholarship, 21,* 98–102.

Ramer, L. (1989). Quantitative versus qualitative research? *JOGNN, 18,* 7–8.

Ross, B. A. (1994). Use of a database for managing qualitative research data. *Computers in Nursing, 12,* 154–159.

Sandelowski, M. (1995a). On the aesthetics of qualitative research. *Image: Journal of Nursing Scholarship, 27,* 205–209.

Sandelowski, M. (1995b). Sample size in qualitative research. *Research in Nursing and Health, 18,* 179–183.

Sandelowski, M. (2000). Combining qualitative and quantitative sampling, data collection, and analysis techniques in mixed-method studies. *Research in Nursing and Health, 23,* 246–255.

Schulte, J. (2000). Finding ways to create connections among communities: Partial results of an ethnography of urban public health nurses. *Public Health Nursing, 17,* 3–10.

Sedlak, C. A. (1997). Critical thinking of beginning baccalaureate nursing students during the first clinical nursing course. *Journal of Nursing Education, 36,* 11–18.

Streubert, H. J., & Carpenter, D. R. (1999). *Qualitative research in nursing: Advancing the humanistic imperative* (2nd ed.) Philadelphia: Lippincott.

Thomas, B. S. (1990). *Nursing research: An experiential approach.* St. Louis: C. V. Mosby.

Wilson, H. S., & Hutchinson, S. A. (1996). *Consumer's guide to nursing research.* Albany, NY: Delmar.

Younger, J. (1985). Practical approaches to clinical research: The case study. *Pediatric Nursing, 11,* 137.

PART IV

Obtaining Study Subjects and Collection of Data

CHAPTER 10

Populations and Samples

✳ OUTLINE

Populations
Samples
Types of Sampling Methods
- Probability Sampling Methods
  Simple Random Sampling
  Stratified Random Sampling
  Cluster Random Sampling
  Systematic Random Sampling
- Nonprobability Sampling Methods
  Convenience Sampling
  Quota Sampling
  Purposive Sampling

Time Frame for Studying the Sample
Sample Size
Sampling Error and Sampling Bias
Randomization Procedures in Research
Critiquing the Sampling Procedure
Summary
Nursing Research on the Web
Get Involved Activities
Self-test

✳ OBJECTIVES

On completion of this chapter, you will be prepared to:

1. Define population and sample
2. Distinguish between target and accessible populations
3. Discuss probability and nonprobability sampling procedures
4. Compare four methods of probability sampling
5. Compare three methods of nonprobability sampling
6. Use a table of random numbers to select a sample
7. Compare longitudinal and cross-sectional studies
8. Enumerate factors to be considered in deciding the size of the sample
9. Discuss sampling error and sampling bias
10. Choose an appropriate sampling method for a selected research study
11. Critique the sampling procedure described in research reports and articles

✖ NEW TERMS DEFINED IN THIS CHAPTER

cluster random sampling
cohort study
convenience sampling
cross-sectional study
disproportional stratified sampling
element
longitudinal study
nonprobability sampling
power analysis
probability sampling
proportional stratified sampling

purposive sampling
quota sampling
sampling bias
sampling error
sampling frame
simple random sampling
snowball sampling
stratified random sampling
systematic random sampling
table of random numbers
volunteers

What have you sampled today? Did you try on some new clothes, taste a new food, or turn on a different TV program than you have ever watched before? Sampling is a part of our everyday life. Frequently, decisions in life are made on limited sampling from all of the available options. If you bought some new clothes today, did you try on all of the clothes in the store before you purchased your selection? Probably not, or you would still be out shopping!

Researchers also make decisions based on data from samples. However, the consequences of basing decisions on inadequate samples may be much more serious for the researcher than for the shopper. If you choose the wrong size or change your mind about the style of a jacket you bought, you are usually allowed to take the jacket back to the store. The researcher is not able to change a decision about the selection of a sample for a study, once the sample has been chosen. Of course, the safest choice then would be to study total populations. Just as it is unlikely that you would buy a whole "population" of clothes, researchers rarely study whole populations of subjects. Therefore, an understanding of the means of selecting samples for research studies is important for nurse researchers.

POPULATIONS

A population is a complete set of persons or objects that possess some common characteristic that is of interest to the researcher. The population for a study usually is described as being composed of two groups—the target population and the accessible population. As mentioned in Chapter 2, the target population is composed of the entire group of people or objects to which the researcher wishes to generalize the findings of a study. The target population consists of people or things that meet the designated set of criteria of interest to the researcher. Examples of target populations might be all people who are institutionalized for psychiatric problems in one state or all the charts from well-child clinics for the year 2000. Because the likelihood of being able to obtain a list of these populations is quite low, the researcher usually samples from an available group, called the accessible population or study population. The need to identify the accessible population is quite important for nurse researchers. By clearly identifying the group from which the study sample was chosen, the investigator allows the readers of a research report to come to their own conclusions about the generalizability of the study findings. The conclusions of a research study are based on data obtained from the accessible population, and statistical inferences (see Chapter 14) should be made only to the group from which the sample was randomly selected.

SAMPLES

Although researchers are always interested in populations, an entire population is generally not used in a research study. The accuracy that is gained when all members are included is often not worth the time and money. In most nursing research studies, a sample or subset of the population is selected to represent the population. When a sample is chosen properly, the researcher is able to make claims about the population based on data from the sample alone. The method of selection and the sample size will determine how representative a sample is of the population.

A single member of a population is called an **element.** The terms *population member* and *population element* will be used interchangeably throughout this chapter. Elements, or members of a population, are selected from a **sampling frame,** which is a listing of all elements of a population. Sometimes listings of populations, such as membership lists, hospital patient census sheets, and vital statistics listings, are readily available. Frequently, the researcher has to prepare a sampling frame by listing all members of the accessible population. This can be a time-consuming task, and care must be taken to delineate the population. For example, you might examine a large group of charts and make a list of all patients who were admitted for their second major surgical procedure within 2 years.

Although examining each member of a population would generally produce more accurate data, occasionally data obtained from a sample are more exact. For example, in large-scale survey studies where many interviewers have to be trained, the quality of the interviews would be difficult to control, and a small number of interviews conducted by a well-trained group of interviewers might produce more accurate data than would be produced by a large group of interviewers. Also, when resources are spread thin, a weak study may result.

TYPES OF SAMPLING METHODS

Samples are chosen through two types of sampling procedures: probability and nonprobability. The various types of probability and nonprobability sampling methods are discussed.

PROBABILITY SAMPLING METHODS

Probability sampling involves the use of a random selection process to select a sample from members or elements of a population. The goal of probability sampling is to examine representative elements of populations.

The term *random* can be confusing to the beginning researcher. The dictionary definition of this word suggests that something occurs haphazardly or without direction. Random sampling, however, is anything but haphazard! It is a very systematic, scientific process. The investigator can specify the chance of any one element of the population being selected for the sample. Each population element has a known chance or probability of being selected for the sample. Selections are independent of each other, and the investigator's bias does not enter into the selection of the sample.

When a random sample is selected, the researcher hopes that the variables of interest in the population will be present in the sample in approximately the same proportions as would be found in the total population. Unfortunately, there is never any guarantee that this will occur. Probability sampling allows the researcher to estimate the chance that any given population element will be included in the sample. When probability samples are chosen, inferential statistics may be used with greater confidence (see Chapter 14). Without the use of random sampling procedures, the ability to generalize the findings of a study is greatly reduced. Four types of random sampling procedures are examined: simple, stratified, cluster, and systematic.

Simple Random Sampling. **Simple random sampling** is a type of probability sampling that ensures that each element of the population has an equal and independent chance of being chosen. This method is generally used in at least one phase of the other three types of random sampling procedures and, therefore, is examined first. The advantages and disadvantages of simple random sampling are listed in Table 10–1.

The word *simple* does not mean easy or uncomplicated. In fact, simple random sampling can be quite complex and time consuming, especially if a large sample is desired.

The first step is to identify the accessible population and enumerate or list all the elements of the population. This listing is called a sampling frame. After the sampling frame is developed, a method must be selected to choose the sample. Slips of paper representing each element in the population could be placed in a hat or a bowl and the sample selected by reaching in and drawing out as many slips of paper as the desired size of the sample.

Although random sampling can be achieved by drawing numbered slips of paper or numbered balls from some type of container, the most commonly used and accurate procedure for selecting a simple random sample is through the use of a **table of random numbers.** A table of random numbers includes a list of numbers that have been generated in such a manner that there is no order or sequencing of the numbers. Each number is equally likely to follow any other number. Today these tables are generated through the use of computers. Tables of random numbers are found in many texts on statistics. An example of a small table of random numbers is shown in Table 10–2.

The thought of using a table of random numbers may seem scary to you. Actually, it is rather easy. It may get a little boring if you have a large number of elements to be selected, but the process is not complicated. Although you will probably never have to select a random sample manually, a step-by-step listing of the procedure for selecting a sample of 15 from a population of 80 is provided for your understanding of the concept of random sampling.

1. Assign a number to each element of the accessible population.
2. Enter the table of random numbers at an arbitrary or random starting point. This can be done through closing your eyes and blindly pointing to a number in the table. That number becomes your first selection. Suppose number 58 is chosen (Table 10–2).

TABLE 10–1. Probability Sampling Chart

Type of Sampling	Description of Methodology	Advantages	Disadvantages
A. Simple random	Assign a number to each member of the population. Select the sample through a table of random numbers.	1. Little knowledge of population is needed 2. Most unbiased of probability methods 3. Easy to analyze data and compute errors	1. A complete listing of population is necessary 2. Time consuming 3. Expensive
B. Stratified	Divide population into strata. Determine number of cases desired in each stratum. Random sample these subgroups.	1. Increases probability of sample being representative 2. Assures adequate number of cases for subgroups	1. Requires accurate knowledge of population 2. May be costly to prepare stratified lists 3. Statistics more complicated
1. Proportionate	Determine sampling fraction for each stratum that is equal to its proportion in the total population.		
2. Disproportionate	Sample is drawn in manner to ensure that each stratum is well represented. Used when strata are very unequal.		
C. Cluster	Groups rather than people are selected from population. Successive steps of selection are done (state, city, county). Then sample is randomly selected from clusters.	1. Saves time and money 2. Arrangements made with small number of sampling units 3. Characteristics of clusters as well as those of population can be estimated	1. Larger sampling errors than other probability samples 2. Requires assignment of each member of population uniquely to a cluster 3. Statistics are more complicated
D. Systematic	Obtain listing of population Determine sample size. Determine sampling interval $(k = N/n)$. Select random starting point. Select every kth element.	1. Easy to draw sample 2. Economical 3. Time-saving technique	1. Samples may be biased if ordering of population is not random 2. After the first sampling element is chosen, population members no longer have equal chance of being chosen

TABLE 10–2. Random Numbers

21	71	89	96	97
82	59	22	78	12
76	93	64	79	28
20	60	70	34	51
93	58	36	93	90
68	63	19	21	91
18	32	36	27	71
58	80	⑤⑧	67	50
66	25	②⓪	31	62
17	25	⓪⑦	94	18
02	29	③⓪	15	92
55	06	②⑤	09	26
38	11	⓪①	47	93
42	47	⑦③	25	84
82	04	②③	08	88
37	24	⑤①	98	05
94	58	85	86	71
37	92	②⑦	20	58
29	64	①③	05	24
85	48	③⑦	37	21
20	56	91	53	66
33	23	13	82	54
62	11	②⑨	17	37
01	57	73	53	97
34	19	⑦⑤	62	16
81	10	⑤⑤	36	36
92	50	32	68	82
37	33	43	20	08
10	50	18	85	27

3. Continue in a systematic way either up, down, to the left, right, or diagonally. The direction is not important, but the decision should be made before the process is started, and this direction should continue until the total sample is selected.

4. Continue to select numbers until 15 numbers have been selected. The numbers are circled in Table 10–2. Notice that numbers 85 and 91 are omitted because they are larger than 80.

5. If a number is encountered more than once, the number is skipped. Notice that numbers 13 and 73 are skipped because they had already been selected.

One table of random numbers may be composed of two-digit numbers, whereas another table may contain three-digit numbers. Some large tables of random numbers may even contain several pages of large-digit numbers. The type of table used will be dictated by the desired sample size. To choose samples from populations containing fewer than 100 members, a two-digit table is most appropriate. Numbers, however, can be randomly selected from any size table. For example, if a four-digit number table is used to obtain a sample from a population containing fewer than 100 elements, the researcher might elect to use only the first two numbers of each four-digit number. The circled numbers might be chosen:

(48)93   (23)21   (86)11   (34)55

(26)11   (34)00   (90)77   (66)33

It would make selecting a sample easier, however, to use a table containing two digits. Remember, if the population size exceeds 100, three digits will be needed to give every member of the population a chance to be chosen. If there are exactly 100 elements in the population, the number 00 can be used to represent 100, rather than shifting to a three-digit table. Although you have been shown how to use a table of random numbers by hand, today it is more likely that a random sample will be generated through the use of a computer-generated list of numbers, as previously mentioned.

> Students from six colleges and universities in a large southeastern city were asked to participate in a study that examined condom use (Dilorio, Dudley, Soet, Watkin & Maibach, 2000). A request was made to each registrar's office for a random sample of students currently enrolled in a degree-seeking program and younger than 25 years. Of the 8118 questionnaires, 2044 were returned (25.2% response rate). Self-efficacy (confidence in one's ability to use a condom in a variety of situations) was directly related to condom use, as had been predicted. However, substance use during sexual encounters was not related to a condom use. The researchers had predicted that college students who reported combining alcohol or drugs with sexual encounters would report less frequent condom use.

Stratified Random Sampling.   In **stratified random sampling,** the population is divided into subgroups, or strata, according to some variable or variables of importance to the research study. After the population is divided into two or more strata, a simple random sample is taken from each of these subgroups.

Many different characteristics of populations may call for the use of stratified sampling. Subject characteristics, such as age, gender, and educational background, are examples of variables that might be used as criteria for dividing populations into subgroups. For example, a school nurse might be interested in studying marijuana usage among high school students. To determine if marijuana usage is different among freshmen, sophomores, juniors, and seniors, the total high school population could be stratified into four separate sampling units and a random sample selected from each grade. If a simple random sample technique is used, the four grades might not be represented in large enough numbers to make valid comparisons. Generally, there are more freshmen than seniors in a school. Some students drop out as they progress through high school. By dividing the total population into the four grades, the school nurse might be more certain that sufficient numbers of students from all four grades will be selected for inclusion in the study.

After dividing the population into subgroups, the researcher must decide how large a sample to obtain from each of these strata. Two approaches may be used. The first is called **proportional stratified sampling** and involves obtaining a sample from each stratum that is in proportion to the size of that stratum in the total population. If there were 400 freshmen, 300 sophomores, 200 juniors, and 100 seniors (highly unlikely!) in a total high school population of 1000 students, the size of the sample from each of these groups should be freshmen, 40%; sophomores, 30%; juniors, 20%; and seniors, 10%. If a sample of 100 students was desired, the selection should include 40 freshmen, 30 sophomores, 20 juniors, and 10 seniors.

What if the school nurse decided that 10 seniors was not a large enough sample to get a clear picture of marijuana usage among that group? She might decide to choose 25 subjects from each class. The selection of members from strata where the number of members chosen from each stratum is not in proportion to the size of the stratum in the total population is called **disproportional stratified sampling.** Whenever disproportional sampling is used, an adjustment process known as weighting should be considered. This process involves simple computations that are described in many texts on sampling procedures. These adjustments will allow a better estimate of the actual population values.

As previously mentioned, simple random sampling is used to obtain the sample elements from each stratum. The advantages and disadvantages of stratified sampling are listed in Table 10–1.

> Estabrooks (1999) selected a proportional stratified sampling method for her study that examined research utilization by nurses in Canada. A random sample of 1500 nurses was drawn from the 15,698 members of the Alberta Association of Registered Nurses (AARN). The sample was stratified so that the size of the sample of home care nurses, public health nurses, and nurses working in nursing homes were proportionate to their numbers in the population of nurses in AARN. Although usable responses were received from only 600 nurses, the sample was determined to be comparable to the population from which it was drawn.

Cluster Random Sampling.   In large-scale studies where the population is geographically spread out, sampling procedures may be difficult and time consuming. Also, it may be difficult or impossible to get a total listing of some populations. Suppose a researcher wanted to interview 100 nurse administrators in the United States. If the 100 names were chosen through a simple random sampling procedure, it is quite likely that the investigator would be faced with traveling to 100 different cities in the United States to conduct the interviews. This would be a very expensive and time-consuming activity. Another approach that might be used to obtain this sample of nurse administrators is cluster sampling. In **cluster random sampling,** large groups or "clusters" become the sampling units. To obtain the sample of nurse administrators, the first clusters to be sampled would be obtained by drawing a simple random sample or stratified random sample of states in the United States. Then cities would be chosen from these states. Next, hospitals from within those cities would be selected, and, finally, the nurse administrators from some of these hospitals would be interviewed. During each phase of sampling from the clusters, either simple, stratified, or systematic random sampling may be used. Because the sample is selected from clusters in two or more separate stages, the approach is sometimes called multistage sampling.

Although cluster sampling may be necessary for large-scale survey studies, the likelihood of sampling error increases with each stage of sampling. A simple random sample is subject to a single sampling error, whereas a cluster sample is subject to as many sampling errors as there are stages in the sampling procedure. To compensate for the sampling error when cluster sampling is used, larger samples should be selected than would normally be chosen for a simple or stratified random sample. In a search of the CINAHL computerized database, no recent nursing research studies were located that mentioned the use of cluster random sampling. A few studies were found in the medical literature in which this sampling process was used. The advantages and disadvantages of cluster sampling are listed in Table 10–1.

Systematic Random Sampling. **Systematic random sampling** involves selecting every *k*th element of the population, such as every fifth, eighth, or twenty-first element. The first step is to obtain a list of the total population (N). Then the sample size (n) is determined. Next the sampling interval width (k) is determined by N/n. For instance, if the researcher was seeking a sample of 50 from a population of 500, the sampling interval would be:

$$k = 500/50 = 10$$

Every tenth element of the population list would be selected for the sample. This method may be used to obtain any sample size from a given population.

This sampling method is the most controversial type of random sampling procedure. In fact, systematic sampling may be classified as either a probability or a nonprobability sampling method. Two criteria are necessary for a systematic sampling procedure to be classified as probability sampling: (a) the listing of the population (sampling frame) must be random with respect to the variable of interest, and (b) the first element or member of the sample must be selected randomly. If either of these criteria is not met, nonprobability sampling occurs.

The first criterion for the inclusion of systematic sampling as a probability sampling method is the requirement that the listing of the population must be in random order. Suppose a researcher were choosing names from an alphabetized list. Certain ethnic groups have large numbers of surnames that begin with the same initial and are grouped together alphabetically. If systematic sampling is used, these ethnic groups may be underrepresented. As another example, the sample to be selected might be patients in hospital rooms. The decision might be made to sample every fifth hospital room. It might happen that every fifth room is a private room. Patients in private rooms may not respond in the same manner that patients in semiprivate rooms might respond.

The second criterion for considering systematic sampling as a type of probability sampling is that a random starting point must be chosen. The best way to obtain this starting point is through a table of random numbers. If the population size is 500 and a sample size of 50 is desired, a number between 1 and 500 is selected as the starting point. Suppose the first number randomly selected is 289. The sampling interval width ($k = 10$) is added to this number (289 + 10 = 299), and the next element selected would correspond to number 299. When 500 is reached, the researcher starts back over at the beginning of the list and continues adding 10 to select each additional element of the sample. An alternate procedure, which is recommended in most texts, is to randomly select the first element from within the first sampling interval. If the sampling interval width is 10, a number between 1 and 10 would be selected as the random starting point. For example, suppose the number 4 is randomly chosen. The next element selected would correspond to number 14 (4 + 10 = 14). Although this latter procedure is technically correct, I prefer choosing a random starting point from across the total population of elements because every element has a chance to be chosen for the sample during the first selection step.

When careful attention is paid to obtaining an unbiased listing of the population elements, and the first element is randomly selected, systematic random sampling is similar to simple random sampling and much easier. Drawing 50 numbers from a table of random numbers is a much more laborious task than choosing 50 numbers through systematic sampling. The advantages and disadvantages of systematic random sampling are listed in Table 10–1. A cursory review of the nursing research literature for the past 5 years revealed few studies in which systematic random sampling was mentioned.

A systematic random sample was used to study family reports of barriers to optimal care of the dying (Tolle, Tilden, Rosenfeld, & Hickman, 2000). All death certificates for deaths that occurred in Oregon between November 1996 and 1997 constituted the sampling frame. A systematic random sample of 1458 was selected from the 24,074 death certificates. Of those families who could be contacted, 475 agreed to participate. The study revealed that barriers to optimal care of the dying remain, including level of pain and pain management and some dissatisfaction with physician availability.

Nonprobability Sampling Methods

In **nonprobability sampling,** the sample elements are chosen from the population by nonrandom methods. Nonrandom methods of sampling are more likely to produce a biased sample than are random methods. The investigator cannot estimate the probability that each element of the population will be included in the sample. In fact, in nonprobability sampling, certain elements of the population may have no chance of being included in the sample. This restricts the generalizations that can be made about the study findings. Despite the limitations of nonprobability sampling, most nursing research studies involve this type of sampling procedure. True random samples are rare in nursing research.

The most frequent reasons for the use of nonprobability samples involve convenience and the desire to use available subjects. Samples may be chosen from available groups of subjects by several different methods, including convenience, quota, and purposive.

Convenience Sampling. **Convenience sampling** is also referred to as *accidental* or *incidental* and involves choosing readily available people or objects for a study. These elements may or may not be typical of the population. There is no accurate way to determine their representativeness. It is easy to see that this may be a very unreliable method of sampling. However, convenience sampling has probably been the most frequently used sampling method in nursing research. A recent review of the nursing research literature confirmed the continued use of convenience samples.

Convenience samples are chosen because of the savings in time and money. The researcher may choose a convenience sample from familiar people, as when a teacher uses students in her or his class, or from strangers, such as might be encountered when a nurse researcher conducts a survey among family members in an intensive care unit waiting room to determine their attitudes about visiting hour limitations.

> A convenience sample of 203 healthy newborns was selected by MacMullen and Dulski (2000) to study factors related to the newborns' sucking ability. The newborns were between 30 minutes and 11 hours of age and between 34 and 42 weeks' gestation. These healthy newborns demonstrated excellent oral motor skills. The larger, full-term infants performed significantly better than the smaller newborns.

Another method of obtaining a convenience sample is through **snowball sampling.** This term is used to describe a method of sampling that involves the assistance of study subjects to help obtain other potential subjects. Suppose the researcher wanted to determine how to help people to stop cigarette smoking. The researcher might know of someone who has been successful in refraining from cigarette smoking for 10 years. This person is contacted and asked if he or she knows others who have also been successful. This type of networking is particularly helpful in finding people who are reluctant to make their identity known, such as substance abusers.

> Snowball sampling was used to locate physicians who had been involved in the resuscitation of extremely low-birth-weight preterm infants (Catlin, 1999). Physicians were sought throughout the United States. The purpose of the study was to examine these physicians' perceptions of their delivery room decisions to resuscitate these types of infants. Two of the main factors affecting their decisions were that they had been trained to save lives and that parents had asked them to do everything possible to save their infant.

Quota Sampling. **Quota sampling** is similar to stratified random sampling in that the first step involves dividing the population into homogeneous strata and selecting sample elements from each of these strata. The difference lies in the means of securing potential subjects from these strata. Stratified random sampling involves a random sampling method of obtaining sample members, whereas quota sampling obtains members through convenience samples.

The term *quota* arises from the researcher's establishment of a desired quota or proportion for some population variable of interest. The basis of stratification should be a variable of importance to the study. These variables frequently include subject attributes such as age, gender, and educational background. The number of elements chosen from each stratum is generally in proportion to the size of that stratum in the total population. For example, if the researcher wanted to determine whether more males or females receive yearly physical examinations, an equal proportion of males and females should be approached for the study. If convenience sampling is used, the two genders may not be equally represented in the sample. If a sample of 100 is desired, a quota of 50% males and

50% females would be set. Then the first 50 males and first 50 females approached by the researcher would be asked to participate in the survey. Of course, because this would not be a probability sample, there is a risk that the sample would not be typical of all males and females.

> The effectiveness of an intervention to prevent abuse to pregnant women was studied by Parker, McFarlane, Soeken, Silva, and Reel (1999). Another purpose of the study was to determine if there were any differences in the amount of abuse reported among women in different ethnic groups. Therefore, a quota sample of equal numbers of African American, Caucasian, and Hispanic women were sought. Significantly less abuse was reported by women in the intervention group than by women in the comparison group. Additionally, African American and Caucasian women reported more physical abuse, and Hispanic women reported more mental abuse.

Purposive Sampling. **Purposive sampling** involves "handpicking" of subjects. This method is also called judgmental sampling. Subjects are chosen that the researcher believes are "typical" or representative of the accessible population, or someone who is believed to be an expert may be asked to select the subjects. This type of sampling is based on the assumption that the researcher or the chosen expert has enough knowledge about the population of interest to select specific subjects for the study.

An investigator might want to determine some of the problems that are experienced by diabetic clients when using insulin pumps. The investigator works in a clinic that services diabetic clients and personally knows several clients who have been experiencing problems with their insulin pumps. These potential subjects are viewed as "typical" cases and are requested to participate in the planned research study. It is evident that bias may enter into the selection of samples through purposive sampling procedures. Researchers, however, may believe that errors in judgment will tend to balance; purposive samples are not uncommon in nursing research. Many qualitative studies use purposive samples.

> A purposive sample was selected by Orne, Fishman, Manka, and Pagnozzi (2000) to study the experiences of medically uninsured working Americans. The purposive sample of 12 was composed of 4 men and 8 women who were recruited through personal and professional contacts. The researchers obtained participants who were currently employed and had been medically uninsured for at least 3 months. The results of this phenomenological study were presented in Chapter 9.

TIME FRAME FOR STUDYING THE SAMPLE

The time frame for selecting and studying subjects in a research study is the criterion by which research studies are classified as longitudinal or cross-sectional. A **longitudinal study** follows subjects over a period of time in the future; a **cross-sectional study** examines subjects at one point in time. There is no agreed upon time period for designating a study as longitudinal. According to Shelley (1984), if subjects are followed for 6 months or longer, the sample can be considered to be longitudinal.

A special type of longitudinal study is a cohort study. In a **cohort study,** persons are studied who have been born during a particular time period. An example of a longitudinal cohort study is the Nurses' Health Study conducted by researchers at Harvard Medical School. This study was begun in 1976. The population to be studied consisted of married, female, registered nurses born between January 1, 1921 and December 31, 1946, and residing in 11 states with the largest number of registered nurses: New York, California, Pennsylvania, Ohio, Massachusetts, New Jersey, Michigan, Texas, Florida, Connecticut, and Maryland. The original sample for this study was composed of more than 100,000 nurses. The study was designed to examine some of the health risks that pose a special threat to women. Included in these risks were cigarette smoking and the use of hair dyes and oral contraceptives. The study was later expanded to examine dietary patterns, stress factors, and the use of prescription drugs. In one of the study's more publicized aspects, nurses were asked to send toenail clippings to determine dietary intakes of selenium. The relationship between selenium intake and cancer was being examined. Nurses were chosen as the subjects for this study, according to Frank Speizer, the principal investigator, because the study called for "a sophisticated group of individuals who could report exposure and diseases more accurately than the general population" ("Massive Nurses' Health Study," 1983, p. 998). The study was originally intended to last for 4 years, but additional funding was received and the study has continued for more than 25 years. A similar but younger cohort group (Nurses Health Study II) has been added to examine the long-term effects of contraceptive use. I am a member of the original sample who sent in their toenails! Do you suppose the Harvard researchers still have them?

In a cross-sectional study, data are gathered on subjects at one specific time, but the data may be collected from groups of people who represent different ages, time periods, or developmental states. Consider the previous example where the school nurse was interested in studying marijuana usage among high school students. She wants to know if changes in usage occur as students progress through high school. A longitudinal study might be conducted in which freshman students from several schools would be followed until graduation, and their marijuana usage would be compared over the 4 years of high school. Because of the time factor and cost involved in such a lengthy study, the nurse researcher might decide to gather all of the data at one time by sampling students in all four grades of high school and comparing the marijuana usage among these groups. Of course, the danger in this type of study is that an assumption must be made that the seniors will reply as the freshmen would have replied at the end of 4 years. This might be a risky assumption. A longitudinal study is a more accurate means of studying changes that occur over time. Cross-sectional studies are conducted, however, because they are less expensive and easier to conduct than longitudinal studies.

A study was conducted to examine women's intentions to use hormones and their actual use of hormones with menopause (Lauver, Settersten, Marten, & Halls, 1999). A cross-sectional sample was selected of 184 premenopausal, perimenopausal, and postmenopausal women. To explain intention to use hormones, data were gathered from 124 participants who were not using hormones. To explain actual use of hormones, data were gathered from 125 perimenopausal and postmenopausal participants. Findings were as follows: (a) anxiety was inversely correlated with use, (b) norms were positively correlated with intentions and use, (c) age was inversely correlated with intentions, and (d) hot flashes were inversely correlated with use.

SAMPLE SIZE

One of the most frequent questions posed to statisticians is "How large should my sample be?" Unfortunately, there is no simple answer.

Generally speaking, large samples are more representative of the population of interest than are small samples. There are no simple rules for determining the desired sample size. Some factors to be considered are the homogeneity of the population, the degree of precision desired by the researcher, and the type of sampling procedure that will be used. If the population is very homogeneous or alike on all variables other than the one being measured, a small sample size may be sufficient. On the other hand, if the researcher wants to be precise in generalizing to the population based on sample data, a large sample may be necessary for the sample to accurately represent the population. Finally, when probability sampling methods are used, smaller samples are required than when nonprobability sampling techniques are employed.

According to Roscoe (1975), there are few instances in behavioral research when a sample size smaller than 30 or larger than 500 can be justified. A sample size of 30 ensures the benefits of the central limit theorem (see Chapter 14). For most behavioral research, a sample size of 30 will be adequate, according to Roscoe (1975).

Large sample sizes may be needed in the following instances:

1. *Many uncontrolled variables are present.* The researcher thinks age may influence study results, but is not able to control for this variable.

2. *Small differences are expected in members of the population on the variable of interest.* Small but important differences between members of the population may not be uncovered when small samples are used.

3. *The population must be divided into subgroups.* Sample sizes must be increased to ensure inclusion of members of each of the subgroups.

4. *Dropout rate among subjects is expected to be high.* This problem is especially likely to occur in longitudinal studies.

5. *Statistical tests are used that require minimum sample sizes.* Certain statistical tests require minimum numbers of responses in each cell of the data.

Although large samples are desirable, the law of diminishing returns applies. A sample of 100, or 10%, may be necessary to obtain the required precision desired for a population of 1000. A 10% sample of a population of 1 million would require 100,000 elements. This would be a huge sample and would be unnecessary. In fact, samples of 2000 or 3000 are often sufficient to estimate the characteristics of the entire population of the United States. A more important issue than the size of the sample is the representativeness of the sample. Election results can be predicted with very small percentages of votes counted because the polled voters have been thoroughly examined for representativeness in voting behavior.

It is always wise to set the sample size a little bit larger than what is actually desired (to allow for nonresponse or subject dropout) and also to establish an absolute minimum size of the sample. Should the study be conducted if only five subjects agree to participate? The researcher must make the decision about the minimum acceptable sample size before data collection begins.

Power analysis is a procedure that can be used to determine the needed sample size for a research study. This procedure is very important in experimental studies. The power of a statistical test is its ability to detect statistical significance in a study, when it is present. When power is low, the likelihood of making a Type II error is high (see Chapter 14). One factor that influences the power of a test is the sample size used in the study. In many studies, researchers erroneously conclude that no significant difference exists between the experimental and the control group when, in fact, a difference would have been detected if the sample had been larger. Polit and Sherman (1990) studied 62 articles that were published in *Nursing Research* and *Research in Nursing and Health* during 1989. They concluded that a substantial number of published studies (and they presumed that even more unpublished studies) had insufficient power because of small sample sizes. However, a recent review of the literature indicates an increasing number of researchers who discuss the use of power analysis to determinine their sample size (Keuter, Bryne, Voell, & Larson, 2000; King, 2000; MacMullen & Dulski, 2000; Neu, Browne, & Vojir, 2000; Parker, McFarlane, Soeken, Silva, & Reel, 1999).

The researcher would be wise to perform a power analysis before conducting a study and make the decision not to conduct a study if the analysis indicates that the needed sample size would be difficult to obtain. External funding sources are increasingly requiring that the researcher determine the sample size needed for a study and, therefore, power analysis is being used more frequently. Although the procedure is not difficult to perform, it is not discussed here. For more information consult Cohen (1988).

Thomas Knapp, a statistician whose articles appear frequently in *Nursing Research,* believes too much emphasis is being placed on this method of determining sample size (Knapp, 1996). He has decried the requirement of nearly all major funding sources that a power analysis be done before the submission of a grant proposal. He cited one researcher's "pink sheet" (notice of denial of funding) that criticized the researcher for the small sample size and for not using power analysis. The researcher had, in fact, used the entire population! Knapp wrote that Jacob Cohen, an expert on power analysis, would never have envisioned that using this technique would be considered more desirable than studying an entire population. Abdellah and Levine (1994) also cautioned about placing too much emphasis on power analysis. They wrote that power analysis does not guarantee a valid study and that "high power cannot in any way compensate for poor data" (p. 80).

Most nursing research studies are limited to small convenience samples. Generalizations to total populations, therefore, are usually difficult to make with any degree of confidence. The use of small sample sizes dictates the need for studies to be replicated. If several investigators find similar results when studying the same topic, generalizations to other populations are more appropriate.

SAMPLING ERROR AND SAMPLING BIAS

Although sampling error and sampling bias are sometimes discussed interchangeably, these two concepts should be considered separately. **Sampling error** may be defined as the difference between data obtained from a random sample and the data that would be obtained if an entire population were measured. Error may be contained in sample data even when the most careful random sampling procedure has been used to obtain the sample. Sampling error is not under the researcher's control; it is caused by the chance variations that may occur when a sample is chosen to represent a population. Table 10–3 demonstrates how random samples vary from the true population values. The table contains pulse measurements on a population of 20 subjects. The mean pulse rate for the population is 71. The mean pulse rate for random sample #3 is also 71. Random sample #1 is considerably below average, and random sample #2 is well above average for the population.

Whereas sampling error occurs by chance, sampling bias is caused by the researcher. **Sampling bias** is that bias that occurs when samples are not carefully selected. If names are written on slips of paper and placed in a hat, each piece of paper would have to be the same size and thickness or bias could occur. Bias could also occur if the slips of paper stuck together in clumps. The literature is replete with examples of bias in sample selections. One of the most famous examples concerns the United States presidential election of 1936. *Literary Digest* magazine conducted a large poll among eligible voters to determine if people planned to vote for Alfred Landon, the Republican candidate, or Franklin Roosevelt, the Democratic candidate. The magazine predicted, on the basis of this poll, that Landon would win by a landslide margin. Roosevelt soundly defeated Landon! It was determined that biased sampling occurred as the result of selecting subjects from the telephone directory and through listings of automobile registrations. Depressed economic conditions were present in 1936, and members of the Republican Party were more likely to own telephones and automobiles than were members of the Democratic Party.

All nonprobability sampling methods are subject to sampling bias. Also, random sampling procedures are subject to bias if some elements of the selected sample decide not to participate in the research study. If questionnaires were sent to a random sample of nurses to examine their knowledge of malpractice issues in nursing, it is possible that nurses who possessed considerable knowledge of malpractice issues would be more likely to return the questionnaire than nurses with little knowledge of this subject.

After the discussion about various types of sampling procedures, it must be pointed out that nursing research studies involve voluntary subjects, regardless of the type of sam-

TABLE 10–3. Sampling Error						
Average pulse rates of a group	66	80	59	70	71	
of cardiac patients	71	63	70	74	55	
	70	65	67	92	83	
	67	79	66	80	72	$\mu = 71$
Random Sample #1	66, 59, 70, 55, 66		$\bar{x} = 63$			
Random Sample #2	80, 92, 83, 79, 80		$\bar{x} = 83$			
Random Sample #3	71, 71, 70, 64, 67		$\bar{x} = 71$			

μ = population mean; $\bar{x}$ = sample mean. (See Chapter 13 for definitions of terms.)

pling procedure that is used. Even if a random sampling method is used to select potential study subjects, the ethics of research requires that subjects must voluntarily agree to participate in research studies. Not all selected subjects may agree to participate in a study. The nurse researcher must always keep in mind that data are based on voluntary responses. Unless all selected members of the sample actually participate in the research study, the potential for a biased sample is present.

Finally, a note of caution is presented about volunteers. **Volunteers** are subjects who approach the researcher asking to participate in the study. This type of sample is to be distinguished from a convenience sample, in which the researcher approaches the potential subjects and asks them to participate in a study. Volunteers may be greater risk takers than nonvolunteers. They also may be motivated to participate by monetary or other types of rewards. Diekman and Smith (1989) cautioned researchers to consider the potential biases of using volunteers when setting up the sampling procedure for a study.

Wewers and Ahijevych (1990) pointed out the differences between random samples and volunteer subjects. They studied the reactions of two groups of adult cigarette smokers to a smoking cessation campaign. One group was obtained through random telephone digit dialing, and the other group was composed of volunteers who registered through the community lung association. Demographic characteristics, such as educational levels, differed between the two groups. The volunteer group was much more successful at attempting and maintaining cessation than the randomly selected group. They confirmed that problems of generalizability exist when nonprobability samples are used in a study.

RANDOMIZATION PROCEDURES IN RESEARCH

Random sampling and random assignment are two areas that seem to cause a great deal of confusion among beginning researchers. These two terms involve quite different aspects of the research process, but both are considered a type of randomization procedure. Random sampling involves the selection of a sample from the population. Random assignment involves the unbiased assigning of subjects from a sample into groups in an experimental study. Random assignment is a necessary condition of a true experimental design and was discussed under experimental studies in Chapter 8. It seems important to discuss this concept again because of the tendency to confuse the two types of randomization procedures. Figure 10–1 depicts the threefold randomization process for experimental studies that would represent the ideal study procedure. First, subjects are randomly selected from the population. Next, subjects are randomly assigned to groups. Finally, experimental treatments are randomly assigned to the groups.

CRITIQUING THE SAMPLING PROCEDURE

The critiquer of a research study should be concerned with the study population and sample. There may be a separate section presented on the population and sample in a research article or report, but usually this information is contained in the methods section. It is generally easy to find the information about the sample, but the population from which the sample was selected may not be discussed.

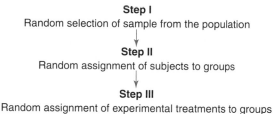

Step I
Random selection of sample from the population

Step II
Random assignment of subjects to groups

Step III
Random assignment of experimental treatments to groups

Figure 10–1. Randomization steps in experimental research.

The reader of a research report would like to know the group to which the investigator wishes to generalize the study results (target population) and the group from which the sample was selected (accessible population). To help the reader determine if the sample is representative of the accessible population, the report should describe the accessible population. The characteristics of the members of this group should be presented, including average age, gender, and educational level. The size of the accessible population should be presented. If there were 100 subjects in a study, the reader of the report would like to know if these 100 subjects represented a fraction of the accessible population or a large portion of this group.

The specific type of probability or nonprobability sampling method should be presented. Although probability sampling is the ideal, most nursing research studies use nonprobability samples. The reader should try to determine how the sample was obtained. Were the subjects volunteers or were they approached and asked to participate in the study? The characteristics of the sample should be described.

The sample size is an important area for critique. Most nursing studies have used small, nonrandom samples. If a small sample size was used, does the researcher present

Box 10–1. Guidelines for Critiquing the Sampling Procedure

1. Is the target population identified?
2. Is the accessible population identified?
3. Was a probability or nonprobability sampling method used?
4. Is the specific sampling method named?
5. Is the sampling technique described?
6. Is the sampling method appropriate for the study?
7. Are the demographic characteristics of the sample presented?
8. Is the sample size adequate?
9. Is the sample representative of the population?
10. Are potential sampling biases identified?
11. Is subject dropout discussed?

the rationale for the sample size? Also, if some of the subjects dropped out of the study, the researcher has the obligation to point out this fact to the reader. Frequently, the reader is made aware of subject dropout when examining the tables. For example, a sample size of $n = 58$ that is presented in a table may not agree with the sample size of 60 that was mentioned in the methods section. Two subjects have mysteriously disappeared! Guidelines for critiquing the sampling section of a research report are presented in Box 10–1.

SUMMARY

Populations are complete sets of people or objects that possess some common characteristic of interest to the researcher. The investigator wishes to generalize study findings to a target population but generally is only able to study an accessible population. Studying entire populations is time consuming and expensive. Samples, or subsets of the population, are usually studied in nursing research. A single member of the population is called an **element,** and these elements are chosen from a **sampling frame** or listing of the population elements.

Samples are chosen through two types of sampling procedures: probability and nonprobability. **Probability sampling** involves random selection of a sample from a population. The four types of probability sampling methods are simple, stratified, cluster, and systematic. **Simple random sampling** ensures that each element of the population has an equal and independent chance of being chosen. A **table of random numbers** may be used to obtain a random sample. **Stratified random sampling** involves dividing the population into subgroups, and then random samples are chosen from these groups. In **proportional stratified sampling,** samples are chosen from each stratum, and these samples are in proportion to the size of that stratum in the total population. When strata are unequal in size, **disproportional stratified sampling** may be used to ensure adequate samples from each stratum. **Cluster random sampling** involves sampling from large groups called clusters. Individual members of clusters are selected in the final stage of the sampling process. Finally, in **systematic random sampling** every kth element of the population, such as every fifth element, is selected.

In **nonprobability sampling,** the sample elements are chosen by nonrandom methods. The types of nonprobability sampling methods are convenience, quota, and purposive. **Convenience sampling** uses readily available people or objects. **Snowball sampling** is a type of convenience sampling in which subjects provide the names of other people they know who meet the criteria for the study. **Quota sampling** is similar to stratified random sampling, except that the desired number of elements for each stratum are selected through convenience sampling. **Purposive sampling** involves "handpicking" of subjects based on the researcher's consideration of the subjects as "typical" of the desired sample.

Longitudinal studies gather data from the same subjects several times to determine change associated with the passage of time. In a **cohort study,** persons are studied who have been born during a particular time period. **Cross-sectional studies** examine several different groups that are thought to be representative of different age groups, time periods, or developmental states.

Generally, large samples are more representative of the population than are small samples. As a rule, a sample size of 30 should be considered the minimum size for each group that is studied. **Power analysis** is a procedure that can be used to determine the optimum sample size for a study, particularly an experimental study.

Sampling error is the difference between data obtained from samples and data that would be obtained if an entire population was studied. This error is due to chance and is not under the researcher's control. **Sampling bias** occurs when samples are not carefully selected by the researcher. **Volunteers** are subjects who approach the researcher asking to participate in a study.

Randomization procedures in research involve random sampling and random assignment. Random sampling concerns selection of a sample from a population. Random assignment involves the unbiased assignment of subjects into groups in experimental studies.

NURSING RESEARCH ON THE WEB

For additional online resources, research activities, and exercises, go to www.prenhall.com/nieswiadomy. Select Chapter 10 from the drop down menu.

✗ GET INVOLVED ACTIVITIES

1. Find a research article that indicates a probability sample was studied. Tell your peers how many studies you had to peruse before finding one that used a probability sampling method. Keep a checklist of the types of nonprobability sampling methods that were used.

2. When examining studies published in the literature, write down the size of the sample that was used in each study. Compare sample sizes of the studies you found with those found by your peers. Determine the smallest and the largest sample sizes that were discussed in the research articles reviewed.

3. Divide into groups. Propose a study idea and identify the type of sampling technique that would be most appropriate.

4. Ask someone to bring a copy of Cohen's book on power analysis to class. Glance through the book and look at the tables that show desired samples sizes and how they are calculated.

✗ SELF-TEST

Write T (True) or F (False) beside the following statements:

_____ 1. The best means of obtaining an unbiased sample of subjects in a community is to select a random sample of names from the telephone directory.

_____ 2. Nonprobability sampling means that there is no probability that the subjects selected will constitute a biased sample.

_____ 3. Researchers generally study samples rather than populations.

_____ 4. A sampling frame is a listing of all elements of a population.

Identify the type of sampling method used in the following examples:

5. The clients in the hypertension clinics of two local hospitals are studied.

6. A total of 20 nursing service administrators are randomly selected from a random sample of 10 hospitals in the state.

7. Every fifth nurse is randomly selected from the mailing list of the American Nurses Association.

8. The first 30 males and first 30 females who are admitted to the hospital for abdominal surgery, during the time of the research study, are asked to participate.

9. To determine the frequency of the recording of nursing diagnoses by nurses, a sample of 100 charts is randomly selected from all of the patients' charts during the previous year.

Circle the letter before the *best* answer.

10. Which of the following is a probability sampling method?
    A. convenience
    B. cluster
    C. quota
    D. purposive

✖ REFERENCES

Abdellah, F. G., & Levine, E. (1994). *Preparing nursing research for the 21st century.* Springer: New York.

Catlin, A. J. (1999). Physicians' neonatal resuscitation of extremely low-birth-weight preterm infants. *Image: Journal of Nursing Scholarship, 31,* 269–275.

Cohen, J. (1988). Statistical power analysis for the behavioral sciences (2nd ed.). Hillsdale, NJ: Lawrence Erlbaum Associates.

Diekman, J. M., & Smith, J. M. (1989). Strategies for recruitment of subjects for nursing research. *Western Journal of Nursing Research, 11,* 418–430.

Dilorio, C., Dudley, W. N., Soet, J., Watkins, J., & Maibach, E. (2000). A social cognitive-based model for condom use among college students. *Nursing Research, 49,* 208–214.

Estabrooks, C. A. (1999). The conceptual structure of research utilization. *Research in Nursing & Health, 22,* 203–216.

Keuter, K., Bryne, E., Voell, J., & Larson, E. (2000). Nurses job satisfaction and organizational climate in a dynamic work environment. *Applied Nursing Research, 13,* 46–49.

King, K. M. (2000). Gender and short-term recovery from cardiac surgery. *Nursing Research, 49,* 29–36.

Knapp, T. R. (1996). The overemphasis on power analysis. *Nursing Research, 45,* 379–380.

Lauver, D. R., Settersten, L., Marten, S., & Halls, J. (1999). Explaining women's intentions and use of hormones with menopause. *Research in Nursing and Health, 22,* 309–320.

MacMullen, N. J., & Dulski, L. A. (2000). Factors related to sucking ability in healthy newborns. *JOGNN: Journal of Obstetric, Gynecologic, and Neonatal Nursing, 29,* 390–396.

Massive nurses' health study in seventh year, reports first findings on disease links in women. (1983). *American Journal of Nursing, 83,* 998–999.

Neu, M., Browne, J. V., & Vojir, C. (2000). The impact of two transfer techniques used during skin-to-skin care on the physiologic and behavioral responses of preterm infants. *Nursing Research, 49,* 215–223.

Orne, R. M., Fishman, S. J., Manka, M., & Pagnozzi, M. E. (2000). Living on the edge: A phenomenological study of medically uninsured working Americans. *Research in Nursing & Health, 23,* 204–212.

Parker, B., McFarlane, J., Soeken, K., Silva, C., & Reel S. (1999). Testing an intervention to prevent further abuse to pregnant women. *Research in Nursing & Health, 22,* 59–66.

Polit, D. F., & Sherman, R. E. (1990). Statistical power in nursing research. *Nursing Research, 39,* 365–369.

Roscoe, J. (1975). *Fundamental research statistics for the behavioral sciences* (2nd ed.). New York: Holt, Rinehart & Winston.

Shelley, S. (1984). *Research methods in nursing and health.* Boston: Little, Brown.

Tolle, S. W., Tilden, V. P., Rosenfeld, A. G., & Hickman, S. E. (2000). Family reports of barriers to optimal care of the dying. *Nursing Research, 49,* 310–317.

Wewers, M. E., & Ahijevych, K. (1990). Differences in volunteer and randomly acquired samples. *Applied Nursing Research, 3,* 166–173.

CHAPTER 11

Measurement and Collection of Data

❊ OUTLINE

❊ OBJECTIVES

On completion of this chapter, you will be prepared to:

1. Demonstrate an understanding of the concept of measurement
2. Differentiate between the four levels of measurement
3. Determine the appropriate level of measurement for data in selected studies
4. Recall questions to be answered in the data-collection process
5. Identify data-collection methods
6. Discuss the selection of a data-collection instrument
7. List criteria for selection of a data-collection instrument
8. Compare and contrast three types of reliability

9. Compare and contrast four types of validity
10. Explain four sources of error that may occur in data collection
11. Critique the data-collection section of research reports

✕ NEW TERMS DEFINED IN THIS CHAPTER

concurrent validity
construct validity
content validity
criterion validity
equivalence reliability
face validity
factor analysis
internal consistency reliability
interobserver reliability
interrater reliability
interval level of measurement

known-groups procedure
measurement
nominal level of measurement
ordinal level of measurement
predictive validity
ratio level of measurement
reliability
research instruments
stability reliability
validity

Many researchers get excited when they talk about the data-collection phase of their studies. This is the time when they get to interact with their subjects on a personal basis or through reading their responses on questionnaires. This is when the real detective work begins!

In any study, the investigator must devise a way to examine or measure the concepts of interest. For example, anxiety could be measured in several ways, such as through galvanic skin response, pulse rates, or self-report questionnaires. The means of measuring variables is determined by the researcher. An understanding of measurement principles and the data-collection process is important for the nurse researcher. Specific types of data-collection methods are discussed in Chapter 12.

MEASUREMENT PRINCIPLES

An understanding of measurement principles is crucial in the data-collection phase of a study. Research variables must be operationally defined. As you recall, operational definitions indicate how variables will be observed or measured.

Measurement is the process of assigning numbers to variables. Ways to assign these numbers include counting, ranking, and comparing objects or events. Mankind has been using some type of measurement system throughout history. Probably fingers and toes were the first method of counting and keeping track of numbers. Measurement, as used in research, implies the quantification of information, that is, the assigning of some type of number to the data. Some qualitative studies gather data in narrative form, and numbers are not associated with these data. These data, therefore, would not be included in the concept of measurement, as it is discussed in this book. If these qualitative data were summarized and placed into categories, they would then fit the criteria for measurement. In the classic sense, measurement implies that some kind of comparison is made between pieces of information. Numbers are the means of comparing this information.

LEVEL OF MEASUREMENT

The types of mathematical calculations that can be made with data depend on the level of measurement of the data. The terms *level of measurement* and *measurement scale* are frequently used interchangeably. Four levels of measurement or measurement scales have been identified: nominal, ordinal, interval, and ratio.

Using the **nominal level of measurement,** objects or events are "named" or categorized. The categories must be distinct from each other (mutually exclusive categories) and include all of the possible ways of categorizing the data (exhaustive categories). There may be only two categories or there may be many categories. Numbers are obtained for this type of data through counting the frequency or percentages of objects or events in each of the categories.

Examples of types of nominal data are gender, religion, marital status, and political party. The researcher could count the number of males and females in a study and report these as percentages or frequencies. No other mathematical operations could be performed with these data. You may have noticed that these types of variables are frequently assigned numbers on questionnaires, such as 1 for males and 2 for females. These numbers are only symbols used for data analysis purposes and have no quantitative meaning. In fact, they would more properly be called numerals rather than numbers.

Some types of nominal data may appear to contain "real" numbers. Examples are zip codes and Social Security numbers. These numbers are symbols and can only be placed into categories. They should not be added or subtracted. The nominal level of measurement is considered the lowest level or least rigorous of the measurement levels.

Data that can be rank ordered as well as placed into categories are considered to be at the **ordinal level of measurement.** The exact differences between the ranks cannot be specified with this type of data. The numbers that are obtained from this measurement process indicate the order rather than the exact quantity of the variables. For example, anxiety levels of people in a therapy group might be categorized as mild, moderate, and severe. It would be appropriate to conclude that those individuals with severe anxiety are more anxious than those individuals with moderate anxiety. In turn, moderate anxiety sufferers in the group could be considered more anxious than group members with mild anxiety. You could not, however, determine the exact difference in anxiety levels according to the different classifications or the quantity of anxiety of any individual within each of the categories. Frequency distributions and percentages are used with this type of data as well as some statistical tests that are discussed in Chapter 14.

Interval data consist of "real" numbers. **Interval level of measurement** concerns data that not only can be placed in categories and ranked, but also the distance between the ranks can be specified. The categories in interval data are the actual numbers on the scale (such as on a thermometer). If body temperature were being measured, a reading of 99.0°F might be one category, 98.6°F might be another category, and 98.2°F might constitute a third category. The researcher would be correct in saying that there is 0.4°F difference between the first and second category and between the second and third category. The researcher could even go one step further and find the average temperature reading.

Data collected at the ratio level of measurement are considered the "highest" level of data. **Ratio level of measurement** includes data that can be categorized and ranked; in addition, the distance between ranks can be specified, and a "true" or natural zero point can be identified. The zero point on the ratio scale means that there is a total absence of the quantity being measured. The amount of money in your bank account could be considered ratio data because it is possible (and quite likely, at times!) to be zero.

If a researcher wanted to determine the number of pain medication requests made by two groups of patients, it would be possible for the subjects in one group to ask for no pain medication. This type of data would be considered ratio data.

There is a debate about classifying some data as interval or ratio. For example, should weight be considered as interval or ratio data? Most authors classify weight as ratio data. However, when measuring humans, can someone have *no* weight?

Although it may be great fun to debate whether a certain piece of data should be classified as interval or ratio, it is really unimportant, for research purposes, to distinguish between these two levels of measurement. The same statistical tests can be used with both types of data. These two types are considered together in Chapters 13 and 14 when discussing analysis of data.

CONVERTING DATA TO A LOWER LEVEL OF MEASUREMENT

Data can always be converted from one level to a lower level of measurement, but not to a higher level. Interval and ratio data can be converted to ordinal or nominal data, and ordinal data can be converted to nominal data. For example, body temperature readings using a Fahrenheit scale could be converted to ordinal data. Subjects with temperatures above 101.0°F could be considered to have high elevations of temperature. Subjects with temperatures between 100.4°F and 101.0°F might be considered to have moderate elevations of temperature. Subjects with temperatures between 99.4°F and 100.2°F might be classified as having mild temperature elevations. Finally, those subjects with temperatures below 99.4°F might be considered to have no temperature elevation. This would be an instance of converting interval data to ordinal data. It would also be possible to change these data to nominal data by classifying the subjects into two groups: those with an elevated temperature and those with no elevation of temperature. The arbitrary cutoff point might be 100.0°F, for example. Rarely do researchers convert higher levels of data to lower levels, however, because precision is always lost.

DETERMINING THE APPROPRIATE LEVEL OF MEASUREMENT

Now that you are familiar with the levels of measurement, you may wonder how the determination is made of which level of measurement to use in a study. If the researcher is concerned about the precision of the data, the interval or ratio level of measurement should be selected, when possible. If ranked or categorized data are sufficient to answer the research questions or test the research hypotheses, ordinal data may be used. Finally, if categories of data are all that is called for, nominal data are appropriate. If the researcher were trying to determine the differences in the number of complications experienced by patients with diabetes who have varying blood glucose levels, accuracy would be important. The two categories of elevated and nonelevated blood glucose levels (nominal data) would not be precise enough for making comparisons among the subjects. In this particular example, the researcher could choose any of the measurement levels because all levels are possible on the variable of blood glucose values. The operational definition of the variable will determine the level of data that will be gathered.

Some variables by their very nature can be measured at only one level. For example, gender can be measured only at a nominal level. A person is either a male or a female. The main considerations in determining the level of measurement for data are (a) the level of measurement that is appropriate for the type of data that is being sought, and (b) the degree of precision that is desired when it is possible to consider the data at more than one level of measurement.

DATA-COLLECTION PROCESS

There are five important questions to ask when the researcher is in the process of collecting data: What? How? Who? Where? When?

What data will be collected? This question calls for a decision to be made about the type of data that is being sought. For example, is the study designed to measure knowledge, attitudes, or behaviors? The type of data that is being sought, of course, will also govern the how, who, where, and when of the data-collection process. The answers to all of these questions are interrelated, and it may be difficult to determine which question should be answered first. The type of data needed to answer the research questions or to test the research hypothesis should be the main consideration in data collection. If the researcher is concerned with the way crises affect people, the "what" of data collection becomes persons' behaviors or responses in crises.

How will the data be collected? Some type of research instrument will be needed to gather the data. This can vary from a self-report questionnaire to the most sophisticated of physiological instruments. Choosing a data-collection instrument is a major decision that should be made only after careful consideration of the possible alternatives. Chapter 12 contains a discussion of some of the types of instruments used in nursing research.

Who will collect the data? If the researcher is going to collect all of the data, this question is easy to answer. However, scientific investigations frequently involve teams of researchers. The decision will then need to be made about who will collect the data. Other people outside the research team may also be used in the data-collection phase; sometimes data collectors are paid for their services. Any time there is more than one person involved, assurances must be made that the data are being gathered in the same manner. Training will be needed for the data collectors, and checks should be made on the reliability of the collected data.

Where will the data be collected? The setting for data collection must be carefully determined. Optimum conditions should be sought. Having subjects fill out questionnaires in the middle of the hallway while leaning up against a wall would definitely not provide the optimum setting. Sometimes it is difficult to decide on the setting. If questionnaires are being used, a researcher might ask respondents to complete the questionnaire while the researcher remains in the same immediate or general area. This procedure will help ensure return of the questionnaires. If subjects happen to be tired or the room is too hot or too cold, however, the answers that are provided may not be valid. If respondents are allowed to complete the questionnaires at leisure, their answers may be more accurate. A disadvantage of using this procedure may be a reduction in the return rate of the questionnaire.

When will the data be collected? The determination will need to be made of the month, day, and somctimes even the hour for data collection. Also, how long will data collection take? Frequently, the only way to answer this question is through a trial run of the procedure by the researcher. If questionnaires will be used, they should be pretested with people similar to the potential research subjects, to determine the length of time for completion of the instrument. The decision may be made to revise the instrument if it seems to take too long for completion. Unfortunately, data collection usually takes longer than you envisioned! But at the conclusion of this step in research, the investigator generally feels a great sense of accomplishment.

DATA-COLLECTION METHODS

The variable or variables of interest to the researcher must be measured in some fashion. This measurement is carried out through various data-collection methods. Data-collection methods are governed by several factors including (a) the research question(s) or hypothesis(es), (b) the design of the study, and (c) the amount of knowledge available about the variable of interest.

There are many alternatives to choose from when deciding on a data-collection method. Self-report questionnaires, interviews, physiological measures, attitude scales, psychological tests, observational methods, and other types of data-collection methods may be selected. Questionnaires have probably been the most frequently reported method of data collection in published nursing studies.

Many studies use more than one data-collection method. In fact, nursing studies are increasingly reporting the use of more than one method of measuring the variable(s) of interest. When several types of data-collection methods produce similar results, greater confidence in the study findings will occur. Chapter 12 presents data-collection methods.

DATA-COLLECTION INSTRUMENTS

Research instruments, also called research tools, are the devices used to collect data. The instrument facilitates the observation and measurement of the variables of interest. The type of instrument used in a study is determined by the data-collection method(s) selected. If physiological data are sought, some type of physiological instrument is needed. If observational data are needed to measure the variable of interest, some type of observational schedule or checklist is called for. One area of the research over which the investigator has a great deal of control is in the choice of the data-collection instrument. Great care should be taken to select the most appropriate instrument or instruments.

USE OF EXISTING INSTRUMENTS

While conducting a review of the literature on the topic of interest, a researcher may discover that an instrument is already available to measure the research variable(s). The use of an already tested instrument helps to connect the present study with the existing body of knowledge on the variables. Of course, the instrument selected must be appropriate to measure the study variable(s).

There are many sources of available instruments to use in nursing research. Some of the best sources are published compilations of instruments. These compilations are particularly useful because they contain discussions of the instruments, such as the reliability and validity of the tools. In some cases, the instrument is printed in its entirety in these sources; in other cases, information as to where a copy of the tool can be obtained is provided. A list of some of the sources of instruments appropriate for nursing research is listed in Appendix B.

A very useful source for nurse researchers is *Instruments for Clinical Health-Care Research* edited by Frank-Stromborg and Olsen (1997). Another well-used source of instruments for nursing research has been the four-volume series edited by Strickland and Waltz (1988, 1990). These volumes, titled *Measurement of Nursing Outcomes,* are devoted to measurement of client outcomes as well as nursing performance outcomes. The titles of each volume are found in Appendix B.

Many of the existing instruments are copyrighted. The copyright holder must be contacted to obtain permission to use such an instrument. Sometimes this permission is given without cost, and sometimes the researcher has to pay for permission to use the instrument or has to purchase copies of the tool. Frequently, instruments developed in research projects supported by public funding remain uncopyrighted and in the public domain. Investigators have free access to this type of instrument.

If an existing instrument will be used, it may be desirable to contact the developer of the instrument to obtain information on its use in past research. This information is usually provided freely. Tool developers are generally pleased when other researchers desire to use their creations. Frequently, the only request is that a copy of the study results and data, particularly data on the reliability and validity of the instrument, be forwarded to the person who developed the instrument.

DEVELOPING AN INSTRUMENT

If no appropriate instrument can be discovered for a particular study, the researcher must develop a new instrument. It may be possible to revise an existing instrument. Caution must be exercised when this approach to instrument development is used. If any items are altered or deleted or new items added to an existing instrument, the reliability and validity of the tool may be altered. New reliability and validity testing will need to be conducted. Also, permission to revise the instrument will have to be obtained from the developer of the tool.

When a completely new instrument is under consideration, a demanding task is faced. Volumes of books have been written concerning tool development. You may consult some of these sources for further information on this subject.

Chapter 12 presents information on the development of questionnaires. Basic material on questionnaire development is included because nearly every nurse will be faced with developing a questionnaire sometime during her or his nursing career, whether for use in research or for some other purpose.

PILOT STUDY

One of the primary reasons a pilot study is conducted is to pretest a newly designed instrument. Whenever a new instrument is being used in a study or a preexisting instrument is being used with people who have different characteristics from those for whom the instrument was originally developed, a pilot study should be conducted.

A pilot study is a small-scale, trial run of the actual research project. A group of people similar to the study subjects should be tested in conditions similar to those used in the actual study. There is no set number of persons needed for a pilot study. A fairly common number is about 10 subjects. Factors such as time, cost, and availability of persons similar to the study subjects will help determine the size of the pilot group.

In an article published in *Applied Nursing Research,* Jairath, Hogerney, and Parsons (2000) discussed the role of a pilot study and gave pointers on the process of conducting a pilot study. They wrote that the researcher may test a long and a short version of the data-collection instrument, try multiple instruments that are purported to measure the same factor or construct, or test various approaches for administering the tools or instruments.

CRITERIA FOR SELECTION OF A DATA-COLLECTION INSTRUMENT

Several criteria must be considered when deciding on a data-collection instrument. These include the practicality, reliability, and validity of the instrument.

PRACTICALITY OF THE INSTRUMENT

Before the researcher examines the reliability and validity of an instrument, questions should be asked about the practicality of the tool for the particular study that is being planned. The practicality of an instrument concerns its cost and appropriateness for the study population. How much will the instrument cost? How long will it take to administer the instrument? Will the population have the physical and mental stamina to complete the instrument? Are special motor skills or language abilities required of subjects? Does the researcher require special training to administer or score the instrument? If so, is this training available? If a psychological instrument such as the Minnesota Multiphasic Personality Inventory (MMPI) will be used, is money available to purchase the instrument, and is someone available to analyze the data? These are important questions; the researcher must attend to the practicality of the instrument before considering its reliability and validity.

RELIABILITY OF THE INSTRUMENT

The researcher is always interested in collecting reliable data. The **reliability** of an instrument concerns its consistency and stability. If you are using a thermometer to measure body temperature, you would expect it to provide the same reading each time it was placed in a constant temperature water bath.

Regardless of the type of research, the reliability of the study instrument(s) is always of concern. Reliability needs to be determined whether the instrument is a mechanical device, a written questionnaire, or a human observer. The degree of reliability is usually determined by the use of correlational procedures. A correlation coefficient is determined between two sets of scores or between the ratings of two judges: The higher the correlation coefficient, the more reliable is the instrument or the judges. Correlation coefficients can range between −1.00 and +1.00. A more thorough explanation of correlation coefficients is presented in Chapter 13.

Correlation coefficients computed to test the reliability of an instrument are expected to be positive correlations. Generally, a correlation coefficient above .70 is considered satisfactory (Polit & Hungler, 1999). Although correlation coefficients are frequently used to determine the reliability of an instrument, when observers or raters are used in a study the percentage or rate of agreement may also be used to determine the reliability of observations or ratings.

In general, the more items that an instrument contains, the more reliable the instrument will be. The likelihood of coming closer to obtaining a true measurement increases as the sample of items to measure a variable increases; however, if a test becomes too long, subjects may get tired or bored.

Caution must be taken concerning the reliability of instruments. Reliability is not a property of the instrument that, once established, remains forever. Reliability must be assessed continually as the instrument is used with different subjects and under different environmental conditions. An instrument to measure patient autonomy might be highly reliable when administered to patients while in their hospital rooms, but it may be unreliable when administered to these same patients while they are lying on a stretcher outside the operating room before surgery.

Strickland (1999) cautioned researchers to be sure they select the most appropriate type of reliability measurement for the instrument that will be used in a study. She stated, "a good instrument could be evaluated as lacking reliability when the real problem is that the wrong reliability assessment approach has been used" (p. 4). Three different types of reliability are discussed: stability, equivalence, and internal consistency.

Stability Reliability. The **stability reliability** of an instrument refers to its consistency over time. A physiological instrument, such as a thermometer, should be stable and accurate. If a thermometer were to be used in a study, it would need to be checked for reliability before the study began and probably again during the study (test-retest reliability).

Questionnaires can also be checked for their stability. A questionnaire might be administered to a group of people, and after a time the instrument would again be administered to the same people. If subjects' responses were almost identical both times, the instrument would be determined to have high test-retest reliability. If the scores were perfectly correlated, the correlation coefficient (coefficient of stability) would be 1.00.

The interval between the two testing periods may vary from a few days to several months or even longer. This period is a very important consideration when trying to determine the stability of an instrument. The period should be long enough for the subjects to forget their original answers but not long enough that real changes may have occurred in the subjects' responses.

If you were interested in developing a test to measure a personality trait, such as assertiveness, you might expect stability of responses. But because there has been a great deal of emphasis on assertiveness training in recent years, subjects might not score the same on an assertiveness test if the period between administrations is more than a few days. Many nursing studies are concerned with attitudes and behaviors that are not stable, and changes would be expected on two administrations of the same questionnaire. Stability over time (test-retest reliability) may therefore not be the appropriate type of reliability to try to achieve for a research instrument.

Meek et al. (2000) compared the test-retest reliability of four instruments to measure fatigue among cancer patients. The four instruments were: Profile of Mood States Short Form fatigue subscale (F_POMS-sf), Multidimensional Assessment of Fatigue (MAF), Lee Fatigue Scale (LFS), and the Multidimensional Fatigue Inventory (MFI). Test-retest correlations for total scores on all four instruments showed good stability. However, some subscales of the LFS and MFI demonstrated marginal stability.

Equivalence Reliability. **Equivalence reliability** concerns the degree to which two different forms of an instrument obtain the same results, or two or more observers using a single instrument obtain the same results. *Alternate forms* or *parallel forms* are terms used when two forms of the same instrument are compared. **Interrater** or **interobserver reliability** are terms applied to the comparisons of raters or observers using the same instrument. This type of reliability is determined by the degree to which two or more independent raters or observers are in agreement.

When two forms of a test are used, both forms should contain the same number of items, have the same level of difficulty, and so forth. One form of the test is administered to a group of people, and the other form is administered either at the same time or shortly thereafter to these same people. A correlation coefficient (coefficient of equivalence) is obtained between the two forms. The higher the correlation, the more confident the researcher can be that the two forms of the test are gathering the same information. Whenever two forms of an instrument can be developed, this is the preferred means for assessing reliability. Researchers, however, frequently find it difficult to develop one form of an instrument, much less two forms!

> Interrater reliability was assessed in a study of mothers' adjustment to caring for medically fragile infants (Miles, Davis, Burchinal, & Nelson, 1999). A rating scale was developed by the researchers. Ratings were done independently by the two members of the research team who had the most contact with the mothers. After they made their ratings, four members of the research team met as a group with the principal investigator. Each rating was discussed. When differences were found, a discussion ensued, and a consensus was reached. An 85% agreement was found at 6 months and an 83% agreement at 16 months.

Internal Consistency Reliability. **Internal consistency reliability,** or scale homogeneity, addresses the extent to which all items on an instrument measure the same variable. This type of reliability is appropriate only when the instrument is examining one concept or construct at a time. This type of reliability is concerned with the sample of items used to measure the variable of interest.

If an instrument were developed to measure depression, all of the items on the instrument must consistently measure depression. If some items measure guilt, the instrument is not an internally consistent tool. This type of reliability is of concern to nurse researchers because of the emphasis on measuring concepts such as assertiveness, autonomy, and self-esteem.

Several procedures can be used to measure the internal consistency of an instrument. One is the split-half method. The items on the instrument are divided into two halves, and the correlation between the scores on the two parts is computed. The halves may be divided by obtaining the scores on the first half of the test and comparing them with the scores on the second half of the test or by comparing odd-numbered items to even-numbered items. Because the reliability of a test is associated with the number of items, split-half procedures tend to decrease the correlation coefficient. Statistical procedures such as the Spearman-Brown prophecy formula are used to determine what the reliability would be if the entire instrument were used.

Before computer usage became prevalent, internal consistency was tedious to calculate. Today, it is a simple process, and more accurate split-half procedures have been developed. A common type of internal consistency procedure used today is the coefficient alpha (α), or Cronbach's alpha, which provides an estimate of the reliability of all possible ways of dividing an instrument into two halves.

Resnick and Jenkins (2000) assessed the internal consistency of their Self-efficacy for Exercise Scale. Preliminary testing provided evidence for the internal consistency of the tool ($\alpha = .92$).

VALIDITY OF THE INSTRUMENT

The **validity** of an instrument concerns its ability to gather the data that it is intended to gather. The content of the instrument is of prime importance in validity testing. If an instrument is expected to measure assertiveness, does it, in fact, measure assertiveness? It is not difficult to determine that validity is the most important characteristic of an instrument.

The greater the validity of an instrument, the more confidence you can have that the instrument will obtain data that will answer the research questions or test the research hypotheses. Just as the reliability of an instrument does not remain constant, neither does an instrument necessarily retain its level of validity when used with other subjects or in other environmental settings. An instrument might measure assertiveness with one cultural group of subjects, and the same instrument might be measuring authoritarianism with another cultural group.

When attempting to establish the reliability of an instrument, all of the procedures are based on data obtained through using the instrument with subjects. On the other hand, some of the procedures for establishing the validity of an instrument are not based on the administration of the instrument. Validity may be established through the use of a panel of experts or through an examination of the existing literature on the topic. Statistical procedures, therefore, may not always be used in establishing validity as they are used in establishing reliability. When statistical procedures are used, they generally are correlational procedures.

Four broad categories of validity are considered: face, content, criterion, and construct. Face and content validity are concerned only with the instrument under consideration, whereas criterion and construct validity are concerned with how well the instrument under consideration compares with other measures of the variable of interest.

Face Validity. An instrument is said to have **face validity** when a cursory examination shows that it is measuring what it is supposed to measure. In other words, on the surface or the face of the instrument, it appears to be an adequate means of obtaining the data needed for the research project. The face validity of an instrument can be examined through the use of experts in the content area or through the use of people who have characteristics similar to those of the potential subjects. Because of the subjective nature of face validity, this type of validity is rarely used alone.

Content Validity. **Content validity** is concerned with the scope or range of items used to measure the variable. In other words, are the number and type of items adequate to measure the concept or construct of interest? Is there an adequate sampling of all the possible items that could be used to secure the desired data? There are several methods of evaluating the content validity of an instrument.

The first method is accomplished by comparing the content of the instrument with the available literature on the topic. A determination can then be made of the adequacy of the measurement tool in light of existing knowledge in the content area. For example, if a new instrument were being developed to measure the empathic levels of nurses in hospice settings, the researcher would need to be familiar with the literature on both empathy and the hospice setting.

A second way to examine the content validity of an instrument is through the use of a panel of experts, which is a group of people who have expertise in a given subject area. These experts are given copies of the instrument and the purpose and objectives of the study. They then evaluate the instrument, usually on an individual basis rather than in a group. These evaluations are compared, and the researcher then determines if additions, deletions, or changes need to be made.

A third method is used when knowledge tests are being developed. The researcher develops a test blueprint designed around the objectives for the content that is being taught and the level of knowledge that is expected (e.g., retention, recall, and synthesis).

The actual degree of content validity is never established. An instrument possesses some degree of validity that can only be estimated.

> Beck and Gable (2000) demonstrated evidence of content validity of their instrument to measure postpartum depression. They based their estimates of content validity on the literature and a panel of five content experts who reviewed the instrument. Four of the five panel members were not only experts in postpartum depression but also had personal experience with this mood disorder. Additionally, a focus group of 15 graduate students in nursing, whose clinical specialties were obstetrics and psychiatry, reviewed the instrument.

Criterion Validity. **Criterion validity** is concerned with the extent to which an instrument corresponds to or is correlated with some criterion measure of the variable of interest. Criterion validity assesses the ability of an instrument to determine subjects' responses at the present time or predict subjects' responses in the future. These two types of criterion validity are called concurrent and predictive validity, respectively.

Concurrent validity compares an instrument's ability to obtain a measurement of subjects' behavior that is comparable to some other criterion of that behavior. Does the instrument under consideration correlate with another instrument that measures the same behavior or responses? For example, a researcher might want to develop a short instrument that would help to evaluate the suicidal potential of people when they call in to the suicide crisis intervention center. A short, easily administered interview instrument would be of great help to the staff, but the researcher would want to be sure that this instrument was a valid diagnostic instrument to assess suicide potential. Responses received on the short instrument could be compared with those received when using an already validated, but longer, suicide assessment tool. If both instruments seem to be obtaining the essential information necessary to make a decision about the suicide potential of a person, the new instrument might be considered to have criterion validity. The degree of validity would be determined through correlation of the results of the two tests administered to a number of people. The correlation coefficient must be at least .70 to consider that the two instruments are obtaining similar data.

The researcher might also be interested in knowing if the suicide potential assessment tool would be useful in predicting actual suicidal behavior in the future. The second type of criterion validity, **predictive validity,** is concerned with the ability of an instrument to predict behavior or responses of subjects in the future. If the predictive validity of an instrument is established, it can be used with confidence to discriminate between people, at the present time, in relation to their future behavior. This would be a very valuable quality for an instrument to possess.

> Criterion-related validity (concurrent) was one of the measures used by Bakas and Champion (1999) to test the 10-item Bakas Caregiving Outcomes Scale (BCOS). Testing of the instrument was conducted with two samples of family caregivers of stroke survivors. Criterion validity was supported in both samples by significant correlations with an existing instrument to measure global well-being, the LIFE-3.

Construct Validity.   Of all of the types of validity, construct validity is the most difficult to measure. **Construct validity** is concerned with the degree to which an instrument measures the construct that it is supposed to measure. A construct is a concept or abstraction that is created or "constructed" by the researcher. Construct validity involves the measurement of a variable that is not directly observable but rather is a construct or abstraction derived from observable behavior. Construct validity is derived from the underlying theory that is used to describe or explain the construct.

Many of the variables that are measured in research are labeled constructs. Nursing is concerned with constructs such as anxiety, assertiveness, and androgyny.

One method to measure construct validity is called the known-groups procedure. In the **known-groups procedure** the instrument under consideration is administered to two groups of people whose responses are expected to differ on the variable of interest. For example, if you were developing an instrument to measure depression, the theory used to explain depression would indicate the types of behavior that would be expected in depressed people. If the tool were administered to a group of supposedly depressed subjects and to a group of supposedly happy subjects, you would expect the two groups to score quite differently on the tool. If differences were not found, you might suspect that the instrument was not really measuring depression.

Another approach to construct validity is called factor analysis. **Factor analysis** is a method used to identify clusters of related items on an instrument or scale. This type of procedure will help the researcher to determine whether the tool is measuring only one construct or several constructs. Correlational procedures are used to determine if items cluster together.

> The **known-groups** method of construct validity was assessed in the development of the Environment-Behavior Interaction Code (EBIC), which was designed to be used in dementia care research (Stewart, Hiscock, Morgan, Murphy, & Yamamoto, 1999). Eighty-two residents

of long-term care facilities were classified as either low risk (n = 27) or moderate-to-high risk (n = 55) for disruptive behavior. The EBIC was able to discriminate between residents according to their risk of disruptive behavior. The researchers contended that the know-groups validity results support the use of the EBIC system in dementia care research.

An instrument to measure professional nursing values was subjected to **factor analysis** by Weis and Schank (2000). A 44-item instrument with a Likert-scale format was administered to 357 baccalaureate students, 125 master's students, and 117 practicing nurses. Eight factors were identified. The two major factors were caregiving and activism.

RELATIONSHIP BETWEEN RELIABILITY AND VALIDITY

Reliability and validity are closely associated. Both of these qualities are considered when selecting a research instrument. Reliability is usually considered first because it is a necessary condition for validity. An instrument cannot be valid unless it is reliable. However, the reliability of an instrument tells nothing about the degree of validity. In fact, an instrument can be very reliable and have *low* validity.

Although reliability was considered first in the discussion of reliability and validity, in actuality, validity is often considered first in the construction of an instrument. Face validity and content validity may be examined, and then some type of reliability is considered. Next, another type of validity may be considered. The process is not always the same. The type of desired validity and the type of reliability are determined, and then the procedures for establishing these criteria for the instrument are determined. A word of caution is issued about using the term *established* in regard to reliability and validity of instruments. Strickland, in an editorial in the *Journal of Nursing Measurement* (1995), stated that reliability and validity cannot be established because there is always an error component in measurement. She wrote that it is more correct to use terms like *supported, assessed,* or *prior evidence has shown* (p. 91).

SOURCES OF ERROR IN DATA COLLECTION

Variations are usually expected in data that are collected from different participants in a study. If the researcher did not expect to find some type of variation in the data, there would probably be no interest in conducting the study. It is hoped that the variations or differences that are found are "real" rather than "artificial." Every researcher must recognize that some error component is likely to exist in the data that are obtained, especially when the data are being collected from human beings and the degree of control that can be placed on the research situation is limited. The errors in data collection can arise from (a) instrument inadequacies, (b) instrument administration biases, (c) environmental variations during the data-collection process, and (d) temporary subject characteristics during the data-collection process.

Instrument inadequacies concern the items used to collect data and the instructions to subjects that are contained within the instrument, such as a questionnaire. Are the items appropriate to collect the data that are being sought? Do the items adequately cover the range of content? Will the order of the items influence subjects' responses? Are the items and directions for completing items clear and unbiased?

Even when there are no errors in the research instrument, biases or errors can occur in the administration of the instrument. Is the instrument administered in the same fashion to all subjects? Are observers collecting data in the same manner?

Environmental conditions during data collection can also influence the data that are gathered. Is the location for data collection the same for all subjects? Are conditions such as temperature, noise levels, and lighting kept consistent for all subjects?

Finally, the characteristics of the subjects during data collection can be a source of error in research data. Are there any personal characteristics of the subjects, such as anxiety levels, hunger, or tiredness, influencing responses? This source of error frequently is called transitory personal factors.

PREPARING DATA FOR ANALYSIS

Once data have been gathered, they must be prepared for analysis. If the computer will be used to analyze data, it is very important that the data are in a form that facilitates entry into the computer. Quantitative data, such as age and weight, may be entered directly into the computer. Qualitative data, such as information obtained from open-ended questions, will need to be transferred into symbols that the computer can understand. Because computer time may be costly, it is important to have data ready for speedy entry. It is not the time to be shuffling back and forth between pieces of paper searching for data. Data coding should be considered, and decisions about missing data made before data entry begins.

USE OF A STATISTICAL CONSULTANT

Many nurse researchers now have personal computers and statistical software packages and are able to do much of their data analysis on their own. However, the use of a statistical consultant is still a much needed part of many research projects. Most research projects require several hours of consultation time. More time will be required if the statistician is asked to do programming or to perform complicated statistical analyses. If you are writing a grant, statistical consultation costs should be included in the budget.

Some researchers visit a statistician after their data are collected to find out what "to do" with their data. This is not the proper way to use the statistician's talents. The time to seek help is in the early planning stages of a study. Shott (1990) has cautioned researchers to seek statistical consultation early in the project to prevent the entire project from "sinking." She wrote that it is too late after the study is completed to find that the data-collection form is a mess and the sample size is much too small.

CODING DATA

Data must be placed in a form that can be easily analyzed. If questionnaires have been used, code numbers may be placed on the margins of the questionnaires. These numbers then will be used when data are entered on the computer or all of the data from the questionnaires may be transferred to a summary sheet. This sheet will be referred to during the data-entry process. A summary sheet entry for one subject might appear like the following:

Column: 1   2   3   4   5   6   7   8   9
          0   1   1   3   5   1   6   1   2

The brackets have been used to show you that the nine entries actually represent only six pieces of information about the subject. The 01 identifies the person as the first subject. The next 1 indicates that the person is a female. The next two numbers (35) are the subject's age. The sixth column is for marital status, and the 1 indicates that the subject is married. In column 7, the 6 denotes that the subject has six children. Finally, the number 12 in columns 8 and 9 indicates the number of years of formal education that the subject has received. An entry such as this would be provided for each subject in the study.

A code book or code sheet should be devised for the researcher to remember what pieces of information are represented by the entries in the columns of the summary sheet. The code sheet may be a single sheet of paper on which has been written:

Columns 1 and 2	Subject identification number
Column 3	1 = female; 2 = male
Columns 4 and 5	Age at last birthday
Column 6	Marital status:
	0 = never married;
	1 = married;
	2 = separated;
	3 = divorced;
	4 = widowed;
	5 = other
Column 7	Number of children
Columns 8 and 9	Number of years of formal education

Although alphabetical symbols may be used in coding schemes, it is better to use numbers. Some software packages will not accept alphabetical coding.

CRITIQUING THE DATA-COLLECTION PROCEDURES

It is important for the reader of a research report to determine if the measurement and collection of data has been conducted in an appropriate manner. This may be a difficult task because the reader will not get to see the instruments. Even when questionnaires are used, they are rarely contained in the research article or report. However, there are some questions that may be asked (Box 11–1) and guidelines that may be used in critiquing the data-collection section of a research report.

The reader first tries to find a section in the research report where the measurement and collection of data are reported. Information that is desired concerns what data were collected, how the data were collected, who collected the data, where the data were collected, and when the data were collected.

A determination is made of the level of measurement that would be appropriate to test the research hypothesis(es) or answer the research question(s). For example, if compliance with diabetic regimen was the dependent variable, has the researcher used a physiological measure of compliance, or has the patient been asked to self-report compliance?

The research instruments should be described clearly and thoroughly. Information should be provided about the reliability and validity of the instruments. The types and degree of reliability and validity should be reported.

Finally, results of the pilot study should be reported. If a pilot study was not conducted, the rationale for failure to do so should be discussed.

SUMMARY

Measurement is the process of assigning numbers to variables. The four levels of measurement are: nominal, ordinal, interval, and ratio. **Nominal level of measurement** produces data that are "named" or categorized. **Ordinal level of measurement** categorizes and ranks the data. The distance between the ranks can be specified with **interval level of measurement.** In addition to these characteristics, **ratio level of measurement** specifies a true zero point.

Five important questions need to be answered concerning the data-collection process: What data will be collected? How will the data be collected? Who will collect the data? Where will the data be collected? When will the data be collected?

There are many alternatives to choose from when selecting a data-collection method. These methods include questionnaires, interviews, physiological measures, attitude scales, psychological tests, and observational measures. The devices used to collect data are called the **research instruments** or tools. The researcher may use an existing instrument or develop a new instrument.

A pilot study should be conducted whenever a new instrument is being developed or when a preexisting instrument is being used with people who have different characteristics from those for whom the instrument was originally developed.

Factors to be considered when choosing a data-collection instrument are the practicality, reliability, and validity of the instrument. The practicality of an instrument concerns its cost and appropriateness for the population. The **reliability** of an instrument determines its consistency and stability. **Validity** concerns the ability of the instrument to gather the data that it is intended to gather.

Types of reliability are (a) stability, (b) equivalence, and (c) internal consistency. The **stability reliability** of an instrument refers to its consistency over time and is usually determined by test-retest procedures. **Equivalence reliability** concerns the degree to which two forms of an instrument obtain the same results or two or more observers obtain the same results when using a single instrument. **Interrater** or **interobserver reliability** is the degree of agreement on ratings or observations made by independent judges. **Internal consistency reliability** addresses the extent to which all items on an instrument measure the same variable.

Types of validity are (a) face, (b) content, (c) criterion, and (d) construct. **Face validity** measures the degree to which an instrument appears, on the surface, to measure the variable of interest. **Content validity** is concerned with the scope or range of items used to measure the variable. **Criterion validity** considers the degree to which an instrument correlates with some criterion measure on the variable of interest. Two types of criterion validity are concurrent and predictive. **Concurrent validity** compares an instrument's measurement of a variable with a criterion measure of the same variable. **Predictive validity** examines the ability of an instrument to predict behavior of subjects in the future. Finally, **construct validity** concerns the measurement of a variable that is not directly observable but rather is a construct or abstraction derived from observable behavior. Two types of construct validity are the **known-groups procedure** and **factor analysis.**

Reliability and validity are closely associated. Reliability is a necessary condition for validity. An instrument, however, can be reliable and not valid.

Errors in the data-collection process can arise from (a) instrument inadequacies, (b) instrument administration biases, (c) environmental variations during the data-collection process, and (d) temporary subject characteristics during the data-collection process.

The researcher must prepare data for analysis. In many studies, nurse researchers use statistical consultants early in the project as well as in the data-analysis phase.

 ## NURSING RESEARCH ON THE WEB

For additional online resources, research activities, and exercises, go to www.prenhall. com/nieswiadomy. Select Chapter 11 from the drop down menu.

✖ GET INVOLVED ACTIVITIES

1. Contact a nurse researcher that you know and ask this person to share with you information about the reliability and validity of an instrument used in her or his research.

2. Examine five research articles in nursing journals. Determine the types of reliability and validity that are discussed in each article. Keep a tally of the different types that you find and the statistics that are presented (such as the reliability coefficients). Bring these to your group for discussion. Make a list on a blackboard or a poster board of each type of reliability and validity that has been discovered and the number of times each one was mentioned in the literature.

3. Based on the preceding information, determine the most common types of reliability and validity that are being used by nurse researchers.

4. Determine the number of research instruments that are mentioned in these articles that have been shown to have a reliability of at least .70.

5. Divide into groups. Discuss an instrument that you might develop for a particular study. Decide the types of reliability and validity that you think would be most appropriate for your instrument.

✖ SELF-TEST

Examine the following statements. Determine the type of reliability or validity that is indicated in each statement.

1. The Assertiveness Inventory was administered to a group of subjects at two different times, with 1 week between the administrations. The correlation between the scores on the two administrations was .85.

2. The items look like they will obtain the data needed to measure assertiveness.

3. The difference between the subjects' scores on assertiveness and submissiveness was highly significant.

4. The correlation between the subjects' assertiveness scores on graduation from nursing school and their leadership ability 2 years after graduation was .70.

5. The correlation between subjects' scores on Form A and Form B of the Assertiveness Inventory was .60.

Examine the following statements concerning reliability and validity and determine if each statement is true (T) or false (F).

_____ 6. The internal consistency of the Assertiveness Inventory is .90. That means that this instrument is a valid measure of assertiveness.

_____ 7. By increasing the number of items on the Assertiveness Inventory from 20 to 30, the reliability of the instrument will probably increase.

_____ 8. An instrument can be reliable without being valid.

_____ 9. If the reliability of the Assertiveness Inventory was determined to be .45, the validity of the instrument would be in serious doubt.

_____ 10. Reliability is the *most* important factor to take into account when considering an instrument for use in research.

✳ REFERENCES

Bakas, T., & Champion, V. (1999). Development and psychometric testing of the Bakas Caregiving Outcomes Scale. *Nursing Research, 48,* 250–259.

Beck, C. T., & Gable, R. K. (2000). Postpartum depression screening scale: Development and psychometric testing. *Nursing Research, 49,* 272–282.

Frank-Stromborg, M., & Olsen, S. (Eds.). (1997). *Instruments for clinical health-care research.* Boston: Jones Bartlett.

Jairath, N., Hogerney, M., & Parsons, C. (2000). The role of the pilot study: A case illustration from cardiac nursing research. *Applied Nursing Research, 13,* 92–96.

Meek, P. M., Nail, L. M., Barsevick, A., Schwartz, A. L., Stephen, S., Whitmer, K., Beck, S. L., Jones, L. S., & Walker, B. L. (2000). Psychometric testing of fatigue instruments for use with cancer patients. *Nursing Research, 49,* 181–190.

Miles, M. S., Holditch-Davis, D., Burchinal, P., & Nelson, D. (1999). Distress and growth outcomes in mothers of medically fragile infants. *Nursing Research, 48,* 129–140.

Polit, D., & Hungler, B. (1999). *Nursing research: Principles and methods* (6th ed.). Philadelphia: Lippincott.

Resnick, B., & Jenkins, L. S. (2000). Testing the reliability and validity of the self-efficacy for exercise scale. *Nursing Research, 49,* 154–159.

Shott, S. (1990). *Statistics for health professionals.* Philadelphia: Saunders.

Stewart, N. J., Hiscock, M., Morgan, D. G., Murphy, P. B. & Yamamoto, M. (1999). Development and psychometric evaluation of the Environment-Behavior Interaction Code (EBIC). *Nursing Research, 48,* 260–268.

Strickland, O. L. (1995). Can reliability and validity be "established?" *Journal of Nursing Measurement, 3,* 91–92.

Strickland, O. L. (1999). When is internal consistency reliability assessment inappropriate? *Journal of Nursing Measurement, 7,* 3–4.

Strickland, O. L., & Waltz, C. F. (Eds.). (1988). *Measurement of nursing outcomes (Vol. 1). Measuring client outcomes.* New York: Springer.

Strickland, O. L., & Waltz, C. F. (Eds.). (1988). *Measurement of nursing outcomes (Vol. 2). Measuring nursing performance: Practice, education, and research.* New York: Springer.

Strickland, O. L., & Waltz, C. F. (Eds.). (1990). *Measurement of nursing outcomes (Vol. 3). Measuring clinical skills and professional development in education and practice.* New York: Springer.

Strickland, O. L., & Waltz, C. F. (Eds.). (1990). *Measurement of nursing outcomes (Vol. 4). Measuring client self-care and coping skills.* New York: Springer.

Weis, D., & Schank, M. J. (2000). An instrument to measure professional nursing values. *Journal of Nursing Scholarship, 32,* 201–204.

CHAPTER 12

Data-Collection Methods

✗ OBJECTIVES

On completion of this chapter, you will be prepared to:

1. Recognize the importance of questionnaires as a data-collection method for nursing research
2. Enumerate the general characteristics of questionnaires
3. Construct items for a questionnaire
4. List the advantages and disadvantages of questionnaires as a data-collection method
5. Identify the importance of interviews as a data-collection method
6. Recognize the necessity for training of interviewers before data collection
7. Differentiate between the three different levels of structure that can be used in interviews
8. List guidelines to be used in the three phases of an interview
9. Recognize the influence of the interviewer on the subjects' responses
10. List the advantages and disadvantages of interviews as a data-collection method
11. Recognize the importance of observation as a data-collection method
12. Determine the need for physiological and psychological data-collection methods
13. Compare and contrast the various types of data-collection methods
14. Critique the data-collection instruments used in research studies reported in the literature

✗ NEW TERMS DEFINED IN THIS CHAPTER

ambiguous questions
attitude scales
attribute variables
closed-ended questions
collectively exhaustive categories
contingency questions
Delphi technique
demographic questions
demographic variables
double-barreled questions
event sampling
filler questions
interview
interview schedule
Likert scale
mutually exclusive categories
nonparticipant observer-covert
nonparticipant observer-overt
observation research

open-ended questions
participant observer-covert
participant observer-overt
personality inventories
physiological measures
preexisting data
probes
projective techniques
Q sort
questionnaire
semantic differential
semistructured interviews
structured interviews
structured observations
telephone interviews
time sampling
unstructured interviews
unstructured observations
visual analogue scale

Questionnaires and interviews are probably the most frequently used data-collection methods in nursing research. Observation is also an important method of testing research hypotheses and seeking answers to research questions. In addition, various physiological and psychological measures are used by nurse researchers. There are numerous other data-collection measures. Some of the more commonly used measures will be discussed in this chapter. Try not to be confused by the wide variety of methods. Once you have had experience in critiquing research studies and in helping to plan research studies, you will be able to select the most appropriate data-collection method more easily. As you read about the various methods presented in this chapter, try to envision a research project that might call for each type of data-collection method that is discussed.

QUESTIONNAIRES

Is there any one of you who has not completed a questionnaire at some time in your life? If so, it is very unusual. A **questionnaire** is a paper-and-pencil, self-report instrument. It contains questions that respondents are asked to answer in writing.

Many people mistakenly believe that the development of a "good" questionnaire is a fairly easy task. Oppenheim (1966) wrote, "The world is full of well-meaning people who believe that anyone who can write plain English and has a modicum of common sense can produce a good questionnaire" (p. vii). This is definitely not true. The development of a reliable and valid questionnaire is a difficult task. Many questionnaires have been used only one time because they were poorly constructed and did not obtain the type of data for which they were designed. There are many available literature resources for use in the construction of questionnaires. Also, help can be sought from experts in the area of questionnaire construction.

Questionnaires can be used to measure knowledge levels, opinions, attitudes, beliefs, ideas, feelings, and perceptions, as well as to gather factual information about the respondents. Of course, the validity of the data obtained through this method is governed by the subjects' willingness or ability to provide accurate information. Nevertheless, questionnaires are extremely important in nursing research and may be the only method of obtaining data on certain human responses. The nurse researcher must therefore be concerned with the construction of questionnaires. More information will be presented on questionnaires than on the other methods of data collection because each one of you will probably be involved in the construction of a questionnaire at some time during your career.

OVERALL APPEARANCE OF QUESTIONNAIRE

The old saying that "first impressions are lasting impressions" may hold true as potential research subjects scan a study questionnaire. I recently received a questionnaire with poor printing and three spelling errors. Remember, a spell-check software program cannot differentiate between words like *hear* and *here.*

There are many methods of duplicating questionnaires, but it is important to use a high-quality printing process and paper. Questionnaires should be neat in appearance and grammatically correct and should contain no typing or spelling errors. The spacing of questions also influences the appearance of the instrument. A questionnaire that has a cluttered or crowded appearance may be difficult and confusing for the subject to complete. Adequate margins and spacing of the questions are needed. It may be better to add another page to the questionnaire than to crowd too many questions on one page. Keep in mind, however, that if the questionnaire seems too long, potential respondents may become discouraged and either discard the questionnaire or fail to answer all of the questions.

LANGUAGE AND READING LEVEL OF QUESTIONS

The questionnaire should be written in the subjects' preferred language (e.g., English, Spanish) and should be appropriate for the knowledge and reading level of the least educated respondents. If the researcher has limited knowledge of the respondents' educational backgrounds, it is wise to write questions aimed at a sixth grade educational level. Glazer-Waldman, Hall, and Weiner (1985) found the average grade equivalent level to be 6.0 among a group of patients in a large public hospital.

In 1993, a group of researchers examined 50 pieces of widely used patient education materials (Albright et al., 1996). Passages of 100 words from each source were computer analyzed. The mean required readability level varied from 8.62 for diabetes educational material to 11.37 for surgery education material. The mean readability for all of the patient education material was 9.84.

French and Larrabee (1999) found the actual reading levels of 50 adult ambulatory clients with hypertension to be 6.57, while their reported years of education was 9.3. They also determined that a hypertension education pamphlet that was being distributed to these clients had a reading level requirement of 12th grade. It is apparent that patients and their families do not understand a lot of health education materials.

When constructing questionnaires, the questions should be made as simple, clear, and specific as possible. Slang expressions, colloquialisms, and medical or nursing jargon should be avoided. Clients may not understand terms such as nursing diagnosis, client-centered goals, and human responses to potential health problems.

LENGTH OF QUESTIONNAIRE AND QUESTIONS

The length of a questionnaire may influence respondents' willingness to participate in the research. Although research results are inconclusive with regard to the length of a questionnaire that is most likely to be returned, generally speaking, short questionnaires are more likely to be returned than are long ones. It would probably be advisable to limit the required completion time to 10 minutes or less. Shelley (1984) cautioned the researcher to limit the questionnaire to two to four pages, unless the topic would be of great interest to subjects.

Questions should be kept as short as possible. Keep in mind that the purpose of the questions is to seek data and not to test the respondents' reading ability and tenacity. A desirable length for a question is less than 20 words. A question may need to be divided into two questions if the length becomes excessive or the question asks the respondent to consider more than one idea at a time.

WORDING OF QUESTIONS

The most difficult aspect of questionnaire construction is the actual wording of individual questions. Some general guidelines are presented.

I. State Questions in an Affirmative Rather than a Negative Manner.

Negative words, such as *never,* may be overlooked, and the respondent will answer the exact opposite of an intended response. Students often complain about the use of negative wording in questions. Multiple choice test questions are frequently written in the following manner:

All of the following criteria should be met in a research study *except:*

A. There is a problem statement or purpose.
B. The references cited in the literature are current.
C. The limitations of the study are acknowledged.
D. The researcher proved the study hypothesis.

You are now going to have revealed to you a well-kept secret of teachers. Questions are written in the preceding manner because it is much easier to write *one* incorrect answer and three correct answers for a question than it is to write *three* plausible incorrect responses and one correct response.

II. Avoid Ambiguous Questions

Ambiguous questions contain words that have more than one meaning or can be interpreted differently by various people. Examples of such words are: *many, usually, few, often, large, several,* and *generally.*

III. Avoid Double Negative Questions

It is difficult for respondents to reply to a question such as: "Don't you disagree with the idea that...."

IV. Questions Should Contain Neutral Wording

Any question that implies the type of answer to be given may result in biased responses. Consider the following question: "Do you believe that smoking is a disgusting habit?" The desired answer is quite obvious. Even if you think that smoking is a disgusting habit, you would not want to bias the answers of respondents. Examples of a neutrally worded question (A), a subtly biased question (B), and a completely biased question (C) follow:

A. What is your opinion about cigarette smoking?
B. Would you say that you are against cigarette smoking?
C. You do not believe that people should smoke cigarettes, do you?

V. Avoid Double-barreled Questions

Double-barreled questions ask two questions in one. An example of such a question might be, "Do you plan to pursue a master's degree in nursing and seek an administrative position upon graduation?" When a question contains "and," it is quite likely that two questions are being asked rather than one.

TYPES OF QUESTIONS

There are many ways to categorize questions. This section examines the following categories of questions: demographic, open-ended, closed-ended, contingency, and filler questions. These types of questions are not mutually exclusive. For example, a demographic question could be written as an open-ended or a closed-ended question.

Demographic Questions. **Demographic questions** gather data on the characteristics of the subjects. These characteristics, sometimes called **demographic variables** or **at-**

tribute variables, include such things as age, educational background, and religion. Nearly every questionnaire will seek some kind of demographic data. These data will be used to describe the study sample. Also, these data may be subjected to statistical analysis to examine relationships between these subject characteristics and other variables of interest in the study.

Open-ended Questions. The researcher asks respondents to complete questions in their own words in **open-ended questions.** Essay and fill-in-the-blank are types of open-ended questions. Open-ended questions may be used in combination with closed-ended questions. After the closed-ended item is presented, a space may be provided for respondents to answer in their own words if none of the choices seem to apply.

Closed-ended Questions. The most structured type of questions are **closed-ended questions** in which the respondents are asked to choose from given alternatives. There may be only two alternatives, as in a true-or-false question, or there may be many, as in a checklist type of question where respondents are asked to check all items that apply to them. Other types of closed-ended questions include multiple-choice questions and matching questions.

When closed-ended items are used on a questionnaire, the response categories must be (a) collectively exhaustive and (b) mutually exclusive. **Collectively exhaustive categories** means that all possible answers are provided, and **mutually exclusive categories** means that there is no overlap between categories. The following example demonstrates categories that are collectively exhaustive and mutually exclusive.

How many apples do you eat each week?

   _____ A.   None
   _____ B.   1–2
   _____ C.   3–4
   _____ D.   More than 4

The following question *violates* the rule concerning collectively exhaustive categories:

Please check your highest level of education:

   _____ A.   Elementary
   _____ B.   High School
   _____ C.   College

How would subjects respond who had not completed elementary school? Other categories are needed to cover all possible answers that subjects might provide. Sometimes researchers find a quick solution to this problem by adding an "other" category. A blank is provided beside the word "other" for respondents' answers.

The researcher also must provide answers that are mutually exclusive. A respondent should be able to check only one response from among a set of alternatives. The following is a sample question that *violates* this rule:

Please check the length of time that you have dieted:

_____ A. 1–4 weeks
_____ B. 4–8 weeks
_____ C. 8–12 weeks
_____ D. More than 12 weeks

A respondent's answer to the preceding question may well depend on the amount of weight loss. If a woman has been on a diet for 4 weeks and is feeling guilty because she has only lost 2 pounds, the 1- to 4-weeks category might be checked, rather than the 4- to 8-weeks category.

Contingency Questions.   Questionnaire items that are relevant for some respondents and not for others are called **contingency questions.** The determination of whether respondents should answer certain questions is dependent or "contingent" on their answers to other questions. For example, a researcher might want to determine if a client has been satisfied with the type of nursing care received during previous hospitalizations. If the client has not been hospitalized previously, an answer could not be provided to this particular question.

1. Have you ever been hospitalized before?
_____Yes   ⟶   How would you rate the care you received during your
                  last hospitalization?
                  ____ Poor ____ Fair ____ Good
_____ No
2. . . .

The arrow indicates that respondents who answer "yes" also should answer the question on the right. Respondents who answer "no" will continue downward on the questionnaire.

Filler Questions.   Occasionally, the researcher wishes to decrease the emphasis on the specific purpose of the study to avoid the tendency for respondents to provide answers that they believe are being sought by the researcher. **Filler questions** are items in which the researcher has no direct interest but are included on a questionnaire to reduce the emphasis on the specific purpose of other questions. For example, if the main purpose of a study was to gain information concerning patients' perceptions of the nursing care that they had received, the researcher also might include a lot of other questions about the food they had been served, visiting hours, and so forth. Subjects might answer more honestly if a few questions about the nursing care they had received were scattered in among a lot of other questions. If the subjects could determine that the only purpose of the study was to obtain their perceptions of nursing care, they might hesitate to criticize the nursing care that they had received.

PLACEMENT OF QUESTIONS

All questions about a certain topic should be grouped together. Also, demographic questions, which ask for factual information about the subject, should be grouped together. There is much discussion about the order or placement of questions in certain areas of the questionnaire, such as at the beginning or at the end. Demographic questions are frequently placed at the beginning of a questionnaire. It may be advantageous to place simple questions such as routine demographic questions at the beginning because these types of questions are easy to answer and may encourage the respondent to continue with the questionnaire. However, the researcher may choose to place the demographic questions at the end of the questionnaire in the belief that some demographic questions, such as those asking for income or age, may be threatening to respondents.

COVER LETTER

A cover letter should accompany all mailed questionnaires and is helpful anytime a questionnaire is administered. The letter should be brief and contain the following information:

1. Identification of the researcher and any sponsoring agency or person
2. Purpose of the research
3. How participant was selected
4. Reason the respondent should answer the questionnaire
5. Length of time to complete the questionnaire
6. How data will be used or made public
7. Deadline for return of questionnaire
8. An offer to inform respondent of results of study
9. Contact phone number, address, or both
10. Personal signature of the researcher

The cover letter is extremely important and may be the single most important factor in motivating respondents to complete questionnaires. When a cover letter is being constructed, the researcher should try to imagine herself or himself as the recipient. What approach or what information would impress you the most and make you want to complete the questionnaire?

COMPLETION INSTRUCTIONS

Information on how to complete the questionnaire must be clear and concise. If all questions are to be answered using the same type of format, a general set of instructions may be written at the top of the questionnaire. Frequently, however, several different types of questions will be included on the instrument, and instructions will need to precede each type of question. It is helpful to provide the respondent with an example of the appropriate way to respond to a particular type of question.

DISTRIBUTION OF QUESTIONNAIRES

There are many methods of distributing questionnaires. They may be given to potential respondents in a one-to-one contact such as might occur when the nurse researcher distributes instruments to hospitalized patients. Researchers may hand out questionnaires to students in a classroom or distribute questionnaires to members of an organization as they come to a meeting. Questionnaires also may be placed in a container in a given location where potential respondents can take one, if they so desire. One of the most frequently used methods of distributing questionnaires is through a mailing system, such as the U.S. Postal Service or a hospital interdepartmental mailing system.

FACTORS INFLUENCING RESPONSE RATES

One serious disadvantage of questionnaires is the low return rate that frequently occurs. Some sources report that a 25 to 30 percent return rate can be expected with mailed questionnaires (Burns & Grove, 1997). Factors that positively influence response rates of mailed questionnaires include (a) information in the cover letter that motivates respondents, (b) mailing at a time other than holiday seasons or popular vacation times, (c) hand-addressed outer envelopes, (d) neatness and clarity of the instrument, (e) time to complete the instrument does not exceed 20 to 25 minutes, (f) ease of completion of the instrument, (g) guarantee of anonymity, (h) personal signature of the researcher, and (i) inclusion of a preaddressed, stamped envelope.

ADVANTAGES OF QUESTIONNAIRES

1. Questionnaires are a quick and generally inexpensive means of obtaining data from a large number of respondents.
2. Questionnaires are one of the easiest research instruments to test for reliability and validity.
3. The administration of questionnaires is less time consuming than interviews or observation research.
4. Data can be obtained from respondents in widespread geographical areas.
5. Respondents can remain anonymous.
6. If anonymity is assured, respondents are more likely to provide honest answers.

DISADVANTAGES OF QUESTIONNAIRES

1. Mailing of questionnaires may be costly.
2. Response rate may be low.
3. Respondents may provide socially acceptable answers.
4. Respondents may fail to answer some of the items.
5. There is no opportunity to clarify items that may be misunderstood by respondents.
6. Respondents must be literate.
7. Respondents must have no physical handicap that would deter them from completing a questionnaire.
8. Respondents may not be representative of the population.

INTERVIEWS

The phone rings and you answer it. A voice on the other end of the line says, "Hello, I'm conducting a research study on _____. It will take only 5 to 10 minutes of your time, and the information that you provide will be very important to the results of this study." Have you ever received such a call? If so, did you provide data or did you hang up the phone? If you have received such a call or have participated in a study in which interviews were conducted, you are already familiar with some of the material on interviews.

An **interview** is a method of data collection in which an interviewer obtains responses from a subject in a face-to-face encounter or through a telephone call. A great deal of information is available in the literature concerning the interview method of data collection. Interviews are frequently used in descriptive research studies and qualitative studies. Also, an experimental study may use an interview in some phase of the study to determine subjects' responses to some treatment. Interviews are used to obtain factual data about people as well as to measure their opinions, attitudes, and beliefs about certain topics. Information will be provided about how to conduct interviews because it is possible that you will be a data collector in a study in the future, even if you never conduct research as the principal investigator.

TYPES OF INTERVIEWS

Interviews can be unstructured or structured. Most interviews, however, range between the two ends of the continuum. For simplification in discussion, interviews are categorized as (a) unstructured, (b) structured, and (c) semistructured.

In **unstructured interviews,** the interviewer is given a great deal of freedom to direct the course of the interview. Although nearly all interviews have a general framework to guide them, unstructured interviews are conducted more like a normal conversation, and topics are pursued at the discretion of the interviewer. Unstructured interviews are particularly appropriate for exploratory or qualitative research studies where the researcher does not possess enough knowledge about the topic to structure questions in advance of data collection. The interviewer may start the interview with a broad opening statement like, "Tell me what it was like for you after your husband had his heart attack." Depending on how the spouse responds to this opening question, further questions are formulated. **Probes** are additional prompting questions that encourage the respondent to elaborate on the topic that is being discussed. When accurate comparisons between subjects are not a critical issue, unstructured interviews produce more in-depth information on subjects' beliefs and attitudes than can be obtained through any other data-gathering procedure.

Structured interviews involve asking the same questions, in the same order and in the same manner of all respondents in a study. Structured interviews are most appropriate when straightforward factual information is desired. The interviewer uses a structured interview schedule that has been planned in detail because one of the main purposes of this type of interview is to produce data that can be compared across respondents. Even subtle changes in the wording of questions may not be permitted in structured interviews.

Interviewers must try to remain objective during the interview and avoid unnecessary interactions with respondents.

The majority of interviews fall somewhere in between the structured and the unstructured types of interviews. During a **semistructured interview,** interviewers are generally required to ask a certain number of specific questions, but additional probes are allowed or even encouraged. Both closed-ended and open-ended questions are included in a semistructured interview. In this type of interview, data are gathered that can be compared across all respondents in the study. In addition, individualized data may be gathered that will provide depth and richness to the findings.

INTERVIEW INSTRUMENTS

Data obtained in interviews are usually recorded on an instrument referred to as an **interview schedule.** The interview schedule contains a set of questions to be asked by the interviewer and space to record the respondents' answers.

Respondents' answers may be entered directly on the interview schedule or recorded on a separate coding sheet such as those that can be tallied by the use of a computer or a grading machine. The process of recording responses should be very clear to the interviewer. The simpler the recording process, the less likely it will be for interviewers to make errors in recording.

Data obtained from an interview also may be recorded on audiotapes or videotapes. Some researchers believe that the written recording of responses jeopardizes rapport and reduces the amount of eye contact that can be established between the interviewer and the interviewee. Also, through tape-recording devices, the total interview process can be captured, and the interviewer is free to observe the respondents. On the other hand, respondents may be reluctant to give permission to be taped. Written permission will be required, and the permission form should indicate how the information will be used and how confidentiality will be maintained.

A major disadvantage to the use of tape recordings is found in the data-analysis phase. The entire tape has to be replayed and transcribed. An interviewer might be inclined to stop using the tape recorder after the first few interviews because of the length of time needed to analyze data.

Videotaping has become an important means of collecting research data. Roberts, Srour, and Winkelman (1996) have written an informative article on the use of this data-collection technique.

Telephone interviews involve the collection of data from subjects through use of phone calls rather than in face-to-face meetings. This data-collection method is a quick and inexpensive means of conducting interviews. Another advantage of telephone interviews is that the respondents' anonymity can be protected. There are several disadvantages associated with telephone interviews. Many people have unlisted numbers. Some people have Caller IDs installed on their phones; they may not answer the phone if they do not recognize the caller's phone number. Also, the interviewer cannot observe nonverbal responses. Majewski (1986) used telephone interviews to obtain data on role conflicts during the transition of women into the maternal role. She suggested that observing the mother with her infant, preferably in the home, would provide valuable nonverbal data that could be used to validate the mother's self-report of her behavior.

One piece of valuable information for interviewers concerns the number of times a phone should be allowed to ring before hanging up. Research has shown that the optimum number is four times. It has been found that 96.7% of people who are at home and who are going to answer the phone will do so within four rings. Approximately 88% will answer within three rings, and 99.2% will answer within five rings ("Ring Policy," 1980). Of course, today, answering machines can be set to pick up a message after a set number of rings. Therefore, this piece of information may not be so valuable after all! (I almost omitted it from this edition of the book.)

INTERVIEW QUESTIONS

The difficulty in developing good items for a questionnaire has been discussed. It might be thought that questions for an interview would be much simpler to construct because the interviewer will be present to explain any unclear items. This may be true to some extent, especially for unstructured interviews. Even items for an unstructured interview, however, must be given thoughtful consideration. Once the data are collected, it is too late to add, subtract, or alter questions.

Items must be clear, unambiguous, and short. When questions are long or complex, it may be difficult to ask them orally. If items cannot be simplified, it may be advantageous to print these questions on cards and have subjects read them before responding. Of course, this procedure would require that subjects can read.

There are two basic categories of questions: open-ended and closed-ended questions. These types of questions were described in the section on questionnaires.

INTERVIEWER TRAINING

The investigator of a study in which interviews will be conducted has the responsibility to provide training for all interviewers who will collect data during the study. The training should be quite rigorous. The research investigator should continue to work closely with the interviewers throughout the course of the study.

Belza (1996, p. 39) described the process she used to train data collectors for her study that involved the collection of data in respondents' homes.

1. The data collector was allowed to provide input into the development of an operations manual, which included a script and scoring guidelines regarding ways to facilitate home visits.
2. The data collector viewed a videotape of an interview being done by a skilled interviewer.
3. The data collector was given practice and feedback in a clinic setting.
4. Rehearsals were done in homes of people who would not be study participants.
5. A videotape was done of the data collector conducting a rehearsal interview.
6. The principal investigator critiqued the data collector's performance on this rehearsal interview.

During the training session(s), the researcher should provide interviewers with a description of the study and its purpose. General procedures are discussed, and the interview schedule is reviewed in detail. The purpose of each question is pointed out, and the meanings of all words are clarified. The process of recording information must be explicitly communicated. Special attention should be given to the use of probes, and any variations that will be allowed in the interview process should be discussed.

Interviewer training should be carried out in groups, so that all interviewers receive the same instructions. Role-playing of interviews helps the interviewer to gain some appreciation of what the actual interviews will be like. Each interviewer should role-play both the interviewer's part and the respondent's part. By acting as a respondent, the interviewer gains a greater insight into the experience of potential study subjects.

TIMING AND SETTING FOR INTERVIEWS

Determining the most appropriate time for conducting an interview can present a real challenge. If home interviews are conducted, the interviewer should try to determine when respondents would be at home. In past years, interviewers found many women at home during the daytime. Increasing numbers of women have entered the work force. Weeks, Jones, Folsom, and Benrud (1980) determined that the optimum time for home interviews is from 5 PM to 9 PM Sunday through Friday and 10 AM to 5 PM on Saturday. Avoid holidays, days when important sporting events are occurring, and times for popular television programs or series.

If hospitalized patients are to be interviewed, the nurse researcher should become familiar with hospital routines and procedures to determine the most convenient times for interviews. Routines to be considered are patient care activities, visiting hours, and physicians' rounds.

Regardless of the setting, the interviewer should attempt to seek as much privacy as possible for the interview. The respondent and interviewer should be alone, and interruptions should be avoided. The television or radio should be turned off.

INTERVIEWER GUIDELINES

Although each interview is unique, some guidelines can be followed in most circumstances. The guidelines are presented in three phases: before the interview, during the interview, and after the interview.

Before the interview is conducted, the interviewer should introduce herself or himself to the potential subject. The purpose of the study should be explained. Potential subjects should be told how they were chosen and how the information will be used. The person should be told how long the interview would last.

Once the person has agreed to the interview, the interviewer should ensure a comfortable interview atmosphere. Subjects should be seated in a comfortable position or lying down, as in some hospital interviews. Unnecessary noises must be controlled as much as possible. The interviewer should use language that is understood by subjects and talk in a conversational tone. Respondents should be informed that there are no right or wrong answers. No pressure should be applied for answers. Questions that are of a sensitive nature should be left until the end of the interview, when rapport may be more fully established.

After the interview has been concluded, subjects should be asked if they have any questions. Further explanations of the study may be made at this time. Common courtesy dictates that respondents be thanked for their participation in the study. In some studies, compensation may be provided. Any time subjects receive compensation for study participation, the possibility of biased data is great. Finally, the interviewer should indicate how study participants may obtain the results of the study.

INFLUENCE OF INTERVIEWERS ON RESPONDENTS

In face-to-face interviews, the interviewer may have a great deal of influence on the outcome. In nonexperimental research, this phenomenon is referred to as the Rosenthal effect. In experimental studies, it is referred to as the experimenter effect. Studies have shown that certain characteristics of the interviewer, such as ethnic background, age, gender, manner of speaking, and clothing, influence the answers provided by respondents. In telephone interviews, the interviewer's verbal mannerisms, such as tone of voice and dialect, may be a positive or a negative factor in soliciting cooperation from respondents.

First impressions are important in face-to-face interviews. If an appointment has been made for the interview, punctuality should be maintained. Interviewers should be neat in appearance, courteous, friendly, and relaxed. Flashy jewelry should be avoided as well as any item that would identify the interviewer with some social group or organization. It is desirable for interviewers to possess similar demographic characteristics and dressing styles as the respondents.

ADVANTAGES OF INTERVIEWS

1. Responses can be obtained from a wide range of subjects.
2. Response rate is high.
3. Most of the data obtained are usable.
4. In-depth responses can be obtained.
5. Nonverbal behavior and verbal mannerisms can be observed.

DISADVANTAGES OF INTERVIEWS

1. Training programs are needed for interviewers.
2. Interviews are time consuming and expensive.
3. Arrangements for interviews may be difficult to make.
4. Subjects may provide socially acceptable responses.
5. Subjects may be anxious because answers are being recorded.
6. Subjects may be influenced by interviewers' characteristics.
7. Interviewers may misinterpret nonverbal behavior.

OBSERVATION METHODS

Although observations can be made through all of the senses, generally speaking, **observation research** is concerned with gathering data through visual observation. Nurses are well qualified to conduct observation research because observations of clients in health care settings are an everyday experience. For the observations to be considered as scientific research, a carefully planned study is necessary. The researcher must decide what behaviors will be observed, who will observe the behaviors, what observational procedure will be used, and what type of relationship will exist between the observer and the subjects.

DETERMINING BEHAVIORS TO BE OBSERVED

The research question or study hypothesis should determine the behaviors that will be observed. Psychomotor skills can be evaluated, such as the ability of clients with diabetes to perform insulin injections. Personal habits, such as smoking and eating behaviors, might be of interest. Nonverbal communication patterns, such as body posture or facial expressions, are frequently observed. The types of observations that are of interest to nurse researchers are quite numerous.

RESEARCH OBSERVERS

If the researcher decides to use other people to collect or help collect data, training sessions will be necessary. It is generally preferable to have more than one observer during training sessions so that estimates of the reliability of the data can be made. Human error is quite likely to occur in visual observations. The reliability of the observations is, therefore, always of utmost importance. Interrater reliability is the degree to which two or more raters or observers assign the same rating or score to an observation. The training of the observers is probably the most crucial phase of observation research.

OBSERVATION PROCEDURES

The researcher must determine how and when observations will be made. The degree of structure of the observations and the period for gathering data must be considered.

Structured and Unstructured Observations. Observations may range from very structured to very unstructured observations. Most observations lie somewhere between these two ends of the continuum. **Structured observations** are carried out when the researcher has prior knowledge about the phenomenon of interest. The data-collection tool is usually some kind of checklist. The expected behaviors of interest have been identified on the checklist. The observer only needs to indicate the frequency of occurrence of these behaviors. In **unstructured observations,** the researcher attempts to describe events or behaviors as they occur, with no preconceived ideas of what will be seen. This requires a high degree of concentration and attention by the observer. Frequently, a combination of structured and unstructured observations is used in research. The observation guide or instrument is designed with some preconceived categories identified, but the observer is also instructed to record any additional behaviors that may occur. This combination of structured and unstructured observations provides the quantitative and qualitative types of data that have become important to nurse researchers.

Event Sampling and Time Sampling. Observation research may be classified as either event sampling or time sampling. **Event sampling** involves observation of an entire event. **Time sampling** involves observations of events or behaviors during certain specified times. If a researcher were interested in determining the ability of nursing students to perform catheterization procedures correctly, event sampling probably would be most appropriate because the entire procedure would need to be observed. If the area of interest was territorial behaviors of families in intensive care unit waiting rooms, it might be more appropriate to conduct time-sampling observations. Some initial trial observation periods probably would be useful to help determine when observations should be made during the 24-hour day, or the researcher might randomly select times to observe family members.

RELATIONSHIP BETWEEN OBSERVER AND SUBJECTS

There are four ways to categorize observation research according to the relationship between the observer and the subjects: (a) nonparticipant observer-overt, (b) nonparticipant observer-covert, (c) participant observer-overt, and (d) participant observer-covert.

As a **nonparticipant observer-overt,** the observer openly identifies that she or he is conducting research and provides subjects with information about the types of data that will be collected. This type of observer might wear a laboratory coat, carry a clipboard and pen, and be clearly identified as a researcher.

The **nonparticipant observer-covert** is one who does not, before the beginning of data collection, identify herself or himself to the subjects who are being observed. Generally this type of research is not ethical. Except for instances of public behavior, observation research should be conducted only when permission has been obtained from those who will be the subjects of the study or with the consent of appropriate persons, such as family members, in the case of children. Public behavior research might involve observations of the number of people who have their seat belts in place while driving on the highway. This type of observation would be ethical.

Nurse researchers must not abuse their privilege as nurses by covertly observing the behaviors of clients. Researchers may contend that concealed observations are necessary because subjects will alter their behavior if they know they are being observed. Although people may initially change their behavior, if an adjustment period is allowed, subjects will generally respond as they normally would.

Such devices as hidden cameras and one-way mirrors may be used as long as subjects are fully informed about them. Therapy groups are frequently observed, with the members' permission, by observers in an adjoining room that contains a one-way mirror.

In some research studies, the observer becomes involved in interactions with the subjects. This interaction may be of an overt or a covert nature. The **participant observer-overt** becomes involved with subjects openly and with the full awareness of those people who will be observed. Margaret Mead conducted many of her famous anthropological field research studies in this manner. She lived with the people, such as the Samoans, and observed their behaviors in their day-to-day living. Participant observation is used frequently in qualitative research.

In contrast, as a **participant observer-covert,** the observer interacts with the subjects and observes their behavior without their knowledge. This type of observer might be disparagingly called a "plant" or a "spy" by people who find out the real purpose of the researcher's behavior. There are very few situations where this type of observation is ethical.

THE ROLE OF THE NURSE VERSUS THE RESEARCHER

Nurse researchers frequently have difficulty maintaining the role of researcher in observation studies. For example, consider the situation where a nurse researcher is sitting in a patient's room observing his or her behavior after some treatment procedure. Will the nurse researcher sit silently and continue with the planned observations if the patient seems to be in pain, if the room seems to be too warm, or if the intravenous bottle is almost empty? It is hoped not! The client's welfare should always take precedence over the gathering of research data. If the researcher varies from the guidelines for the data-collection procedure, however, the accuracy of the data may be in question.

PHYSIOLOGICAL MEASURES

Physiological measures involve the collection of physical data from subjects. These types of measures are generally more objective and accurate than many of the other data-collection methods. It is much more difficult for subjects to intentionally or unintentionally provide biased data on physiological measures than on self-report measures.

One of the greatest advantages of physiological measures is their precision and accuracy. One of the greatest disadvantages is that special expertise may be necessary to use some of these devices. Another disadvantage is that the presence of certain data-collection instruments may adversely influence the subjects. For example, the process of applying the equipment to measure a person's blood pressure may, in fact, cause the blood pressure readings to be elevated.

In the past, only a small percentage of nursing studies have examined physiological variables. Pugh and DeKeyser (1995) searched the research reports published between 1989 and 1993 in four broad-based nursing research journals (*Image: Journal of Nursing Scholarship, Nursing Research, Research in Nursing and Health,* and *Western Journal of Nursing Research).* Of the 763 reports, only 114 (15%) examined physiological variables.

A recent review of two nursing research journals (*Nursing Research* and *Applied Nursing Research)* revealed an increasing number of studies in which physiological instruments were used. Lee and colleagues (2000) used echocardiography to measure cardiac function in patients after myocardial infarction. Lee had trained at the Echocardiography Laboratory of the University of California at San Francisco Medical Center for 2 years before the study. In a study by Hill, Kurkowski, and Garcia (2000), sucking patterns of preterm infants were measured with the Whitney Mercury Strain Gage (WMSG), which uses stretch-sensitive gauges that are appropriate for the size of the infant. In this same study, the Nonin 8800 Cardiorespiratory Oximeter (NCO) was used to determine cardiopulmonary functions. To study the energy costs of T'ai Chi C'hih exercise, expired breath-by-breath analysis was performed by Fontana (2000) using the Quinton Q-Plex metabolic cart and indirect calorimetry.

Some nurses have called for caution in the use of physiological measures for nursing research. Holden (1996) wrote that some of the confusion regarding physiological research comes from nursing's struggle to gain autonomy from medicine. As an attempt has been made to develop a unique body of knowledge, nursing has claimed psychosocial issues as within its realm of independent study. Therefore, many studies have concerned psychosocial variables. A recent review of the nursing research literature uncovered a large number of studies in which psychosocial variables were the only study variables.

It appears that the time has come for nurses to be more involved in physiological research. Funding for this type of research has increased a great deal in recent years. The National Institute for Nursing Research and Sigma Theta Tau, as well as many other organizations, provide funds for studies that are concerned with physiological variables.

Increasing numbers of published studies are reporting on data that have been collected from both physical measures and self-report measures. The use of multiple data-collection instruments provides a more valid measure of a variable than when only one of these types of instruments is employed.

ATTITUDE SCALES

Attitude scales are self-report data-collection instruments that ask respondents to report their attitudes or feelings on a continuum. Attitude scales are composed of a number of related items, and respondents are given a score after the item responses are totaled. Respondents' attitudes may be compared by examining the scores that are obtained for each person or for each group. The most commonly used attitude scales are the Likert scale and the semantic differential scale.

LIKERT SCALES

The **Likert scale** was named after its developer, Rensis Likert. These scales usually contain five or seven responses for each item, ranging from strongly agree to strongly disagree. Figure 12–1 provides an example of a Likert scale.

Some researchers prefer to eliminate the "uncertain" category and force respondents into some form of agreement or disagreement with the items. When the "uncertain" option is eliminated, however, respondents may be forced to select answers that are really not of their choice.

An approximately equal number of positively and negatively worded items should be included on a Likert instrument. This requires that respondents read each question carefully and prevents the respondents from rapidly completing an instrument by checking one category of responses all the way through the instrument.

If five responses are used, scores on each item generally range from 1 to 5. A score of 1 is usually given to "strongly disagree," a score of 2 to "disagree," a score of 3 to "uncertain," a score of 4 to "agree," and, finally, a score of 5 to "strongly agree." Usually,

Nursing Diagnosis Questionnaire

Please read the following items and indicate your agreement or disagreement by checking the appropriate category.

SD = Strongly disagree
 D = Disagree
 U = Uncertain
 A = Agree
SA = Strongly agree

	SD	D	U	A	SA
1. Nursing diagnoses should be written on all nursing care plans.	____	____	____	____	____
2. The use of nursing diagnoses allows nurses to be autonomous health care professionals.	____	____	____	____	____
3. The medical diagnosis is more important in determining clients' health care needs than is the nursing diagnosis.	____	____	____	____	____
4. Nursing care should be based on the nursing diagnosis.	____	____	____	____	____
5. Nurses waste valuable time in trying to formulate nursing diagnoses.	____	____	____	____	____
6. The term *nursing* diagnosis is a popular phrase that will soon become forgotten.	____	____	____	____	____

Figure 12–1. Example of a Likert scale.

negatively worded items are reverse scored: "Strongly disagree" responses to negative items would receive a score of 5 rather than 1. If 20 items were included on an instrument, the total score could vary from 20 to 100.

Although data from a Likert scale are generally at the ordinal level of measurement, some statistical texts indicate that arithmetic operations may be performed with this type of data and, therefore, the more powerful parametric statistical tests may be used in analyzing the data (see Chapter 14). In an article in *Nursing Research,* Wang, Yu, Wang, & Huang (1999) discussed the pros and cons of treating ordinal data as interval data.

Beck and Gable (2000) described the development of the Postpartum Depression Screening Scale (PDSS). The PDDS uses a Likert scale response format. The instrument was administered to 525 new mothers. These women were asked to indicate their agreement with each item on a scale of 1 (strongly disagree) to 5 (strongly agree). All items on the tool were derived from actual quotes of women who had experienced postpartum depression.

SEMANTIC DIFFERENTIAL SCALES

Although not as commonly used as the Likert scale, the semantic differential is a useful attitude scale for nurse researchers. The **semantic differential** asks subjects to indicate their position or attitude about some concept along a continuum between two adjectives

Evaluation of Clinical Instructor

Each item below concerns characteristics of instructors. Words are presented in pairs and represent opposite characteristics. Please place a (✓) above the line on the scale at the place which you believe comes the closest to describing your evaluation of the instructor.

Example:
Kind _____ ✓_____ _____ _____ _____ _____ Unkind

1. Friendly _____ _____ _____ _____ _____ _____ Unfriendly
2. Sensitive _____ _____ _____ _____ _____ _____ Insensitive
3. Praises _____ _____ _____ _____ _____ _____ Criticizes
4. Caring _____ _____ _____ _____ _____ _____ Uncaring
5. Flexible _____ _____ _____ _____ _____ _____ Inflexible
6. Helpful _____ _____ _____ _____ _____ _____ Unhelpful

Figure 12–2. Example of a semantic differential scale.

or phrases that are presented in relation to the concept being measured. The technique was developed by Osgood, Suci, and Tannenbaum (1957) to measure the psychological meaning of concepts. They used the term *semantic differential* to indicate that the difference in subjects' attitudes could be compared by examining their responses in "semantic space" or attitudinal space.

Usually, subjects are asked to describe or evaluate a particular situation or experience. This technique also may be used to evaluate a setting, a person, a group, or an educational course. The positions along the continuum or scale are assigned numerical values. The number of positions on the continuum varies from five to nine, with seven being used commonly. Scores are then calculated for all subjects. Scores are derived much the same way as in the Likert procedure. An example of a semantic differential scale is presented in Figure 12–2.

The semantic differential scale is generally easier for subjects to complete than a Likert scale. Subjects, however, may not understand the adjectives that are used on a semantic differential scale or may become bored with the format of the items and select the middle scale position throughout the entire instrument.

The Organizational Climate for Service Semantic Differential (OCSSD) was used by Niedz (1998) in her study of patient satisfaction with nursing care. The eight-item scale measures patients' perception of the organizational climate for service in hospitals. Adjective pairs on the instrument included "good-bad," "flexible-inflexible," and "helpful-unhelpful." Patient satisfaction with nursing care and patients' perceptions of organizational climate for service were both positively related to patients' perceptions of the quality of the service they received.

PSYCHOLOGICAL TESTS

Researchers have devised many methods to assess the personality characteristics of people. Personality inventories and projective techniques are two of these methods.

PERSONALITY INVENTORIES

Personality inventories are self-report measures used to assess the differences in personality traits, needs, or values of people. These inventories seek information about a person by asking questions or requesting responses to statements that are presented. Scores are then derived for each person for the trait being measured. Many of the personality inventories have preprinted scoring guides that allow comparisons between subjects and also allow comparisons with a "norm" or "average" group. Because these devices are of a self-report nature, they are accurate to the extent that subjects respond honestly to the items.

Some of the more commonly used personality inventories are the Minnesota Multiphasic Personality Inventory (MMPI), Edwards Personal Preference Schedule (EPPS), and Sixteen Personality Factor Questionnaire (16 P.F.). The MMPI contains 550 affirmative statements that require an answer of True, False, or Cannot Say. This test is composed of 10 subdivisions, including areas such as depression, paranoia, and hysteria. The MMPI has been used with people considered normal and those with psychological problems. The EPPS contains 15 scales that measure concepts such as autonomy and dominance. The 16 P.F. measures personality dimensions such as reserved versus outgoing, practical versus imaginative, and relaxed versus tense.

PROJECTIVE TECHNIQUES

One of the criticisms of self-report psychological measures is that they may elicit socially acceptable answers or answers desired by the researcher rather than the true feelings or attitudes of the subjects. A data-collection method that is believed to be more accurate in gathering psychological data is the projective method. In the various **projective techniques,** a subject is presented with stimuli that are designed to be ambiguous or to have no definite meaning. Then the person is asked to describe the stimuli or to tell what the stimuli appear to represent. The responses reflect the internal feelings of the subjects that are projected onto the external stimuli.

Probably the most famous of all the projective measures is the Rorschach Inkblot Test. Subjects are presented with cards that contain designs, which are actually inkblots rather than true pictures or drawings. One person might interpret a card to be two figures dancing, while another person might describe the same scene as two people fighting. Of course, only specialists should make the interpretation of this type of data.

Another commonly used projective test is the Thematic Apperception Test. This test consists of a set of pictures about which subjects are asked to tell a story involving what they think is happening in the pictures. The projective tests are particularly useful with small children because of their limited vocabularies. Children may be given dolls and asked to arrange the dolls in a particular setting that is provided by the researcher. Children also may be given finger paint, crayons, or clay to use in telling a story.

A group of children with sickle cell disease and their nonaffected siblings participated in a research study that sought to describe how these children problem solve and cope with social and academic stress at school (Lee, Phoenix, Brown, & Jackson, 1998). Pictures were used to evoke story telling. Results revealed that problem solving and coping methods were similar among children with sickle cell disease and their nonaffected siblings. Both groups of children used direct action in stressful situations.

Q SORT

The **Q sort,** also called Q methodology, is a means of obtaining data in which subjects sort statements into categories according to their attitudes toward, or rating of, the statements. Subjects are presented with a number of words or statements that are written on cards or pieces of paper. The number of items to be placed into each category or pile by the subjects is predetermined by the researcher. This forced-choice arrangement usually calls for piles to be distributed in the form of a bell-shaped curve. If 100 items were being used, the distribution might be:

1   4   11   21   26   21   11   4   1

The respondents are asked to arrange the items from left to right in front of them according to their attitude or belief about the items. The first pile should contain the item about which the subject has the most positive attitude or the strongest belief about the importance of the item to the topic of interest, and the last pile on the right should contain the item about which the subject has the most negative attitude or the weakest belief about the importance of the item. The other piles will contain items of varying intensity of attitudes or beliefs. This type of data-collection procedure may present a difficult task for respondents. Therefore, clear instructions must be provided.

A Q sort was used by Kovach and Krejci (1998) to study factors that might facilitate positive changes in dementia care. Employees of long-term care facilities (n = 181) were presented with 50 facility factors and 50 personal factors. Each of these factors was printed on a 2 × 4 card. The respondents were asked to place each of the facility cards in one of five piles (from greatest to least importance). The procedure was repeated for the personal factor cards. The factors cited as most important in making positive changes in dementia care concerned teamwork, administrative support, staff attitude, and knowledge.

DELPHI TECHNIQUE

The **Delphi technique** is a data-collection method that received its name from the famous Greek oracle at Delphi. As you may remember, the ancient Greeks sought answers to important questions from the deities. Today, the term Delphi technique is used to describe a data-collection method that uses several rounds of questions to seek a consensus on a particular topic from a group of experts. The purpose is to obtain group consensus from the panel of experts without bringing this group together in a face-to-face meeting. This type of procedure is appropriate to examine the opinions, beliefs, or future predictions of knowledgeable people on some special topic of interest.

The simplest way to explain this procedure is to describe a study conducted by Lindeman (1975). The purpose of this study was to determine priorities for clinical nursing research in the future. Of the 433 leaders in nursing who were originally contacted, 341 experts responded to all four rounds of questionnaires.

The first questionnaire asked for the identification of five areas where clinical nursing research was needed in the future. More than 2000 priorities were listed on the returned questionnaires. The 150 most frequently mentioned areas were placed on the second questionnaire. Respondents were asked to examine these 150 areas according to the importance of the item for patient welfare and the nursing profession. Also, respondents were asked to decide whether nursing should assume the primary responsibility for research in this area.

The third round of the study provided subjects with a summary of all responses received in the second round of data collection. They were asked to respond again to the same 150-item questionnaire. Respondents were asked to make comments if their choices were different from the majority of the other experts. Experts thus were faced with examining the responses of their colleagues and making a decision to stick with their own ideas or to become more in agreement with the other experts.

In the fourth and final round of the survey, respondents were again asked to complete the 150-item questionnaire after reviewing the results of Round 3 and the comments of a minority opinion report. These comments were made by experts who chose answers that were in disagreement with the majority of the other respondents.

The results indicated that the most important priority for clinical nursing research was the development of valid and reliable indicators of quality nursing care. Other important areas of needed research were identified as (a) effective ways to decrease the psychological stress experienced by patients, (b) means of enhancing the quality of life for the aged, and (c) interventions to manage pain.

A Delphi technique was used by Fochtman and Hinds (2000) to determine research priorities for pediatric oncology nursing. The study was sponsored by the Pediatric Oncology Group (POG). Nurses in this group conduct clinical nursing research that will improve the care of pediatric oncology patients and their families. A total of 57 unique research ideas were generated in Round 1. The top 10 nursing research priorities were determined in Round 2. Important research topics included caregiver burden, quality of life, disease response, and cost when care is provided on an outpatient versus inpatient basis.

VISUAL ANALOGUE SCALE

The **visual analogue scale** (VAS) presents subjects with a straight line drawn on a piece of paper. The line is anchored on each end by words or short phrases that represent the extremes of some phenomenon, such as pain. Subjects are asked to make a mark on the line at the point that corresponds to their experience of the phenomenon. Frequently, the line is 100 mm long, which simulates a 0 to 100 rating scale. From their review of the literature, Huang, Wilkie, and Berry (1996) have concluded that the VAS is a "simple, reliable, reproducible, valid, and sensitive tool" (p. 370).

A caution is issued if you are trying to photocopy a visual analogue scale for use in a study. The length of the line may change slightly (lengthen) during the photocopying process and you will not end up with a 100-mm line. The VAS line may be drawn either horizontally or vertically on the paper. Some authors have suggested that the vertical scale is easier for subjects to use (Flaherty, 1996). It appears that it is universally recognized that the bottom of a vertical scale is low and the top of a vertical scale is high. However, not all cultural groups view the far left on a horizontal scale as indicating low and the far right as indicating a high score.

The Short-Form McGill Pain Questionnaire (SF-MPQ) contains present pain intensity items (PPI) and a horizontal version of a visual analogue scale (VAS). Stephenson and Herman (2000) decided to compare the horizontal version of the VAS with a newly devised vertical form. They found the vertical form to have a higher correlation with the PPI than did the horizontal form.

The visual analogue scale is being used with increasing frequency in nursing research studies. It has been found to be particularly useful with patients who are experiencing discomfort, such as nausea, pain, fatigue, and shortness of breath.

Yoos and McMullen (1999) used a visual analogue scale to measure children and their parents' report of the severity of asthma in these children. The 100-mm line was anchored on each end with the phrases "best breathing could ever be" and "worst breathing could ever be."

PREEXISTING DATA

Nurse researchers have available a wealth of data that may be used for research. As a data-collection method, **preexisting data** involve the use of existing information that has not been collected for research purposes. Patients' charts are a valuable source of data.

Lee and Mills (2000) examined the records of 244 home health care patients to identify the most commonly used medical diagnoses, nursing diagnoses, and nursing interventions for these patients. Common medical diagnoses were infectious and parasitic disease, disease of the circulatory system, and neoplasms. Common nursing diagnoses were alteration in mobility, alteration in cardiac status, and alteration in comfort: pain. Teaching was the most commonly used nursing intervention.

Other sources of existing data include records from agencies such as hospitals, the United States government, local public health departments, churches, licensing bureaus, and professional organizations. Personal documents, such as diaries and letters, may be examined, as well as almanacs and professional journals.

Yoos and McMullen (1999) used diaries (as well as a visual analogue scale) to gather data in their study of childhood asthma. The children and their parents were asked to independently record symptom severity and peak expiratory flow rates (PEFR) in a diary each morning and evening for 2 weeks.

CRITIQUING DATA-COLLECTION METHODS

In the previous chapter, some general guidelines were presented concerning the data-collection process that is reported in a research report. The specific data-collection method that is used also needs to be critiqued. Some general guidelines for critiquing data-collection methods and some specific questions to ask about questionnaires and interviews are presented in Box 12–1.

If a questionnaire was used in a study, sufficient information should be provided to allow the reader to determine if it was appropriate for use in the study. The manner in which the questionnaire was developed, the reliability and validity of the instrument, the number of questions, how the instrument was scored, and the range of possible scores should be presented. Assurance of subject anonymity or confidentiality should be addressed.

When an interview has been used, the reader needs information about how long the interviews took, who conducted the interviews, and how the interviewers were trained. Means of ensuring confidentiality should be presented.

Observation research requires that the reader be able to determine how observations were made, who made the observations, and how data were recorded. Were subjects aware that they were being observed?

Box 12–1.   Guidelines for Critiquing Data-collection Methods

General Criteria

1. Were the data-collection methods described thoroughly?
2. Were the data-collection methods appropriate to test the research hypotheses or answer the research questions?
3. Was a self-report or psychological method used when a physiological method might have gathered more valid data?
4. How many methods were used to collect data? If only one method was used, would the study have benefited from more than one method?

Questionnaires

1. Was information provided on the number of questions, the length of the questionnaire, and how long it would take to complete the questionnaire?
2. Was the response rate provided for the return of the questionnaires?
3. Were sampling biases discussed?
4. Was anonymity or confidentiality ensured?

Interviews

1. Was information provided on how long the interview would take?
2. Was information provided about training for the interviewers?
3. Was confidentiality assured?

If physiological instruments were used, the accuracy of these data-collection measures needs to be addressed. Does it appear that the researcher would have had the expertise to use these instruments?

The researcher may have used a psychological data-collection method, such as an attitude scale or a personality test. The reader will need to determine the appropriateness of these instruments and the qualifications of the researcher to use them.

The reader may not be familiar with data-collection methods, such as the Delphi technique or Q Sort, which are mentioned in research articles. It would be advisable to consult research textbooks to learn more about the data-collection methods that have been mentioned in research reports.

SUMMARY

A **questionnaire** is a paper-and-pencil, self-report instrument. Factors to consider in constructing questionnaires are (a) overall appearance, (b) language and reading level, (c) length of questionnaire and questions, (d) wording of questions, (e) types of questions, and (f) placement of questions.

Ambiguous questions contain words that have more than one meaning. **Double-barreled questions** ask two questions in one. **Demographic questions** concern subject characteristics. These subject characteristics are called **demographic variables** or **attribute variables. Open-ended questions** allow respondents to answer questions in their own words, whereas **closed-ended questions** are very structured, and respondents are asked to choose from given alternatives. The term **collectively exhaustive categories** indicates that a category is provided for every possible answer. **Mutually exclusive categories** are categories that are uniquely distinct; no overlap occurs between categories. **Contingency questions** are items that are relevant for some respondents and not for others. **Filler questions** are items in which the researcher has no direct interest but are included on a questionnaire to reduce the emphasis on the specific purpose of other questions.

A cover letter should accompany all mailed questionnaires. Questionnaires may be distributed in a one-to-one contact, through group administration, or through a mailing system. Response rates of questionnaires are frequently low.

There are many advantages and disadvantages in using questionnaires as a method of data collection. The researcher considers each of these factors in determining if questionnaires are an appropriate type of research instrument for a particular study.

An **interview** is a data-collection method in which an interviewer obtains responses from a subject in a face-to-face meeting or from **telephone interviews.** Data are recorded on an **interview schedule** or may be tape-recorded. **Unstructured interviews** contain open-ended questions and are appropriate for exploratory studies where the researcher possesses little knowledge of the study topic. **Probes** are additional prompting questions that encourage the respondent to elaborate on a certain topic. **Structured interviews** use closed-ended questions and are generally used to obtain straightforward, factual information. **Semistructured interviews** contain both open-ended and closed-ended questions. The majority of interviews are of the semistructured type.

Observation research gathers data through visual observations. In **structured observations,** the expected behaviors have been predetermined, and the frequency of occurrence is noted during data collection. In **unstructured observations,** the researcher describes events or behaviors as they occur, with no preconceived ideas of what will be seen. **Event sampling** involves observation of an entire event, while **time sampling** concerns events or behaviors during certain specified times.

As a **nonparticipant observer-overt,** the observer openly identifies that research is being conducted. The **nonparticipant observer-covert** does not identify herself or himself as a researcher. This type of observation is quite likely to be unethical. The **participant observer-overt** becomes involved with subjects openly and with the full awareness of those people who will be observed in their natural settings. In contrast, the **participant observer-covert** interacts with subjects and observes their behavior without their knowledge. Again, this type of observation may be unethical.

Physiological measures involve the collection of physical data from subjects. These measures are generally quite accurate.

Attitude scales ask respondents to report their attitudes or feelings on a continuum. The scales are composed of a number of related items, and respondents are given a score after the item responses are totaled. The **Likert scale** and the **semantic differential** are two commonly used types of attitude scales.

Personality inventories are self-report measures that seek information about someone's personality traits, needs, or values by asking questions or requesting responses to statements that are presented.

In the various **projective techniques,** subjects are presented with stimuli that are designed to be ambiguous. Responses reflect the internal feelings of the subjects that are projected on the external stimuli.

When a **Q sort** is used**,** subjects are asked to sort statements into categories according to their attitudes toward, or rating of, the statements. The statements are written on cards or pieces of paper, and respondents are asked to arrange the items in piles according to the intensity of their attitudes or beliefs about the items.

A **Delphi technique** uses several rounds of questionnaires to seek consensus on a particular topic from a group of experts. This procedure is appropriate for examining the opinions, beliefs, or future predictions of knowledgeable people on a topic of interest.

The **visual analogue scale** (VAS) presents subjects with a straight line drawn on a piece of paper. Subjects are asked to make a mark on the line at the point that corresponds to their experience of pain, for example.

Preexisting data are data from records of agencies such as hospitals, the United States government, and public health departments that have not been collected for research purposes. Also, diaries, letters, almanacs, and professional journals may be examined.

 ## NURSING RESEARCH ON THE WEB

For additional online resources, research activities, and exercises, go to www.prenhall. com/nieswiadomy. Select Chapter 12 from the drop down menu.

✕ GET INVOLVED ACTIVITIES

1. Read through research articles in the library until you find at least three articles that have used some data-collection method other than a questionnaire. Make a list of these different data-collection methods.

2. Divide into groups. Pretend that you are designing some demographic questions for a questionnaire that you will administer in a study. Design a question to obtain marital status and one to obtain educational level. You will find that both of these variables present a challenge when trying to choose categories that are mutually exclusive and collectively exhaustive.

3. Divide into pairs. One person will serve as an interviewer and the other person will serve as the respondent. The interviewer will ask the respondent to provide information on what she or he ate during the last week. Switch roles. The interviewer will ask the respondent to describe the last movie that he or she viewed. Hopefully, this exercise will help you to experience some of the feelings that accompany these two roles in research.

4. From a bowl containing pieces of paper on which are written all of the data-collection methods listed in this chapter, draw one method and develop an idea for a study in which this method would be used.

✕ SELF-TEST

1. Examine the following question and determine if any errors exist in the construction of the question:

What is your age category?

_____ 6–20

_____ 20–25

_____ 25–30

_____ 30 and above

Circle the letter before the *best* answer.

2. Which of the following is an *advantage* of an interview method of data collection versus a questionnaire?

  A. Data are less expensive to obtain.
  B. The collected data tend to be more complete.
  C. Data collectors do not need to be trained.
  D. Data may be collected more easily from a widespread geographical area.

3. A purpose of observation research is to:

  A. determine beliefs of people.
  B. examine attitudes of people.

    C. obtain examples of peoples' behaviors.

    D. analyze personal experiences of people.

4. A researcher wants to determine future priorities for research in psychiatric nursing. The participants will be clinical specialists in psychiatric nursing. Which of the following data-collection methods would probably be used?

    A. projective technique

    B. observation

    C. Delphi technique

    D. semantic differential

5. Which of the following data-collection methods is *most* likely to obtain objective data?

    A. observational methods

    B. questionnaires

    C. physiological measures

    D. interviews

6. Which of the following data-collection methods is *most* likely to prevent subjects from providing socially acceptable responses to questions?

    A. attitude scales

    B. projective techniques

    C. self-report questionnaires

    D. interviews

Choose the letter of the data-collection method that matches the method described in statements 7 to 10 below.

    A. semantic differential

    B. projective technique

    C. Q Sort

    D. Likert scale

_____ 7. Presents statements to which respondents indicate level of agreement or disagreement along a continuum.

_____ 8. Contains sets of bipolar adjectives; asks respondents to select a point on a scale between two adjectives.

_____ 9. Participants are asked to place statements into categories according to their attitudes toward or rating of the statements.

_____ 10. Subjects are asked to look at pictures and tell what meaning the pictures have for them.

✁ REFERENCES

Albright, J., Guzman, C., Acebo, P., Paiva, D., Faulkner, M., & Swanson, J. (1996). Readability of patient education materials: Implications for clinical practice. *Applied Nursing Research, 9,* 139–143.

Beck, C. T., & Gable, R. K., (2000). Postpartum depression screening scale: Development and psychometric testing. *Nursing Research, 49,* 272–282.

Belza, B. (1996). Conducting research in respondents' homes: Benefits, problems, and strategies. *Applied Nursing Research, 9,* 37–44.

Burns, N., & Grove, S. K. (1997). *The practice of nursing research: Conduct, critique and utilization* (3rd ed.). Philadelphia: Saunders.

Flaherty, S. A. (1996). Pain measurement tools for clinical practice and research. *Journal of the American Association of Nurse Anesthetists, 64,* 39.

Fochtman, D., & Hinds, P. S. (2000). Identifying nursing research priorities in a pediatric clinical trials cooperative group: The Pediatric Oncology Group experience. *Journal of Pediatric Oncology Nursing, 17,* 83–87.

Fontana, J. A. (2000). The energy costs of a modified form of T'ai Chi exercise. *Nursing Research, 49,* 91–96.

French, K. S., & Larrabee, J. H. (1999). Relationships among educational material readability, client literacy, perceived beneficence, and perceived quality. *Journal of Nursing Care Quality, 13,* 68–82.

Glazer-Waldman, H., Hall, K., & Weiner, M. (1985). Patient education in a public hospital. *Nursing Research, 34,* 184–185.

Hill, A. S., Kurkowski, T. B., & Garcia, J. (2000). Oral support measures used in feeding the preterm infant. *Nursing Research, 49,* 2–10.

Holden, J. E. (1996). Physiological research is nursing research. *Nursing Research, 45,* 312–313.

Huang, H., Wilkie, D. J., & Berry, D. L. (1996). Use of a computerized digitizer to score and enter visual analogue scale data. *Nursing Research, 45,* 370–372.

Kovach, C. R., & Krejci, J. W. (1998). Facilitating change in dementia care. *Journal of Nursing Administration, 28,* 17–27.

Lee, E. J., Phoenix, D., Brown, W., & Jackson, B. S. (1998). Sickle cell disease: Problem solving/coping methods among affected children and their non-affected siblings. *Journal of School Health, 14,* 24–28.

Lee, H., Kohlman, G. C. V., Lee, K., & Schiller, N. B. (2000). Fatigue, mood, and hemodynamic patterns after myocardial infarction. *Applied Nursing Research, 13,* 60–69.

Lee, T. T., & Mills, M. E. (2000). The relationship among medical diagnosis, nursing diagnosis, and nursing intervention and the implications for home health care. *Journal of Professional Nursing, 16,* 84–91.

Lindeman, C. (1975). Delphi survey of priorities in clinical nursing research. *Nursing Research, 24,* 434–441.

Majewski, J. (1986). Conflicts, satisfactions, and attitudes during transition to the maternal role. *Nursing Research, 35,* 10–14.

Niedz, B. A. (1998). Correlates of hospitalized patients' perceptions of service quality. *Research in Nursing & Health, 21,* 339–349.

Oppenheim, A. (1966). *Questionnaire design and attitude measurement.* New York: Basic Books.

Osgood, C., Suci, G., & Tannenbaum, P. (1957). *The measurement of meaning.* Urbana, IL: University of Illinois Press.

Pugh, L. C., & DeKeyser, F. G. (1995). Use of physiologic variables in nursing research. *Image: Journal of Nursing Scholarship, 27,* 273–276.

Ring policy in telephone surveys. (1980). *Public Opinion Quarterly, 44,* 115–116.

Roberts, B. L., Srour, M. I., & Winkelman, C. (1996). Videotaping: An important research strategy. *Nursing Research, 45,* 334–337.

Shelley, S. (1984). *Research methods in nursing and health.* Boston: Little, Brown.

Stephenson, N. L., & Herman, J. (2000). Pain measurement: A comparison using horizontal and vertical visual analogue scales. *Applied Nursing Research, 13,* 157–158.

Wang, S., Yu, M., Wang, C., & Huang, C. (1999). Bridging the gap between the pros and cons in treating ordinal scales as interval scales from an analysis point of view. *Nursing Research, 48,* 226–229.

Weeks, M., Jones, B., Folsom, R., & Benrud, C. (1980). Optimal time to contact sample households. *Public Opinion Quarterly, 44,* 101–114.

Yoos, H. L., & McMullen, A. (1999). Symptom perception and evaluation in childhood asthma. *Nursing Research, 48,* 2–8.

PART V

Data Analysis

CHAPTER 13

Descriptive Statistics

OUTLINE

OBJECTIVES

On completion of this chapter, you will be prepared to:

1. Recognize statistical symbols for population parameters and sample statistics
2. Identify the two broad classifications of statistics
3. Discuss four major groups of descriptive statistics
4. Compare categories within each of the four major groups of descriptive statistics
5. Determine appropriate descriptive statistics to use in presenting selected data
6. Construct graphs to present selected descriptive statistics
7. Critique descriptive statistics presented in research reports

✖ NEW TERMS DEFINED IN THIS CHAPTER

bar graph	negatively skewed
bimodal	nonsymmetrical distributions
class intervals	normal curve
coefficient of determination	normal distribution
contingency table	parameters
descriptive statistics	percentage
frequency distribution	percentile
frequency polygon	positively skewed
histogram	range
inferential statistics	scatter diagram
interquartile range	scatter plot
mean	scattergram
measures of central tendency	semiquartile range
measures of relationships	skewed
measures of variability	standard deviation
measures to condense data	statistics
median	symmetrical distributions
modal class	unimodal
mode	variance
multimodal	z-score

You have been excitedly waiting to read this chapter and the next one. Is that correct? The two chapter titles, "Descriptive Statistics" and "Inferential Statistics," provide enough information for you to know that you are going to enjoy the contents. (Oh sure!) If you are one of those people who try to avoid anything involving mathematics, rest assured that only minimal math skills are necessary to understand the material in these chapters. According to Norwood (2000), all that is needed is basic arithmetic and logical thinking skills. Does that make you feel better? Rather that understanding each of the various statistical tests, it is much more important that you are familiar with the type of data that you have collected or that someone else has collected and the types of statistical tests that might be appropriate for these data. Also you really do not need to know how to calculate statistics. In this age of computers, it is quite unlikely that you will ever have to hand-compute any statistics.

The word *statistics* is derived from the Latin word for state. In the mid-18th century, the term was used in a political context to describe the resources of states and kingdoms. The term is used much more broadly today, and statistics are used by many disciplines. Statistics as a singular noun is a branch of knowledge that is used to summarize and to present numerical data. As a plural noun, statistics are numerical characteristics of samples. According to Polit and Hungler (1999), statistical procedures allow the researcher to "reduce, summarize, organize, evaluate, interpret, and communicate numeric information" (p. 439).

This chapter and the next chapter present a review of statistical concepts. If you need more information, there are many statistics textbooks available. One that may be of particular interest to you is *Statistics for the Terrified* by Gerald Kranzler and Janet

Moursund (see Amazon.com for more information). Some free textbooks can now be found online. The Web addresses, as of January 2001, of three of these statistics textbooks are listed below:

http://www.psychstat.smsu/edu/introbook/sbk00m.htm
http://ebook.stat.ucla.edu/textbook/
http://www.statsoft.com/textbook/stathome.html

STATISTICAL SYMBOLS

When discussing numerical characteristics of populations, the word **parameters** is used. When discussing numerical characteristics of samples, the term **statistics** is used. An easy way for you to recall this information is to remember that population and parameter both begin with a *p*, and sample and statistics both begin with an *s*. You, therefore, have population *p*arameters and *s*ample statistics. Different symbols are used to depict parameters and statistics.

	Population Symbols	Sample Symbols
Mean	μ	$\overline{X}$
Standard deviation	σ	s, SD
Variance	σ^2	s^2, SD^2

Greek letters such as mu (μ) are used to designate population parameters, and English letters such as s and SD are used to indicate sample statistics. When you encounter these symbols in descriptions of research studies and in tables that accompany studies, you will be able to quickly determine which type of data is being reported. In many research articles, words are used instead of symbols. A recent review of the literature revealed that words and letters rather than symbols are used frequently to depict population parameters and sample statistics. For example, in reviewing some recent research articles, the word "mean" or "average" and the letter "M" were found more frequently than the $\overline{X}$ symbol to depict the mean.

CLASSIFICATIONS OF STATISTICS

There are two broad classifications of statistics—descriptive and inferential. **Descriptive statistics,** are those statistics that organize and summarize numerical data gathered from populations and samples. **Inferential statistics** are concerned with populations and use sample data to make an "inference" about a population. Inferential statistics help the researcher to determine if the difference that is found between two groups, such as an experimental and a control group, is a real difference or is only a chance difference that occurred because an unrepresentative sample was chosen from the population. Any time sample data are used to estimate the characteristics of a population, there is a chance that the estimate will be inaccurate. Inferential statistics are used to determine the likelihood that the sample that is chosen for a study is actually representative of the population.

DESCRIPTIVE STATISTICS

Descriptive statistics allow the researcher to examine the characteristics, behaviors, and experiences of study participants (Polit, 1999). There are many different ways to categorize descriptive statistics. In this book, they have been divided into four classifications: (a) measures to condense data, (b) measures of central tendency, (c) measures of variability, and (d) measures of relationships.

MEASURES TO CONDENSE DATA

When the researcher is faced with analyzing a large amount of data, some method is needed to condense the data into a more understandable form. **Measures to condense data** are statistics that are used to summarize and condense data. Some of the various ways to condense or summarize the data include frequency distributions, graphic presentations, and percentages.

Frequency Distributions.   One of the simplest ways to present data is through frequency distributions. Frequencies are obtained by simply counting the occurrence of values or scores represented in the data. Frequency distributions are appropriate for reporting all level of data (nominal, ordinal, interval, ratio). In a **frequency distribution,** all values or scores are listed, and the number of times each one appears is recorded. Values may be listed from highest to lowest or from lowest to highest.

It is helpful to use the familiar slash method of recording frequencies: Four vertical lines are listed for the first four occurrences of a score, and a slash line is used to indicate the fifth occurrence (*HHt*). This procedure is repeated until all scores are recorded.

Frequency distributions present useful summaries of data. For example, the reader will get a much clearer picture of students' scores on a test or the pulse rates of a group of patients.

If the range of scores in a frequency distribution is small, say less than 20, each score may be listed individually, as in Table 13–1. When the range of scores is large, it may be helpful to group the scores before counting frequencies, as is seen in Table 13–2. Groups of scores in a frequency distribution are called **class intervals.** These intervals are arbitrarily chosen to depict the data in the most meaningful way. Class intervals may be in units of 3, 5, 10, and so forth. The intervals must be exhaustive (include all possible values) and mutually exclusive (no overlapping of categories). Of course, when data are grouped, some information is lost. Consider the following examples:

EXAMPLE A			EXAMPLE B	
Score	*Frequency*		*Score*	*Frequency*
20	3		20–22	14
21	5			
22	6			
	14			

TABLE 13–1. Frequency Distribution of Respiration Rates

Respiration	Rate Tallies	Frequency
14	///	3
15	//	2
16	////	5
17	////	4
18	///	3
19	//	2
20	/	1
		20

In example A, you can determine exactly how many people received a score of 20, 21, or 22. In example B, you are able to determine only that 14 people scored between 20 and 22. This loss of information is the price that is paid when data are summarized into groups or classes.

Frequency distributions may be described according to their shape. Distribution shapes may be characterized as either symmetrical or nonsymmetrical. **Symmetrical distributions** are those in which both halves of the distribution are the same. If the left half of the distribution was to be folded over the right half, the two halves would match. **Nonsymmetrical distributions,** also called **skewed,** are those in which the distribution has an off-center peak. If the tail of the distribution points to the right (Figure 13–1), the distribution is said to be **positively skewed;** if the tail of the distribution points to the left (Figure 13–2), the distribution is said to be **negatively skewed.** An example of a variable that

TABLE 13–2. Frequency Distribution of Pulse Rates

Pulse Rate	Tallies	Frequency
56–60	//	2
61–65	//	2
66–70	////	5
71–75	//// //	7
76–80	//// ///	8
81–85	//// ////	10
86–90	//// //	7
91–95	////	5
96–100	////	4
		50

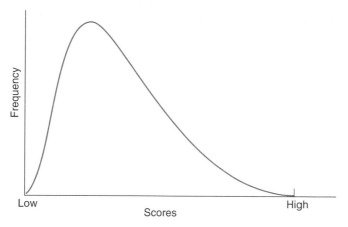

Figure 13–1. Positively skewed distribution.

tends to be positively skewed is personal income. A lot of people have small or middle incomes, while a few people have large incomes. An example of a negatively skewed distribution would be the age of people who have chronic illnesses. A few young and middle-aged men and women have chronic illnesses, but many more elderly people have chronic conditions.

A theoretical frequency distribution of particular importance in statistics is the normal distribution. The **normal distribution** is a symmetrical distribution that has one central peak or set of values in the middle of the distribution. The **normal curve** is a bell-shaped curve that graphically presents a normal distribution. The normal distribution is a theoretical, mathematical construct that was developed by Carl Gauss. The normal curve is sometimes called the Gaussian curve. As with all graphic presentations of frequency distributions, the values of the distribution are placed on the horizontal axis, and the frequency of the values is placed on the vertical axis. The one difference in this type

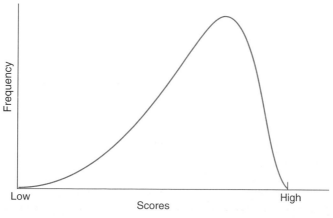

Figure 13–2. Negatively skewed distribution.

of graph compared with a histogram or frequency polygon is that the vertical axis is usually not displayed. The actual frequency of the values is therefore not depicted on the graph of a normal curve.

Normal is a mathematical rather than a medical or psychological term and is used in the sense that a normal distribution is frequently found in many happenings in nature. Such variables as height and weight are normally distributed in the population. For example, most people are of average height. There are a few very short and a few very tall people, but most people are within a few inches of each other in height. For a frequency distribution to approximate the normal curve, a fairly large number of values are needed. However, the normal curve will be closely approximated with sample sizes of at least 30 (Roscoe, 1975; Shott, 1990).

Characteristics of the normal curve include the following:

1. It is bell-shaped, with a symmetrical distribution, and the maximum height being the mean.
2. The mean, median, and mode are the same value.
3. Most of the values cluster around the mean.
4. A few values occur on both extreme ends of the distribution curve.
5. The point where the curve begins to grow faster horizontally than vertically is called an inflection point and lies at 1 SD above and below the mean.
6. The tails of the curve never touch the base because the distribution is theoretical, rather than empirical.

In the normal curve, 50% of the values lie on the left half of the distribution, and 50% lie on the right half. Other percentages can be determined by assessing the distances of various values from the mean. For example, 34.13% of the area under the curve lies between the mean and +1 SD from the mean. Because the distribution is symmetrical, 34.13% of the area under the curve lies between the mean and −1 SD from the mean. Therefore, 68.26% of the distribution lies between ±1 SD from the mean, 95.44% of the distribution lies between ±2 SD, and 99.72% lies within ±3 SD of the mean. Although theoretically the curve never touches the base, nearly 100% of the values lie between −3 SD and +3 SD. Only 0.14% of the values lie above +3 SD and 0.14% below −3 SD. Figure 13–3 depicts the areas under the normal curve.

The percentages under the normal curve may be thought of as probabilities. These probabilities are usually stated in decimal form. For example, 34.13% of the area under the normal curve lies between the mean and +1 SD. When this percentage is converted to a decimal, it becomes .3413. The probability that a value in a normal distribution lies between the mean and +1 SD is .3413. The probability that a value lies above +1 SD is .1587 (.5000 − .3413 = .1587). An understanding of probabilities is important when considering inferential statistics and are discussed more in Chapter 14.

Graphic Presentations. Data may be presented in a graphic form that makes the frequency distribution of the data readily apparent. Graphic presentations also have a visual appeal that may cause the reader to analyze the data more closely than would be the case

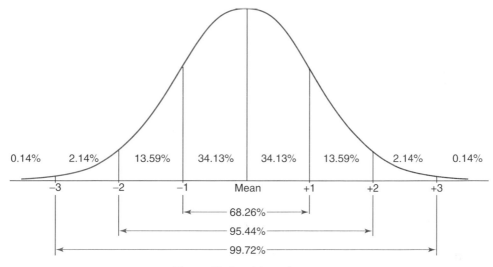

Figure 13–3.   Normal curve.

if a written description of the data were presented. Various graphic displays are appropriate according to the level of measurement of the variable to be presented. A graphic display is called a *figure.*

Bar Graph.   A **bar graph** is a figure used to represent a frequency distribution of nominal data and some types of ordinal data. The bar graph is especially useful when the categories of the variables are qualitative rather than numerical. As can be seen in Figure 13–3, the lengths of the bars represent the frequency of occurrence of the category. Bar graphs may be drawn with the bars extending in a horizontal direction (as in Figure 13–4) or with the bars extending in a vertical direction. To show that the data being represented

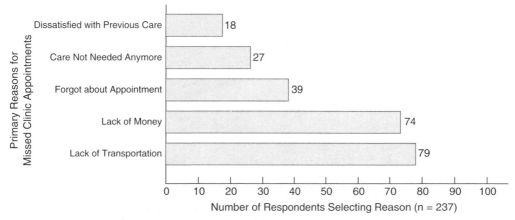

Figure 13–4.   Bar graph of reasons for missed clinic appointments.

are separate categories, the bars do not touch each other. Data are presented on only one variable in a bar graph. In Figure 13–4, the variable is "reasons for missing clinic appointments." Each of the reasons given by the respondents represents a separate category of the variable being measured.

Histogram. A **histogram** is a graph that uses bars to represent the frequency distribution of a variable that is measured at the ordinal, interval, or ratio level (Figure 13–5). Data are presented on only one variable in a histogram. The bars in a histogram are of equal width and touch each other to indicate that data are being presented on a continuum. The width of the bar represents the size of the class interval. The height of the bar represents the frequency of occurrence of each class interval. To construct a histogram, two axes are drawn—a vertical and a horizontal axis. The vertical axis is called the ordinate, and the horizontal axis is called the abscissa. Beginning at 0, the ordinate axis is marked off in equal intervals up to the highest possible frequency of the category being measured. The abscissa is marked off with the class intervals or categories of the variable. For good graphic proportions the vertical axis is generally drawn about two-thirds the length of the horizontal axis.

Frequency Polygon. A **frequency polygon** is a graph that uses dots connected with straight lines to represent the frequency distribution of ordinal, interval, or ratio data (Figure 13–6). A dot is placed above the midpoint of each class interval; these dots are then connected. Although not strictly correct, it is customary to bring the distribution down to the horizontal axis by adding a 0 frequency at each end of the distribution.

As is the case with histograms, the class intervals of the variable are represented on the horizontal axis of the frequency polygon, and the frequency of the class intervals is represented on the vertical axis. The height of each dot indicates the frequency of a particular class interval.

Percentages. A **percentage** is a statistic that represents the proportion of a subgroup to a total group, expressed as a percentage ranging from 0 to 100. A percentage is the number of parts per hundred that a certain portion of the whole represents. The size of the total

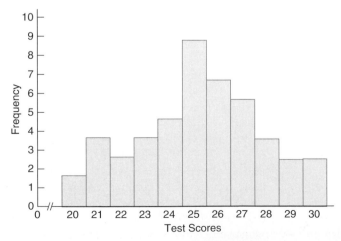

Figure 13–5. Histogram of test scores.

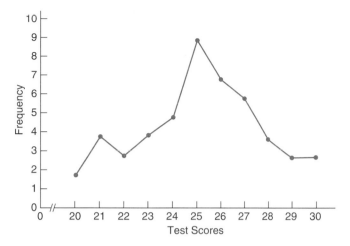

Figure 13–6. Frequency polygon of test scores.

group on which a percentage is based should be reasonably large for the percentage to be a useful or valid statistic. The minimum number for the computation of percentages should be at least 20. This number ensures that each element in a group represents only 5% of the total group. To illustrate the need for fairly large numbers of scores or values when computing percentages, consider the following example. A friend comes up to you and says, "I just heard that they conducted a survey, and 60% of the students interviewed said they thought another year should be added to our educational program." If you were a student in the program, your first instinct might be to go find the "traitors" and give them a piece of your mind. First, however, it would be wise to ask how many students were interviewed. If told that only five students were interviewed, you would probably not consider the sample to be very representative of the student population and would probably not worry about the survey's results.

Measures of Central Tendency

In many cases, the condensing of data will not be of as much interest or importance as the average value of a distribution. **Measures of central tendency** are statistics that describe the average, typical, or most common value for a group of data. *Central* refers to the middle or average value, and *tendency* refers to the general trend of the numbers to cluster in a certain way. A measure of central tendency summarizes a frequency distribution by the use of a single number.

Nurse researchers are frequently interested in such questions as these: What is the average level of anxiety of nursing students before an examination among those who practiced progressive relaxation before the exam compared with those who did not practice progressive relaxation? Of course, the frequency distribution of the anxiety scores would be of interest, but the average anxiety level would provide a much more succinct indication of any difference that might exist in the anxiety levels of the two groups.

Although average is frequently used to indicate the arithmetic mean, there are also two other measures of central tendency—the mode and the median. The level of measurement of the data determines which measure of central tendency should be used in presenting the average value of a set of data.

Mode. The **mode,** sometimes abbreviated as Mo, is the category or value that occurs most often in a set of data under consideration. It may be thought of as the most representative category or value in the group. The mode is determined by visually analyzing and counting data.

The mode is the only measure of central tendency appropriate for nominal data. When the data are only categories rather than actual numbers, as is the case with nominal data, the category with the greatest frequency is called the **modal class.** For example, if a sample were composed of 50 nurses, 40 occupational therapists, 35 dental technicians, and 30 physical therapists, the modal class would be nurses.

The mode may also be reported for ordinal, interval, or ratio data. In the following distribution of scores, the mode is 13 because it appears twice and the other six numbers appear only once:

$$16 \quad 15 \quad 13 \quad 13 \quad 12 \quad 9 \quad 6 \quad 4$$

If the distribution of the values is symmetrical in a frequency distribution, the mode will be the same value as the median and the mean. A set of data with one value that occurs most frequently is called **unimodal.** If two values have the same high frequency, the distribution is called **bimodal.** If more than two values have the same high frequency, the distribution is said to be **multimodal.** Although the mode is an interesting statistic, it is rarely reported in the literature because it is only a crude estimate of the average value of the data.

Median. The **median,** sometimes abbreviated as Md or Mdn, is the middle score or value in a group of data. With interval and ratio data, the median divides the frequency distribution of the data in half. If the number of scores or values is uneven, the median is the middle value. If the number of scores is even, the median is the midpoint between these two middle values and is found by averaging these two values. Consider the following examples:

Uneven Number of Scores		**Even Number of Scores**	
16		16	
15		15	
13	50% of values	13	50% of values
13		13	
12	Median	(12.5)	Median
9		12	
6		9	
4	50% of values	6	50% of values
3		4	

The median is appropriate for ordinal, interval, and ratio data. When ordinal data are analyzed, the average category can be identified. For example, if anxiety levels were classified as mild, moderate, severe, and panic, the average category chosen might be moderate. When percentiles are being calculated, the median is the 50th percentile. If grouped data from a frequency distribution are being used, a formula is needed to compute the median. One of the most valuable qualities of the median is that it is not influenced by extreme values. The median is frequently used in reporting average income because extremely high or low incomes do not affect the median, as would be the case if the mean were calculated.

Mean. The **mean,** sometimes abbreviated as M or presented as $\overline{X}$, is the average sum of a set of values found by adding all values and dividing by the total number of values. This measure of central tendency is also called the arithmetic mean. Whereas the mode and median indicate the position of certain values in a distribution, the mean considers all of the values as a whole.

The mean is appropriate for interval and ratio data. It is considered the most stable measure of central tendency for these levels of data if the distribution is normal. If the distribution is not normal and extreme values are present, the mean will not present an accurate picture of the distribution. As mentioned under the discussion of the median, if average income were reported as the mean, a few extremely wealthy people could make the rest of us appear rich.

The symbol for a sample mean is $\overline{X}$ and the symbol for the population mean is μ. The mean is figured in the following manner:

$$\overline{X} = \frac{\Sigma X}{N}$$

where X = score; Σ = a summation sign, indicating that all scores are added; and N = total number of scores.

$$
\begin{array}{c}
16 \\
15 \\
13 \\
13 \\
12 \\
9 \\
6 \\
\underline{4} \\
\Sigma X = 88
\end{array}
$$

$$\overline{X} = \frac{\Sigma X}{N} = \frac{88}{8} = 11$$

MEASURES OF VARIABILITY

Measures of variability describe how spread out values are in a distribution of values. Although measures of central tendency are very important, sometimes it may be of more interest to know how spread out the values are in a distribution. Consider the following pulse rates:

Group A	Group B
80	100
79	90
78	80
78	70
75	50
$\Sigma X = 390$	$\Sigma X = 390$
X = 78	X = 78

As can be seen, the mean of both groups of pulse rates is the same. However, pulse rates of people in Group A are homogeneous, or alike, while pulse rates of people in Group B are heterogeneous, or dissimilar. This information would be very important because the arithmetic mean is not appropriate to use in describing Group B or to use in comparing the two groups of pulse rates. The most common measures of variability are range, percentile, standard deviation, variance, and z-scores.

Range. The distance between the highest and lowest value in a group of values or scores is called the **range.** The range is the simplest measure of variability. It is presented as a single number. Frequently, the word *range* is used incorrectly to indicate the lowest and highest values. For example, a statement might be made: "The scores ranged from 40 to 60." Although this type of statement is fairly common, technically the range for these scores is 20 (60 − 40 = 20). The range is a measure that may be used to gain a quick picture of the dispersion of the data. It has limited usefulness because one extreme score can change the range drastically.

To correct for the influence of extreme scores or values, the interquartile range (IQR) may be reported. The **interquartile range** contains the middle half of the values in a frequency distribution.

$$IQR = Q_3 - Q_1$$

where Q_3 = the point below which three fourths of the distribution lies, and Q_1 = the point below which one fourth of the distribution lies.

The **semiquartile range** (SQR) is found by dividing the interquartile range in half. SQR = IQR/2.

Percentile. A **percentile** is a datum point below which lies a certain percentage of the values in a frequency distribution. If you score at the 80th percentile on a test, it means that 80% of the other students received lower scores. You might also say that 20% of the other students scored higher (it depends on whether you are an optimist or a pessimist!)

The median of a frequency distribution lies at the 50th percentile. Percentile is a common statistic used to allow people to compare their performance with that of others. Raw scores, or untreated data, are transformed into percentile ranks. For an explanation of how to compute percentiles, consult a statistics book.

Percentiles are used a great deal in the assessment of infants and children. Imagine that you read a child's chart and find out that for his age group he is at the 95th percentile in height and at the 15th percentile in weight. What would you expect the physical appearance of this child to be like in height and weight? Tall and skinny, right?

An anxiety test used frequently in nursing research is the State-Trait Anxiety Inventory by Spielberger (1983). Spielberger views state anxiety as a current feeling of emotional and physical uneasiness, whereas trait anxiety refers to a person's anxiety proneness and is considered to be a relatively stable personality trait. The test booklet that accompanies this anxiety test provides information about the test and furnishes percentile ranks for groups on which the test was normed. The lowest possible score is 20 and the highest possible score is 80 on the two scales that measure state and trait anxiety. You might think that an average anxiety score would be 50, which is half way between 20 and 80. Not so! A raw score of 50 on the state anxiety scale is at the 82nd percentile when compared with a group of female college students who were used in establishing norms for the test. A score of 66 is at the 99th percentile.

Standard Deviation. The standard deviation is the most widely used measure of variability when interval or ratio data are obtained. This statistic describes how values vary about the mean of the distribution. The word *standard* is used to mean average. The **standard deviation,** abbreviated SD or s, is a measurement that indicates the average deviation or variation of all the values in a set of values from the mean value of those data. Like the arithmetic mean, the standard deviation considers all the values in a distribution. The actual definition of the standard deviation is difficult to understand. Mathematically, the standard deviation is equal to the square root of the sum of the squared deviations about the mean divided by the total number of values. The formula for calculating the standard deviation is:

$$s = \sqrt{\frac{\Sigma(X - \overline{X})^2}{N}}$$

where s = standard deviation, $\sqrt{}$ = square root, $\Sigma(X - \overline{X})^2$ = sum of the squared deviations about the mean, and N = number of values.

Because a sample is a biased estimation of the population, N-1 should be used in the formula when estimating a population standard deviation from sample data. The use of N-1 makes the value obtained a more accurate estimate of the population standard deviation.

The following steps are used in calculating the standard deviation:

1. Add each score or value in the distribution (ΣX)
2. Find the mean (ΣX/N = $\overline{X}$)
3. Find the deviation score by subtracting the mean from each score (X – $\overline{X}$)
4. Square each of the deviation scores (X – $\overline{X}$)^2
5. Add all of the squared deviation scores [Σ(X – $\overline{X}$)^2]
   This value is called the sum of squares

6. Find the mean of the squared deviation scores $\dfrac{[\Sigma(X - \overline{X})^2]}{N}$

   This value is called the variance

7. Find the square root of the mean of the squared deviation scores

$$\sqrt{\dfrac{\Sigma(X - \overline{X})^2}{N}}$$

   This value is called the standard deviation

Examples of the calculation of a standard deviation will be shown so you can get a better understanding of the meaning of this important measure of variability. Table 13–3 presents the calculation of two standard deviations. For ease of calculation, only five values are presented in each set of data.

Note that the average pulse rate is the same for both groups, but the standard deviations are much different. The pulse rates are much more varied in Group B.

Several formulas may be used to calculate the standard deviation. The formula that is used in Table 13–3 gives a clear conceptual picture of the standard deviation. Some of the other formulas are easier to use if a calculator or computer is available.

TABLE 13–3.   Calculation of Standard Deviation

Pulse Rates (X)	Deviation Scores $(X - \overline{X})$	Squared Deviation Scores $(X - \overline{X})^2$
Group A		
75	$75 - 78 = -3$	9
80	$80 - 78 = 2$	4
79	$79 - 78 = 1$	1
78	$78 - 78 = 0$	0
78	$78 - 78 = 0$	0
$\Sigma X = 390$		$\Sigma(X - \overline{X})^2 = 14$
$\overline{X} = 390/5 = 78$	$s = \sqrt{14/5} = \sqrt{2.8} = 1.67$	
Group B		
100	$100 - 78 = 22$	484
90	$90 - 78 = 12$	144
80	$80 - 78 = 2$	4
70	$70 - 78 = -8$	64
50	$50 - 78 = -28$	784
$\Sigma X = 390$		$\Sigma(X - \overline{X})^2 = 1480$
$\overline{X} = 390/5 = 78$	$s = \sqrt{1480/5} = \sqrt{296} = 17.2$	

You may wonder when you would ever use the standard deviation in nursing. All of you are familiar with critical pathways. They are useful in planning care for a group of patients with the same condition and who have a predictable course of recovery. If, for example, the SD for length of stay for a group of patients with a certain serious condition is 5.2 days, it might be difficult to develop a critical pathway. It appears that there may be too much variability in recovery time for one plan of care to be suitable for all patients with this condition.

Variance.   The variance is a measure that is used in several inferential statistical tests. It is the value obtained in step 6 of the calculation of the standard deviation. In other words, the **variance** is the standard deviation squared.

Mathematically, the variance is equal to the sum of the squared deviations about the mean divided by the total number of values. The variance is discussed infrequently in descriptive statistics because it is not in the same unit of measurement as the variable that is being examined. For example, in Table 13–3 pulse rates are the variable of interest. If the variance were presented, it would be in units of "pulse rates squared." It is difficult to think in terms of squared pulse rates. The standard deviations of 1.67 and 17.2 in Table 13–3 are in actual pulse rate units.

z-Scores.   A *z-score* is a standard score that indicates how many standard deviations from the mean a particular value lies. A *z*-score is called a standard score because it is interpreted in relation to standard deviation units above or below the mean. The formula for calculating *z*-scores is:

$$z = \frac{X - \overline{X}}{s}$$

where z = z-score, X = score or value, $\overline{X}$ = mean of scores or values, and s = standard deviation.

The *z*-score is a very useful statistic for interpreting a particular value in relation to the other values in a distribution. Also, *z*-scores allow you to compare the performance of someone on nonequivalent tests. If a score is 1 SD above the mean, it has a *z*-score of 1. Consider the following example. You received a raw score of 92 on a test where there were 110 questions. The mean raw score was 98, and the SD was 3. How well did you score on the test compared with others who took the examination?

$$\frac{92 - 98}{3} = \frac{-6}{3} = -2.0$$

You did not do too well! Your *z*-score is −2.0. This means that only 2.28% of the group scored lower than you did. Review Figure 13–3 again, and you will see that 2.14% of the values lie between −2 SD and −3 SD, and 0.14% of the values lie beyond −3 SD. Thus, 2.28% of the values lie beyond −2 SD (2.14 + .14 = 2.28). Tables are available in statistical texts if you wish to determine the percentage of a distribution above and below any given *z*-score.

MEASURES OF RELATIONSHIPS

So far, the material in this chapter has been concerned with the analysis of data on one variable at a time. The frequency distributions that have been discussed might be referred to as univariate frequency distributions. In nursing research, however, we are frequently concerned with more than one variable. **Measures of relationships** concern the correlations between variables. As you recall, a correlation concerns the extent to which values of one variable (X) are related to values of a second variable (Y). You might want to determine if there is a correlation between the amount of time spent with a patient and the number of requests for pain medication made by that patient. A record might be made of the total time nurses spent in a patient's room during a given period of the day and the number of requests for pain medication made by the patient during that time. These data would be gathered on a group of patients. You would want to know if these two values seemed to vary together. When the time spent with the patient increased, did the number of requests for pain medications increase or decrease? There are several ways to examine a relationship such as this. Correlation coefficients, scatter plots, and contingency tables are discussed. Also, various types of correlational procedures are presented.

Correlation Coefficients. Correlations are computed through pairing the value of each subject on one variable (X) with the value on another variable (Y). As you will recall from the discussion of correlational studies in Chapter 8, the magnitude and direction of the relationship between these two variables are presented through a measurement called a correlation coefficient. The correlation coefficient can vary between −1.00 and +1.00. These two numbers represent the extremes of a perfect relationship. A correlation coefficient of −1.00 indicates a perfect negative relationship, +1.00 indicates a perfect positive relationship, and 0 indicates the absence of any relationship. Correlation coefficients are frequently symbolized by the letter r.

An $r = +.80$ indicates that as the value of one variable (X) increases, the value of the other variable (Y) tends to increase. It also means that as the value of one variable decreases, the value of the other variable tends to decrease. In other words, a positive relationship means that the two variables tend to increase or decrease together. Although a plus sign has been included to show a positive relationship (+.80), the sign is usually not included and the assumption is made that the relationship is positive if no sign is present (.80). An $r = -.80$ denotes a negative (inverse) relationship and indicates that as one variable increases, the other variable tends to decrease.

A positive relationship might be found between anxiety levels and pulse rates. As anxiety levels increase, pulse rates increase. A negative relationship might be found between anxiety levels and test scores. As anxiety levels increase, test scores decline.

Whereas the sign of the correlation coefficient shows the direction or nature of the relationship (positive or negative), the size of the correlation coefficient indicates the magnitude or strength of the relationship. An $r = .80$ denotes a stronger relationship than an $r = .60$. Also, an $r = -.50$ indicates a stronger relationship than an $r = .40$. Remember, the sign only indicates the direction of the relationship.

Generally, correlation coefficients are calculated on measurements obtained from each subject on two variables. Correlation coefficients, however, may be calculated on the measurements of one variable that are obtained from two groups of matched subjects, such as fathers and sons. A researcher might want to determine if there is a relationship between the height of fathers and their sons. Also, as was discussed in Chapter 11, correlation coefficients may be used to measure reliability. For example, the reliability of an instrument may be determined by examining subjects' scores at Time 1 versus scores at Time 2. This is called test-retest reliability.

Caution must be exercised in interpreting correlations. It cannot be emphasized too much that correlation does not equate with causation. If a strong positive relationship is found between anxiety levels and pulse rates, you should not conclude that the anxiety levels caused the pulse rates to go up. It is possible that the pulse rates increased and then the anxiety levels increased or that some other variable caused the pulse rates to rise and also increased anxiety.

You may wonder how to determine if a correlation is weak or strong. Is $r = .30$ a mild or a moderate relationship? There are no set criteria to evaluate the actual strength of a correlation coefficient. The nature of the variables being studied will help determine the strength of the relationship. According to Polit (1996), correlations between psychosocial variables rarely exceed .50. Roscoe (1975) has written, "a correlation of .70 between scholastic aptitude in the first grade and grade point average in college would be phenomenal" (p. 101). He cautioned, however, that a correlation of .70 between two tests that were supposedly equivalent would be too low.

The coefficient of determination is a statistic that should be calculated after the computation of a correlation coefficient. The **coefficient of determination** is obtained by squaring the correlation coefficient (r^2, R^2) and is interpreted as the percentage of variance shared by the two variables. The coefficient of determination for an $r = .50$ would be .25 ($.50 \times .50 = .25$), which would then be multiplied by 100 and read as 25%.

Suppose that a correlation of .60 were obtained between anxiety scores and pulse rates. The coefficient of determination would be .36, which would mean that these two variables share a common variance or overlap of 36%. If you knew a person's anxiety score, you would have 36% of the information needed to predict that person's pulse rate. Because the coefficient of determination is reversible, you would have 36% of the information needed to predict that person's anxiety level, if you knew his or her pulse rate. Of course, you would still be lacking 64% of the knowledge needed to predict one of these variables based on knowledge of the other variable. Table 13–4 displays the percentage of variance explained by different correlation coefficients. An $r = .708$ is necessary before 50% of the variance is explained. Perhaps researchers will begin to report this statistic more often because it gives a much clearer picture of the value of a correlation coefficient than the tests of significance of correlation coefficients, which will be discussed in Chapter 14. It is possible for a very low correlation coefficient, such as .20 or even lower, to be statistically significant when a large sample size is used. Only 4% of the shared variance of two variables is explained by a correlation coefficient of .20. If the coefficient of determination is not presented in a research article in which correlation coefficients are presented, you can quickly do the calculation yourself.

Scatter Plots. A **scatter plot,** also called a **scatter diagram** or a **scattergram,** is a graphic presentation of the relationship between two variables. The graph contains variables on an X axis and a Y axis. The X variable is plotted on the horizontal axis, and the Y variable is plotted on the vertical axis. The scatter plot is a visual device that can be

TABLE 13–4.   Percentage of Variance Explained by Correlations

Correlation Coefficient (r)	Coefficient of Determination (r^2)	Percentage of Variance Explained
.950	.9025	90
.850	.7225	72
.750	.5625	56
.708	.5013	50
.650	.4225	42
.550	.3025	30
.450	.2025	20
.350	.1225	12
.250	.0625	6
.150	.0225	2

used to eyeball a correlation between two variables. The magnitude of the relationship as well as the direction of the relationship can be determined.

Pairs of scores are plotted on a graph by the placement of dots to indicate where each pair of Xs and Ys intersects. For a positive correlation, the lowest score or value for each variable is placed at the lower left corner of the graph. Values increase as they go up the vertical axis and as they go toward the right on the horizontal axis. If the dots seem to be distributed from the upper left corner down toward the lower right corner, a negative correlation is said to exist (Figure 13–7).

This graph depicts chemistry and physics examination scores. One student's score is plotted on the graph (Figure 13–7A). As can be seen, the student, Ann, scored a 7 on both tests. If each student receives the same score on both tests (5 and 5, 6 and 6), a perfect positive correlation is said to exist, and the dots would all fall on a straight line drawn from the lower left corner of the graph to the upper right corner. Figure 13–7B shows the placement of the dots for eight students' scores (note the name of the person who scored the highest!).

Generally you will not find a perfect correlation as seen in Figure 13–7B. Figure 13–8 depicts varying degrees of correlations. The closer the dots are to a straight line, the higher the correlation. When the dots are scattered all over the graph, there is an indication that no relationship exists between the two variables.

Contingency Tables.   If data are nominal or categorical, relationships cannot be depicted on a scatter plot. No actual scores are available for nominal data; rather, the frequencies of the occurrences of the values are presented. A **contingency table,** also called a cross-tabulation table, is a means of visually displaying the relationship between sets of nominal data. For example, the researcher might wish to determine if there is a relation-

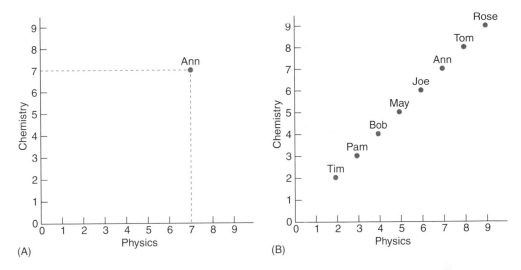

Figure 13–7. Scatter plots of chemistry and physics test scores for one student (**A**) and for eight students (**B**).

ship between gender and exercise behavior. Table 13–5 depicts the data that were gathered on 50 male and 50 female subjects.

The data from Table 13–5 seem to indicate that more males than females participate in regular exercise programs. The chi-square statistic (see Chapter 14) may be calculated to determine if there is a significant relationship between these variables. If a significant relationship is found, the researcher cannot conclude that gender "causes" one to participate in an exercise program. The reason for the existence of the relationship would still remain unknown.

Table 13–5 is called a 2×2 table because there are two variables and each variable has two categories. If exercise had been divided into three categories, such as (a) never exercises, (b) exercises occasionally, and (c) exercises frequently, the table would have been called a 2×3 table.

Types of Correlational Procedures. The most common correlational procedures used in nursing research are the Pearson product-moment correlation (Pearson r), Spearman's rho, and the contingency coefficient. The Pearson r, symbolized by the letter r, is the appropriate correlation statistic for two sets of interval or ratio data. Spearman's rho, symbolized by r_s, r_{rho}, or rho, is used with two sets of ordinal data. Finally, the contingency coefficient, symbolized by C, is used with nominal data. The calculation of the chi-square statistic (χ^2) (see Chapter 14) is necessary before computing the contingency coefficient.

In this chapter, correlations are discussed as a type of descriptive statistics. In the next chapter, correlations will be taken a step further and discussed under inferential statistics.

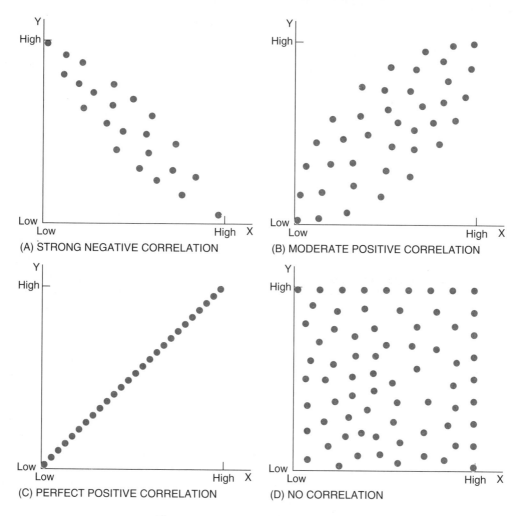

Figure 13–8. Scatter plots of correlations.

TABLE 13–5.	Example of Contingency Table		
	Exercise Regularly	**Do Not Exercise Regularly**	**Total**
Males	35	15	50
Females	10	40	50
Total	45	55	100

INTRAOCULAR METHOD OF DATA ANALYSIS

The researcher should always use the "intraocular method" when analyzing data. What is the intraocular method? It is a humorous term used to indicate that you should "eyeball" your data. Many mistakes could be avoided in data analysis if the researcher's eyes and common sense were used. For example, imagine that the following group of scores were obtained: 78, 79, 80, 76, and 74. When the average is calculated, it is found to be 68. The intraocular method should tell the researcher that a mistake has been made in calculation. After glancing at the data, an estimate should be made of the results of data analysis. This procedure provides a checks-and-balances system that frequently pays off in the detection of an error in calculations or an error in the data entry process.

CRITIQUING DESCRIPTIVE STATISTICS IN RESEARCH REPORTS

It is often difficult for the beginning reader of research reports to critique the statistical content of these reports. The reader may not have taken a basic statistics course. Even if such a course has been completed, the content may not have been remembered or even understood at the time the course was taken. Therefore, many consumers of research examine the study statistics with "fear and trembling."

It is desirable to have some background in statistics before reading research reports. However, the background knowledge needed to critique most reports is not extensive. Knowledge of a few statistical concepts will go a long way toward helping the reader understand data analysis presented in research articles and other types of research reports. Some guidelines for critiquing descriptive statistics are found in Box 13–1.

The first task is to identify the various descriptive statistics used to analyze data. Nearly every research study will use descriptive statistics to present the demographic characteristics of the sample. For example, the ages, educational levels, and incomes of the subjects may be presented through descriptive statistics. If the mean was used to present the average income, the reader should try to determine if the median would have

---

Box 13–1.   Guidelines for Critiquing Descriptive Statistics

1. What types of descriptive statistics are included in the research report?
2. Were the descriptive statistics appropriate for the level of measurement of the variable(s)?
3. Were measures of central tendency and variability both presented?
4. Do the descriptive statistics clearly present the demographic characteristics of the subjects?
5. Are the descriptive statistics clearly presented in the text? In tables and graphs?
6. Do the descriptive statistics presented in the text agree with those presented in the tables?

been a more appropriate measure of central tendency. This would be true if some of the subjects reported extremely high or low incomes.

The level of measurement of each variable should be determined, if possible, and then a decision made about the appropriateness of the descriptive statistics that were reported. Was gender treated as a nominal variable or reported as an interval variable? It makes no sense to see gender reported as an average of 1.2. This might occur if the researcher had assigned a value of 1 to women and 2 to men. The best way to determine the level of measurement for variables is to search for the researcher's operational definitions. These are frequently found in the discussion of the instruments that were used in the study.

Were the descriptive data presented both in the text of the report and in tables and graphs? If so, do the data agree? If the data were not presented in tables or graphs, would the use of these methods of reporting data have made the material more easily understood?

Descriptive statistics should be presented in a manner that can be understood by the average practicing nurse. If this is not done, the results of the study will not be considered for implementation in practice.

SUMMARY

Statistics is a branch of knowledge that is used to summarize and to present numerical data. Numerical characteristics of populations are called **parameters;** numerical characteristics of samples are called **statistics.**

Statistics can be classified as descriptive and inferential. **Descriptive statistics** are those that organize and summarize numerical data from populations or samples. **Inferential statistics** are concerned with populations and use sample data to make an "inference" about a population. Types of descriptive statistics are (a) measures to condense data, (b) measures of central tendency, (c) measures of variability, and (d) measures of relationships.

Measures to condense data are statistics that summarize and condense data. Included in this category are frequency distributions, graphic presentations, and percentages. **Frequency distributions** are used with all levels of data. Groups of scores in a frequency distribution are called **class intervals.**

Distribution shapes may be classified as symmetrical or nonsymmetrical. **Symmetrical distributions** are those in which both halves of the distribution are the same. **Nonsymmetrical distributions,** also called **skewed** distributions, are those in which the distribution has an off-center peak. The tail of the distribution points to the right in a **positively skewed** distribution and to the left in a **negatively skewed** distribution. The **normal distribution** is a symmetrical distribution that has one central peak or set of values in the center of the distribution. The **normal curve** is a bell-shaped curve that graphically presents a normal distribution. The distribution is *symmetrical,* with 50% of the values contained on the left half of the curve, and 50% on the right half. Approximately 68% of the distribution of a normal curve lies between ±1 SD of the mean. Approximately 95% of the distribution lies between ±2 SD, and about 99% lies within ±3 SD.

Graphic presentations include bar graphs, histograms, and frequency polygons. A **bar graph** is used to depict nominal data and some types of ordinal data. A **histogram** and a **frequency polygon** are used to display ordinal, interval, and ratio data.

A **percentage** is a statistic that represents the proportion of a subgroup to a total group, expressed as a percentage ranging from 0 to 100.

Measures of central tendency are used to describe the average value of a set of values. The **mode** is the category or value that occurs most often in a set of data. **Modal class** is the category of nominal data with the greatest frequency. A frequency distribution that contains one value that occurs more frequently than any other is called **unimodal.** If two values have the same high frequency, the distribution is **bimodal.** If more than two values have the same high frequency, the distribution is **multimodal.**

The **median** is the middle score or value in a group of data, and the **mean** is the average sum of a set of values.

Measures of variability describe how spread out values are in a distribution of values. Measures of variability are range, percentile, standard deviation, variance, and z-score. The **range** is the distance between the highest and lowest value in a group of values. The **interquartile range** contains the middle half of the values in a frequency distribution. The **semiquartile range** is found by dividing the interquartile range in half. A **percentile** is a data point below which lies a certain percentage of the values in a frequency distribution. The **standard deviation** is a measure that indicates the average deviation or variability of all the values from the mean of a set of values. The standard deviation is the most widely used measure of variability when interval or ratio data are described. The **variance** is the standard deviation squared. A **z-score** is a standard score that indicates how many standard deviations from the mean a particular value lies.

Measures of relationships are concerned with the correlation between variables. Correlation coefficients, scatter plots, and contingency tables are means of presenting correlations.

The magnitude and direction of a relationship between two variables are presented through a correlation coefficient that varies between −1.00 and +1.00. The **coefficient of determination** is a statistic obtained through squaring a correlation coefficient. This statistic is interpreted as the percentage of variance shared by two variables.

A **scatter plot,** also called a **scatter diagram** or a **scattergram,** is a graphic presentation of the relationship between two variables. Pairs of scores are plotted on a graph by the placement of dots to indicate where each pair of Xs and Ys intersects.

A **contingency table** is a means of displaying the relationship between two sets of nominal data. There are no actual scores presented; rather, the frequency of occurrence of the categories of data is included in the table.

The most common correlation procedures used in nursing research are the Pearson product-moment correlation (Pearson *r*), Spearman's rho, and the contingency coefficient. The Pearson *r* is used with interval and ratio data, Spearman's rho is used with ordinal data, and the contingency coefficient is appropriate for nominal data.

 ## NURSING RESEARCH ON THE WEB

For additional online resources, research activities, and exercises, go to www.prenhall. com/nieswiadomy. Select Chapter 13 from the drop down menu.

✕ GET INVOLVED ACTIVITIES

1. Write down all of the different kinds of descriptive statistics found in this chapter. Also, list the various types of figures discussed in this chapter. Take these two lists to

the library. Examine the first five research articles that you locate in nursing journals. Place a check mark on your list beside each type of descriptive statistic that is mentioned in the articles. Also, place a check mark beside each type of figure that you observe in these articles.

2. Bring your list to class and compare it with the lists compiled by your classmates or colleagues. Determine the most common descriptive statistic that is reported in nursing research articles. Determine the most common type of figure displayed in these research articles.

3. Divide into two debate groups. Select a variable and debate whether it is more appropriate to use the mean or the median when reporting the data on this variable. Examples of variables that might be selected are height, weight, or age of clients in a particular clinic population. Each side should present specific circumstances that would indicate the need for either the mean or the median to be used.

✕ SELF-TEST

Circle the letter before the *best* answer.

1. Which type of statistics is used to examine the characteristics of samples?
   A. descriptive statistics
   B. inferential statistics
   C. parametric statistics
   D. nonparametric statistics

2. What is the mode of the following group of vision test results? 20/20; 20/30; 20/40; 20/30; 20/50; 20/40; 20/100; 20/30
   A. 20/20
   B. 20/30
   C. 20/40
   D. 20/50
   E. 20/100

3. Which of the following measures of central tendency would be appropriate to describe the average pulse rates of a group of surgical patients?
   A. mode
   B. median
   C. mean

4. The standard deviation is a measure of:
   A. skewness.
   B. correlation.
   C. central tendency.
   D. variability.

5. What does it mean if a person's score is 3 standard deviations above the mean on a test?

    A. All of the scores on the test are high.

    B. The person has an unusually high score compared with others who took the test.

    C. An error has been made in recording the score.

    D. The score is 30% higher than the mean.

6. As a nurse researcher conducting a research study with a group of children, you discover that the average weight of the subjects is at the 95th percentile for their age. Which of the following statements would be correct?

    A. The subjects are not eating enough.

    B. The subjects are 5% above the average weight for their age.

    C. The subjects are 5% below the average weight for their age.

    D. The subjects are well above the average weight for their age.

7. Which of the following statements is true?

    A. The most reliable and accurate measure of central tendency is the mode.

    B. The standard deviation indicates how spread out scores are in a distribution.

    C. The type of graph that shows the relationship between two variables is a histogram.

    D. The range of a group of scores is figured by adding the highest and lowest numbers.

8. Correlation is a procedure used to determine if:

    A. X comes before Y.

    B. X causes Y.

    C. X and Y are different.

    D. X and Y vary together.

9. A nurse researcher examines the correlation between anxiety levels and pain. She calculates a correlation coefficient of 2.19. The size of this correlation indicates:

    A. a strong positive relationship.

    B. a significant correlation.

    C. an error in calculation.

    D. no relationship between the two variables.

10. Which of the following correlation coefficients would indicate the strongest relationship between anxiety and the ability to concentrate?

    A. $r = -.03$

    B. $r = +.30$

    C. $r = -.35$

    D. $r = +.57$

    E. $r = -.60$

✕ REFERENCES

Norwood, S. L. (2000). *Research strategies for advanced practice nurses.* Upper Saddle River, NJ: Prentice Hall Health.

Polit, D. F. (1996). *Data analysis & statistics for nursing research.* Stamford CT: Appleton & Lange.

Polit, D. F., & Hungler. B. P. (1999). *Nursing research: Principles and methods* (6th ed.). Philadelphia: Lippincott.

Roscoe, J. (1975). *Fundamental research statistics for the behavioral sciences* (2nd ed.). New York: Holt, Rinehart & Winston.

Shott, S. (1990). *Statistics for health care professionals.* Philadephia: W. B. Saunders.

Spielberger, C. (1983). *Manual for the state-trait anxiety inventory.* Palo Alto, CA: Consulting Psychologists Press.

CHAPTER 14

Inferential Statistics

OUTLINE

Purposes of Inferential Statistics
- Estimating Population Parameters
  - Sampling Distribution of the Mean
  - Confidence Intervals
- Testing Hypotheses
  - The Study Hypothesis
  - Choosing a Statistical Test
  - Level of Significance
  - One-tailed and Two-tailed Tests
  - Calculating the Test Statistic
  - Comparing Calculated Value and Critical Value
  - Support for the Study Hypothesis

Type I and Type II Errors
Parametric and Nonparametric Statistical Tests
Power of a Statistical Test
Statistical Tests Used in Nursing Research
- *t*-Test
- Analysis of Variance
- Chi-square

Testing the Significance of Correlation Coefficients
Advanced Statistical Tests
Critiquing Inferential Statistics in Research Reports
Summary
Nursing Research on the Web
Get Involved Activities
Self-test

OBJECTIVES

On completion of this chapter, you will be prepared to:

1. Recall the two purposes of inferential statistics
2. Discuss the sampling distribution of the mean
3. Define terms used in inferential statistics
4. Distinguish between a one-tailed and a two-tailed test
5. Describe Type I and Type II errors
6. Differentiate between parametric and nonparametric statistical tests
7. Discuss the power of a statistical test
8. List criteria for selecting a statistical test
9. Identify statistical tests commonly reported in nursing studies
10. Critique the inferential statistics section of research reports

✕ NEW TERMS DEFINED IN THIS CHAPTER

analysis of covariance	multiple regression
analysis of variance	multivariate analysis of variance
canonical correlation	nonparametric tests
central limit theorem	one-tailed test of significance
chi-square	parametric tests
confidence interval	power of a statistical test
critical region	region of rejection
critical value	sampling distribution
degrees of freedom	standard error of the mean
dependent *t*-test	*t*-test
independent *t*-test	two-tailed test of significance
level of significance	Type I error
meta-analysis	Type II error

The material in this chapter is not really difficult to understand, but if you have not been exposed to the material before or did not absorb the content during a statistics class, you may think it is "tough." If so, take it as a challenge to understand the material. It is hoped your efforts will gain for you a greater appreciation of the value of statistics in making decisions about data obtained in research studies.

Chapter 13 discussed descriptive statistics. These types of statistics are used to present the characteristics of samples or populations. This chapter discusses inferential statistics, which are those statistics that use sample data to make decisions or "inferences" about a population. Populations are the group of interest when inferential statistics are used, even though data are analyzed from samples.

Inferential statistics are based on the laws of probability. The word *chance* is used in discussing probability. Other terms that are sometimes used interchangeably in the literature are *sampling error* and *random error.* All inferential statistical tests are based on the assumption that chance (sampling error, random error) is the only explanation for relationships found in research studies. For example, if one group scores higher than another group on a test, the assumption is made that the difference is due to chance. Reread that sentence several times. The concept of chance will be used throughout this chapter. A researcher wants to demonstrate that chance is *not* the reason for the relationships that are found in research.

The larger the difference that is found between groups, the lower the probability that the difference occurred by chance. In other words, the groups really are different in regard to the variable that is being measured. The same can be said of tests that examine the significance of correlations: The larger the correlation between variables measured on members of the sample, the greater the likelihood that the variables are, in fact, correlated in the population.

Inferential statistics are based on the assumption that the sample was randomly selected. As you remember from Chapter 10, when a random sample is selected, each member of the population has an equal chance of being selected. At this point, you may be wondering how inferential statistics can be useful because random samples are generally not obtained. Some of the reasons for using nonprobability samples involve time, money, and ethical issues. Spatz and Johnston (1984) presented the rationale for the use of inferential statistics with nonrandom samples. "Usually, the results based on samples that are unsystematic (but not random) are true for other samples from the same population" (p. 162). Shott (1990) stated that it is appropriate to make a statistical inference from a nonrandom sample to the population, as long the researcher does not deliberately select a biased sample. Polit (1996) agreed that inferential statistics can be used with nonrandom samples but cautioned the researcher to be conservative in interpreting study findings.

The use of a nonrandom sample greatly reduces the ability to generalize study results. You may now be able to better understand the need for replication studies in nursing. Agreement among the findings of several similar studies conducted with nonrandom samples allows conclusions to be derived from the data that are similar to the conclusions that could be made if one random sample were used.

PURPOSES OF INFERENTIAL STATISTICS

There are two broad purposes of inferential statistics: (a) estimating population parameters from sample data, and (b) testing hypotheses. The second purpose has been of more interest to nurse researchers, but estimating population parameters, which involves determining confidence intervals, is also an important purpose of inferential statistics.

A distinguishing point between the two purposes is the time of data collection. The estimation of population parameters is considered after the data are collected, whereas the testing of hypotheses is considered before data collection. Hypotheses are formulated before the data collection begins. Of course, the decision to support or not support the hypothesis is made after the data are analyzed.

A brief explanation of the use of estimation procedures is presented. A more thorough discussion of hypothesis testing procedures is made because, at present, the testing of hypotheses seems to be of more concern to nurse researchers.

ESTIMATING POPULATION PARAMETERS

To estimate population parameters from sample data, an understanding of sampling error and sampling distribution is necessary. Whenever a sample is chosen to represent a population, there is some likelihood that the sample will not accurately reflect the population. Even when a true random sample is chosen, the sample may not be an average or representative sample. Sampling error occurs when the sample does not accurately reflect the population. Reexamine the example in Table 10–3. The table contains pulse measurements on a population of 20 subjects. The mean pulse rate for the population is 71. One sample of five subjects drawn from the population is shown to have an average pulse rate of 71. Another sample of five subjects has an average pulse rate of 63, and still another sample has an average pulse rate of 83. These last two samples demonstrate what sampling error means. The pulse rates of these two samples of subjects do not accurately reflect the average pulse rate of the population.

An interesting phenomenon may be observed about sampling error. The majority of the samples chosen from a population will accurately reflect the population. In the previous example, if an infinite number of separate samples were chosen from the population, the majority of the mean pulse rates of these samples would be close to the population average pulse rate of 71. Most of the samples would have average rates such as 69, 70, 71, 72, and 73. A few samples would have average rates that were quite different from the population mean, like the previously mentioned 63 and 83. The light bulb is probably turning on in your head right now, and the idea of the normal distribution is flashing before your eyes. The phenomenon in which sample values tend to be normally distributed around the population value is known as the **central limit theorem.**

Whenever a large number of sample values are arranged in a frequency distribution, those values will be normally distributed, even if the original population of values was not normally distributed. This may be hard to believe, but it has been demonstrated to be true, if the sample size is fairly large. The sampling distribution of the mean approximates the normal curve when samples contain 100 or more observations or values. Sample sizes as small as 30 are generally adequate to ensure that the sampling distribution of the mean will closely approximate the normal curve (Shott, 1990).

A theoretical frequency distribution, based on an infinite number of samples, is called a **sampling distribution.** This distribution is said to be theoretical because you never actually draw an infinite number of samples from a population. Instead, decisions are made based on one sample. The concept of sampling distributions, however, is used over and over in inferential statistics. The researcher works with one sample, but inferential statistics are based on the idea of what would occur if the researcher had actually drawn an infinite number of samples from the population. You may want to reread that sentence again. The reason the concept of sampling distributions is difficult for some people to understand is that it deals with "what ifs" rather than actual data. Sampling distributions are based on mathematical formulas and logic. You will never have to calculate or plot out sampling distributions. Statisticians figured out these theoretical distributions years ago (Thank goodness!).

Every inferential statistical test uses the concept of sampling distributions, and each test has its own particular set of sampling distributions that are referred to when analyzing the data obtained in a study. The sampling distribution of the mean is a sampling distribution that is used quite often in inferential statistical tests.

Sampling Distribution of the Mean.   As discussed in Chapter 13, when scores or values are normally distributed, approximately 68% of the values lie between ±1 SD, and approximately 95% lie between ±2 SD. To be exact, 95% of the values in a normal distribution lie between ±1.96 SD from the mean. That figure of 1.96 will become more important as you read on in this discussion about the use of inferential statistics to estimate population parameters, but it will be even more important during the discussion of hypothesis testing.

Let us turn now to the theoretical sampling distribution of the mean. The standard deviation of any sampling distribution is called the standard error (rather than the standard deviation). The standard deviation of the sampling distribution of the mean is called the **standard error of the mean** ($s_{\bar{x}}$). The term *error* indicates that when a theoretical sampling distribution of the mean is used to estimate a population mean, some error is likely to occur in this estimate. The smaller the standard error of the mean, the more confidence you can have that the mean from a sample is an accurate reflection of the population mean. How can you tell how much error is likely to exist in your estimate of the population mean based on only one sample? There is a simple formula that allows you to calculate the $s_{\bar{x}}$.

$$s_{\overline{x}} = \frac{SD}{\sqrt{n}}$$

where SD = standard deviation of sample and n = sample size.

Suppose 25 subjects have taken a test. Their average raw score is 70. The standard deviation is 10. Plug these data into the formula for $s_{\bar{x}}$.

$$s_{\overline{x}} = \frac{10}{\sqrt{25}} = \frac{10}{5} = 2$$

The standard error of the mean ($s_{\bar{x}}$) is 2. You can now determine that there is about a 68 percent likelihood that the population mean lies between 68 and 72 (70 ± 2). Also, there is about a 95 percent likelihood that the population mean lies between 66 and 74 (70 ± 4).

Confidence Intervals. Although the value of a sample mean may be chosen as the value that is most likely to be the actual population mean, most researchers are not very comfortable with this choice. As you recall, any one sample that is chosen from a population may or may not be an accurate representation of the population. Researchers establish a range of values within which the population parameter is thought to occur. A **confidence interval** (CI) is a range of values that, with a specified degree of probability, is thought to contain the population value. Confidence intervals contain a lower and an upper limit. The researcher asserts with some degree of confidence that the population parameter lies within those boundaries.

Suppose a nurse researcher named Joan wishes to determine how knowledgeable the nurses in her state are about legal responsibilities in their practice. A test is located (or she develops one) that measures knowledge of legal issues in nursing practice. Joan is able to obtain the mailing list for all the 10,000 registered nurses in her state. When she examines her financial situation, the cost of mailing a questionnaire to all of the nurses will not fit in her budget. She decides to select a random sample of 100 nurses from the list. Let us assume that all 100 of the nurses return the questionnaire (which is highly unlikely). Data analysis shows the mean score of this group to be 31 (of a possible 35 points), with a standard deviation of 3. The mean score is rather encouraging. Joan decides that the nurses in her state are fairly knowledgeable about legal issues. Excitedly, she reports the results to a friend. The friend says, "How can you be so confident about your results? There were only 100 nurses in the sample. I don't think you would find an average score of 31 if you tested all of the nurses in the state." Feeling somewhat deflated, Joan decides to determine how much confidence to place in the results. This is done by estimating the knowledge level of the total population of nurses in the state based on the sample of 100 nurses. She decides that she wants to be 95% confident about her estimation when she goes back to talk to her friend again. First she determines the standard error of the mean ($s_{\bar{x}}$).

$$s_{\overline{X}} = \frac{3}{\sqrt{100}} = \frac{3}{10} = 0.3$$

Next, she inserts 0.3 into the formula for obtaining the 95% confidence interval (LL = lower limit, UL = upper limit).

$$LL = \overline{X} - 1.96 \ (s_{\overline{x}})$$
$$UL = \overline{X} + 1.96 \ (s_{\overline{x}})$$
$$LL = 31 - 1.96 \ (0.3)$$
$$31 - 0.588 =$$
$$30.412$$
$$UL = 31 + 1.96 \ (0.3) =$$
$$31 + 0.588 =$$
$$31.588$$

Joan then determines the 95% confidence interval to have a lower boundary of 30.41 and an upper boundary of 31.59. She was right after all! Her estimation of the knowledge of legal issues in nursing practice among the total population of nurses in her state indicates that their knowledge levels would be quite close to the mean of her sample of 100 nurses. She can be 95% confident that if she had selected another sample of 100 nurses from the mailing list, the mean score would be between 30.41 and 31.59. Another way to state this is that she is 95% confident that the interval of 30.41 to 31.59 contains the population mean. If she wanted to be 99% confident of her estimate, she would replace 1.96 in the formula with the figure 2.58.

$$LL = 31 - 2.58 \ (0.3) =$$
$$31 - 0.774 =$$
$$30.226$$
$$UL = 31 + 2.58 \ (0.3) =$$
$$31 + 0.774 =$$
$$31.774$$

Joan is now 99% confident that the mean of the population lies between 30.23 and 31.77. With this statistical ammunition she can again approach her friend and see if she is any more successful in convincing this friend that nurses in her state are fairly knowledgeable about legal issues in nursing practice.

Imagine that you were asked to be a subject in a weight loss study. The researcher tells you that you will lose significantly ($p < .05$) more weight on this new diet than you did on the one you had previously tried. Wouldn't you also want to know how *much* weight you would lose? If the researcher said, "I am 95% sure that you will lose between 10 and 15 lbs in 6 weeks," she would be giving you a confidence interval.

For some reason, confidence intervals have not been reported very often in nursing studies. Generally, only significance levels are reported for hypothesis-testing studies. Many medical studies report both of these statistics. Nurse researchers should become aware of the value of reporting confidence intervals in their research reports. In an article in *Journal of Nursing Scholarship,* Rothstein and Tonges (2000) contended that confidence interval analysis is a "useful approach to quantify the effect of an intervention and predict the results that can be expected from implementation" (p. 69).

A recent review of research journals showed some nurse researchers are beginning to report confidence intervals. Bliss, Johnson, Savik, Clabors, and Gerding (2000) reported CIs in their study of fecal incontinence in hospitalized patients who are acutely ill. CIs were also reported by Defloor (2000) in his study to determine which position and type of mattress resulted in the lowest pressures to the skin of persons lying in bed.

TESTING HYPOTHESES

As previously mentioned, the testing of hypotheses is important to nurse researchers. Steps in testing hypotheses include the following:

1. State the study hypothesis (generally, a directional research hypothesis).
2. Choose the appropriate statistical test.
3. Decide on the level of significance (alpha level).
4. Decide if a one-tailed or two-tailed test will be used.
5. Calculate the test statistic, using the research data.
6. Compare the calculated value to the critical value for that particular statistical test.
7. Reject or fail to reject the null hypothesis.
8. Determine support or lack of support for the research hypothesis.

The Study Hypothesis. A researcher should take great pains in formulating the hypothesis(es) for a study. The hypothesis should be based on the theoretical/conceptual framework of the study; therefore, the hypothesis should generally be a directional research hypothesis that predicts the results of the study.

Although the research hypothesis is of primary interest to an investigator, this hypothesis is never tested statistically. The null hypothesis (H_0) is the one that is subjected to statistical analysis. The null hypothesis states that no difference exists between the populations from which the samples were chosen or no correlation exists between variables in the population. Because this is not what the researcher expects to find, why is the null hypothesis necessary? Statistical tests are set up to test the null hypothesis. Remember, all inferential statistical tests are based on the assumption that no difference or relationship (correlation) exists. If small differences or low correlations are found, chance is considered to be the reason, and the null hypothesis is not rejected. If the results of the analysis show that the difference or correlation is too large to be the result of chance, the null hypothesis is rejected. Of course, rejection of the null hypothesis provides support for the research hypothesis. Researchers are never able to say that they "proved" their research hypotheses. It is possible for them to say, however, with a specified degree of certainty, how likely it is that the null hypothesis is false.

The null hypothesis is frequently depicted using the following symbols:

$$H_0 : \mu_A = \mu_B$$

The symbols are those used for population parameters. Remember that statistical inference uses data from samples to draw conclusions about populations. The null hypothesis in the preceding formula indicates that there is no difference in the two populations from which the samples were drawn. Even if the two samples were drawn from the same population, for statistical purposes the samples are assumed to have come from two separate populations concerning the variable of interest. For example, suppose a group of patients was divided into two treatment groups by a random assignment procedure. The null hypothesis assumes that these two groups have been selected from one hypothetical population. Although this idea is somewhat difficult to understand or to visualize, the concept is used in all of the inferential statistical tests that examine differences between groups. If the null hypothesis is rejected, the statistical decision is made that the two samples came from two hypothetical populations that were different on the variable being measured. If the null hypothesis is not rejected, the statistical decision is made that the two samples came from the same hypothetical population with respect to the variable being studied.

The correct words to use when discussing the results of testing the null hypothesis are *reject* or *fail to reject. Retain* is also an acceptable word to use when the null hypothesis is not rejected. Although you will also see the word *accept* used in the literature, technically you never accept the null hypothesis. As Elzey (1974) has remarked, "We can only 'not reject' the hypothesis that there is no difference. We are not justified in concluding that there is no difference" (pp. 36–37).

When discussing the research hypothesis, it is correct to say that the hypothesis was *supported* or *not supported.* You do not *reject* the research hypothesis because it was never actually tested. These points may seem minor and nitpicking, but if you learn to use the correct terminology in the beginning of your research career, you will not have to change bad habits later on.

Choosing a Statistical Test.

Being able to choose an appropriate statistical test to use in analyzing your data and knowing the rationale for this choice are more important than being able to calculate the statistic. Currently, many of the actual numerical calculations are done by computer. Although it is important to be familiar with the theoretical principles behind formulas that are used in the various tests, there is no need to memorize these formulas. Frequently, when students take a statistics course, they are so concerned with being able to perform mathematical calculations that they lose sight of the purposes of the various statistical tests and of how the choice of a particular test is made.

Basically, there are two types of inferential procedures—those that search for differences in sets of data and those that search for correlations between sets of data. Are you trying to determine if there is a significant difference between groups, or do you want to know if there is a significant correlation between variables within one group?

The choice of a statistical test is based primarily on the hypothesis for the study or the research questions. The hypothesis will indicate, for example, that the pain level of one group of subjects is going to be measured before and after some specific nursing intervention to relieve pain. The study design based on this hypothesis (one group, pretest and posttest) tells you that you will have two sets of dependent data. The data are considered dependent or related because the same subjects are measured both times. If the level of measurement of the dependent variable (pain) is interval or ratio, the most appropriate statistical test is a paired *t*-test.

Some of the questions that need to be answered when choosing the appropriate inferential procedure include:

1. Are you comparing groups or sets of scores? Are you correlating variables?
2. What is the level of measurement of the variables (nominal, ordinal, interval/ratio)?
3. How large are the groups (sample size)?
4. How many groups or sets of scores are being compared?
5. Are the observations or scores dependent or independent?
6. How many observations are available for each group?

Level of Significance. After analyzing data from a study, the decision must be made whether to reject or fail to reject the null hypothesis. The researcher wants to know how likely it is that a wrong decision has been made when two groups are said to be different or when an independent variable is said to cause the change in the dependent variable. To make this decision, the researcher must decide how certain or how accurate the decision must be. In other words, how willing is the researcher to be wrong when declaring that one group really is different from the other group on the variable being measured? The **level of significance** can be defined as the probability of rejecting a null hypothesis when it is true, and it should not be rejected. The difference or relationship that is found is caused only by chance or sampling error, and the researcher has mistakenly said that the difference is due to the treatment variable.

The level of significance, represented by the Greek letter alpha (α), is an extremely important concept in inferential statistics. No matter what statistical test is used, a decision must be made about whether or not the specified level of significance was reached and, therefore, whether or not to reject the null hypothesis.

The letter *p* and the symbol α are used to symbolize the probability level that is set. The most common level of significance that is found in nursing studies is $p = .05$. Traditionally, this value has been set by scientists as a cutoff point for testing the null hypothesis. A significance level of .05 means that the researcher is willing to risk being wrong 5% of the time, or 5 times out of 100, when rejecting the null hypothesis. If the decision needs to be much more accurate, such as deciding whether a drug is effective, the level of significance might be set at .01 or even at .001. With a .01 level of significance, the researcher stands the risk of being wrong 1 time out of 100 when rejecting the null hypothesis. At the .001 level of significance, the risk of error is 1 time out of 1000.

An argument is occasionally made for setting a less stringent level of significance, such as .10. In research where no great harm would come from rejecting a true null hypothesis, a .10 level of significance might be acceptable. Again, nursing has accepted the .05 level as the standard in most studies. It is stressed that the researcher must decide how accurate the decision should be concerning the hypothesis.

It is important not to confuse level of significance with clinical significance or clinical importance. Although findings that are statistically significant are more likely to be clinically significant than findings that are not statistically significant, the two do not always go together hand-in-hand. Findings that are statistically significant may not be clinically significant. The reverse situation is also possible.

One-tailed and Two-tailed Tests. A research hypothesis may be stated in the directional form (the degree of difference or type of correlation is predicted) or in the nondirectional form (a difference or correlation is predicted, but the degree of difference or type of correlation is not indicated). Directional research hypotheses should be based on a sound conceptual or theoretical framework. In other words, the rationale for the prediction contained in a directional research hypothesis should be quite clear.

If the researcher has stated a directional research hypothesis, it is appropriate to use a one-tailed test of significance. When a **one-tailed test of significance** is selected, differences or correlations will be sought in only one tail of the theoretical sampling distribution (either the right or the left tail). The word *tail* is used to indicate the values on each end of the distribution. A **two-tailed test of significance** is used to determine significant values in both ends of the sampling distribution. The nondirectional research hypothesis is therefore considered to be a two-tailed hypothesis.

The type of research hypothesis that is chosen determines the significance level needed to reject the null hypothesis. It is much easier to reject the null hypothesis when a one-tailed test rather than a two-tailed test is used. The entire area of rejection of the null hypothesis is in one tail, rather than being split between the two tails, as would be necessary if a two-tailed test were used. If a two-tailed test is used, and the .05 level of significance is chosen, the .05 must be divided into .025 in each tail of the distribution. For a one-tailed test, the region of rejection is all in one end of the distribution, and the entire .05 is sought in one tail. A *z*-score of 1.65 is significant at the .05 level for a one-tailed test. A *z*-score of 1.96 is necessary for significance at the .05 level for a two-tailed test. Figure 14–1 shows the area of significant values for a one-tailed and a two-tailed test when the probability level is set at .05.

To illustrate the use of a one-tailed test, consider the following example. The framework for a study indicates that play is an effective means of introducing children to unfamiliar environments or unfamiliar equipment. The hypothesis for the study is: Four-year-old children who have played with physical examination equipment, including a stethoscope and a tongue blade, before a physical examination are more cooperative during the examination than children who have had no such previous play experience. This hypothesis would allow the researcher to expect higher cooperation scores for the experimental group who had had experience with physical examination equipment than for the control group. The entire .05 probability level will be sought in the right tail or the positive end of the distribution. Suppose that the mean cooperation score of the experimental group was higher than the mean score of the control group. If a *z*-score of 1.65 or higher was obtained for the difference between the means of the experimental and control groups, the researcher would conclude that the children in the experimental group were significantly more cooperative than the children in the control group.

Nursing research that is based on a conceptual or theoretical framework allows the prediction of the results. One-tailed tests are therefore appropriate for studies based on a sound study framework.

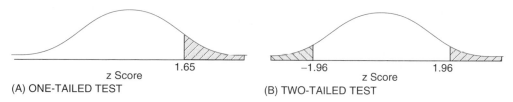

Figure 14–1. Significant values for one-tailed and two-tailed tests at α = .05.

Calculating the Test Statistic. Although this step in hypothesis testing may seem like the most difficult, today you will rarely have to do any hand calculations. Numerous statistical software programs are available. Of course, a nurse researcher may want to take advantage of a statistician.

Comparing Calculated Value and Critical Value. Critical values may be determined by consulting tables found in the back of statistics textbooks. However, today computer printouts generally provide critical values with which to compare the statistical results. A **critical value** is a scientific cutoff point. It denotes the value in a theoretical distribution at which all obtained sample values that are equal to or beyond that point in the distribution are said to be statistically significant. Critical values are found in the tails of a distribution. All values beyond the critical value are said to lie in the **critical region** or **region of rejection.** The critical value is determined by the level of significance chosen and the degrees of freedom. If the computed value of a statistic is less than the critical value, the null hypothesis is not rejected; if the computed value is equal to or greater than the critical value, the null hypothesis is rejected.

The interpretation of a statistical test is dependent on the degrees of freedom (df). **Degrees of freedom** concerns the number of values that are free to vary. Although the degrees of freedom indicate the number of values that can vary, the concern is really focused on the number of values that are not free to vary. Procedures to calculate the degrees of freedom for a particular statistical test are usually included in the description of that test. Degrees of freedom are generally denoted by the letters df and a number (e.g., df = 2). The concept of degrees of freedom is somewhat complex. A simplified example may help you to gain a basic understanding of this concept. Suppose you were told to pick a number between 1 and 10. You would have 10 degrees of freedom because you could pick any of 10 numbers. Now imagine that you are told to pick three numbers that add up to 10. After you have picked the first two numbers, the third number is not free to vary. For example, if you chose the numbers 3 and 5, the third number would have to be 2 to arrive at a sum of 10. You were thus allowed two degrees of freedom in this calculation.

Support for the Study Hypothesis. If a directional research hypothesis has been formulated for a study, support for this hypothesis is based on whether the null hypothesis is rejected. In nearly every study, the goal of the researcher is to reject the null hypothesis. Occasionally, the null hypothesis is actually a statement of the researcher's expectation. For example, in a study to determine if an inexpensive educational program was as effective as an expensive program, the researcher's prediction or expectation might be that there would be no difference in the effectiveness of these two programs. Again, as previously mentioned, the researcher generally hopes to be able to reject the null hypothesis. After examining the obtained p value, if it is less than the level of significance that was set for the study (generally $p = .05$), the researcher rejects the null hypothesis. Conversely, if the p value is greater than the set level of significance, the researcher must fail to reject the null hypothesis.

TYPE I AND TYPE II ERRORS

Four possible decisions may be made concerning the null hypothesis. Two of the decisions are correct. If the null hypothesis is actually false and you reject the null, you have made a correct decision. If the null hypothesis is actually true and you fail to reject it (retain the null), you have made a correct decision. There are, however, two mistakes that can be made. These mistakes are called Type I and Type II errors. If the null hypothesis is actually true and you reject it, you have made a **Type I error.** If the null hypothesis is actually false and you fail to reject it, you have made a **Type II error.** Figure 14–2 depicts these four decisions. Because sample data are used to make a decision about a population, you never know for sure if you have made the correct decision.

As the probability of a Type I error increases, the probability of a Type II error decreases and vice versa. The level of significance (α) set for a study determines the probability of a Type I or alpha error. For example, if the level of significance for a study is set at .05, the probability of a Type I error is .05 or 5%. The probability of a Type II or beta error (β) can be controlled by using power analysis (see Chapter 10).

Type I errors in research findings usually result in unnecessary changes being instituted, whereas Type II errors result in failure to institute needed changes. Both of these errors may be serious. In general, however, researchers are more concerned with a Type I error than a Type II error. A Type I error seems to be more embarrassing to the researcher because something is said to exist when it does not actually exist. For example, a signifi-

ACTUAL SITUATION IN POPULATION
Null Hypothesis

	True	False
Null Rejected	Type I Error	No Error
Null *Not* Rejected	No Error	Type II Error

(Statistical Decision)

Figure 14–2. Type I and Type II errors in hypothesis testing.

cant difference might be said to exist between an experimental and a control group when, in fact, the difference that was found was due to chance.

PARAMETRIC AND NONPARAMETRIC STATISTICAL TESTS

Inferential statistical tests may be classified as parametric and nonparametric. As the term implies, **parametric tests** are concerned with population parameters, and these tests make assumptions about the population from which a sample was drawn. **Nonparametric tests** are less stringent in the requirements for their use and do not make assumptions about the population from which a sample is selected. The assumptions of parametric statistical tests include (a) the level of measurement of the data is interval or ratio, (b) data are taken from populations that are normally distributed on the variable that is being measured, and (c) data are taken from populations that have equal variances on the variable that is being measured.

Because nonparametric tests make no assumptions about the distribution of the population, they are often called distribution-free statistics. Nonparametric statistical tests may be used with nominal and ordinal data, and sample sizes may be small.

There has been a growing body of research that suggests that violations of the assumptions of parametric tests do not adversely affect statistical decisions. The parametric tests are quite "robust," which means that these tests are not influenced by violations of the assumptions. Some researchers therefore routinely use parametric tests if data are at the interval or ratio level of measurement.

Because it appears that nonparametric tests have fewer restrictions, you may ask why these types of tests are not used when analyzing all data. The answer lies in the power of the tests. If the assumptions of parametric tests are met, these types of statistical tests are more powerful than nonparametric tests. However, if the assumptions are violated, it is possible that a nonparametric test might be more powerful.

POWER OF A STATISTICAL TEST

The **power of a statistical test** is defined as the ability of the test to reject a null hypothesis when it is false. In other words, the more powerful a test, the more likely it will detect a significant difference between groups or a significant correlation between variables. The power of a statistical test is dependent on the sample size and the level of significance that is chosen. The larger the sample that is chosen, the more power the statistical test will have. The higher the level of significance that is selected (.05 rather than .01, for example), the more power the statistical test will have. A test will also be more powerful if a one-tailed test rather than a two-tailed test is used.

STATISTICAL TESTS USED IN NURSING RESEARCH

Three of the most common statistical tests used in nursing research are discussed: the *t*-test, analysis of variance, and chi-square.

t-TEST

The *t*-test is a parametric test that examines the difference between the means of two groups of values. It is one of the most popular statistical tests. The *t*-test is appropriate for samples of nearly any size but is particularly useful with small sample sizes (<30). Because the test compares means, interval or ratio data are required. Also, because the *t*-test is a parametric test, the sample data are assumed to have been selected from populations that are normally distributed and have equal variances on the variable that is being measured.

Another name for the *t*-test is Student's *t*-test. This name was derived from the pseudonym used by the originator of the test, William Gosset. Gosset worked for a brewery in Dublin, Ireland. To maintain brewing secrets, there was a company policy that prohibited publications by employees. Gosset chose to secretly publish his mathematical formulas under the pseudonym of Student.

The *t*-test uses a *t*-distribution. Actually, there is a set of *t*-distributions, one for each different degree of freedom. As the number of degrees of freedom decreases, the shape of the distribution flattens from that of the normal curve. As the number of degrees of freedom increases, the more the distribution shape resembles the normal curve.

There are two forms of the *t*-test. One form is used with independent samples, and the other is used with dependent samples. An independent sample is one in which there is no association between the scores of the groups that are being observed; for example, an experimental group and a control group are compared. The test for independent samples is called an **independent *t*-test** or *independent samples t-test.* The **dependent *t*-test,** also called *correlated samples t-test* and *paired t-test,* is used when scores or values are associated. For example, anxiety scores of mothers and daughters might be compared. If each mother is matched with her daughter on some variable such as age or weight, the sets of values are dependent data. Dependent data are also obtained when the same subjects are measured before and after they receive an experimental treatment.

Separate formulas are used to calculate the independent *t*-test and the dependent *t*-test. These can be found in statistics textbooks. The *t*-value that is obtained is compared with the critical value associated with the *t*-distribution appropriate for the data (based on the degrees of freedom). If the *t*-value that is obtained is greater than the critical value, the null hypothesis is rejected, and the mean scores or values for the groups are considered to be significantly different.

ANALYSIS OF VARIANCE

The *t*-test is a very useful technique to determine the significance of the difference between two means. However, many studies compare more than two groups. For example, a researcher might want to compare the effectiveness of four different methods of teaching clients how to give insulin injections (four levels of the independent variable). The dependent variable might be the number of correct insulin injections that patients are able to perform in a given time period. If four groups were being compared, six separate *t*-tests would have to be computed. Suppose Groups A, B, C, and D were being compared. The following pairs would result: A and B, A and C, A and D, B and C, B and D, and C and D (for a total of six comparisons). Whenever the researcher wishes to compare the difference among more than two means, the appropriate statistical test is the **analysis of variance** (ANOVA—pronounced un-nóv-uh). ANOVA allows the researcher to simultaneously analyze the difference between several means at one time.

ANOVA is a parametric statistical test and, therefore, is based on the assumption that data are interval or ratio level and that the data have been selected from populations that are normally distributed and have equal variances on the variable that is being measured.

ANOVA uses the F-distribution, which was named after Sir Ronald Fisher. As is true with the t-distribution, there is more than one F-distribution. Each F-distribution is based on the degrees of freedom.

As the name of the statistic indicates, analysis of variance examines the variance in data obtained. Two types of variation are examined—variation between the means of the groups and variation of individual scores within each of the groups. These two types of variation are called mean square between groups and mean square within groups. These terms are symbolized by MS_B and MS_W.

You may wonder why the difference between the means of the groups does not provide enough information to make a decision about the difference between the groups. It has been determined that the variability of the scores or values in the population affects the mean. By only examining the differences among the means of the samples, the researcher might falsely conclude that there is a true difference between the populations that are represented by the sample data when, in actuality, this seeming difference has occurred because there is a great deal of variability within the samples. To avoid rejecting a true null hypothesis, the ANOVA examines two types of variability—the variability between the groups and the variability within each of the groups. The means of each of the groups are compared with the grand mean of all of the groups combined. Then each value within a group is compared with the mean value for that particular group. These two estimates of population variation are then compared by dividing the "between" estimate by the "within" estimate. An F-ratio is obtained. This F-ratio is symbolized by:

$$F = \frac{MS_B}{MS_W} \quad \begin{array}{l} \text{(Between group variance)} \\ \text{(Within group variance)} \end{array}$$

If the null hypothesis is true, these two measures of variability should be very similar, and the result of the division will be a value less than 1. If the null hypothesis is false, a value greater than 1 will occur. The larger the F-value, the greater is the variation or difference between the groups as compared to the variation within the groups. The significance of the F-value or F-ratio is determined by consulting an F-table in a statistics textbook to ascertain the critical value for F. If a computer program is used to analyze the data, the computer printout will usually provide the obtained value and the critical value.

If the difference or variation between the groups is significantly greater than the difference within the groups, the null hypothesis is rejected. In contrast, if the between-groups variation is not significantly greater than the within-groups variation, the null hypothesis is not rejected.

If the F-value is significant, the researcher knows that there is a significant difference between the means of at least two of the groups. The F-statistic, however, does not tell exactly where the difference occurs. Other statistical procedures are necessary. You might think that the appropriate statistic to calculate would be *t*-tests between all of the various pairs of groups. This technique will result in an increased likelihood of a Type I error. The more comparisons that are made, the more likely that one of the comparisons will be significant, by chance. For example, if 20 *t*-tests were run and the level of significance was set at .05, the researcher could expect to find statistical significance in at least one of these tests, even if there was no true difference between the means of any of the groups that were being compared. Several multiple comparison tests may be used to decrease the probability of making a Type I error. These tests include the Neuman Keul's test, Tukey's B, and the Scheffé test.

CHI-SQUARE

Statistical tests that were previously discussed, the *t*-test and ANOVA, are appropriate for interval data. The **chi-square test** is a nonparametric inferential technique that is appropriate for comparing sets of data that are in the form of frequencies or percentages (nominal data). The chi-square statistic (χ^2) is probably the most commonly used statistic with nominal data.

Using the chi-square technique, the researcher compares the frequencies that are obtained or observed in categories with the frequencies that would be expected to occur if the null hypothesis is true. Observed frequencies are compared with expected frequencies. If the observed frequencies are quite different from the expected frequencies at a specified level of significance (such as .05), the null hypothesis is rejected.

The chi-square distribution is the theoretical sampling distribution that is used when the chi-square statistic is calculated. Actually, there is a set of chi-square distributions. The shape of each of these distributions is governed by the degrees of freedom. To consult a chi-square table, you will need to know the degrees of freedom, just as you do when examining a *t*-distribution table or an *F*-distribution table.

Although the chi-square distribution may be used for several purposes, probably the most common use is with the *chi-square test for independence,* also called the *chi-square test for contingency tables.* Chapter 13 described contingency tables as those tables used to illustrate data that are presented in frequencies. The chi-square test for contingency tables is used to analyze the data that are displayed in contingency tables. The observed and expected frequencies in each cell of the table are compared.

Examine the data in Table 14–1. The research problem of the study was to determine whether nurses are more or less likely to smoke than occupational therapists. There are 100 nurses in the sample and 100 occupational therapists. The data show that half of the total sample, or 100 subjects, are smokers and 100 subjects are nonsmokers. The data also show that 60 nurses smoke, and 40 nurses do not smoke. The figures are reversed for the occupational therapists. The number 50 that is displayed in the upper right corner of each cell in the table is the number of smokers and nonsmokers that would be expected in each group if these two variables were not related.

The chi-square distribution will be used to determine if the observed values might have occurred by chance. If many samples, each containing 100 nurses and 100 occupational therapists, were chosen from the population, how many times would this size difference between groups occur by chance? To make this decision, the obtained value is

TABLE 14–1. **Smoking Behavior of Nurses and Occupational Therapists**			
	Smokers	Nonsmokers	Total
Nurses	50 60	50 40	100
Occupational therapists	50 40	50 60	100
Total	100	100	200

compared with the critical value. In this case the obtained value for χ^2 is 8.00, and the critical value is 3.84. The null hypothesis would therefore be rejected, and the researcher would conclude that this large a difference would occur by chance less than 5 times out of 100. There is a significant difference in the smoking behavior of the two groups. Because the chi-square test that was used is called the chi-square test of independence, another way to state the results is that smoking behavior is dependent on the type of health care profession to which one belongs. The null hypothesis says that smoking behavior and type of health care profession to which a person belongs are independent and, therefore, there will be no difference between the observed frequencies and the expected frequencies in the cells of the table. Rejection of the null hypothesis indicates that these two variables are dependent or related.

TESTING THE SIGNIFICANCE OF CORRELATION COEFFICIENTS

In Chapter 13, correlation coefficients were discussed as descriptive statistics. A correlation coefficient presents the degree to which the values of one variable (X) are related to the values of another variable (Y). The closer the correlation coefficient is to +1.00 or −1.00, the greater is the relationship between these two variables. Although the size of the correlation coefficient gives some indication of the degree to which two variables are related, an inferential statistical procedure is necessary to determine whether this correlation coefficient is the result of chance (sampling error) or whether there is a true relationship between these variables in the population.

In testing the significance of a correlation coefficient, the researcher wants to determine if the obtained *r,* based on sample data, came from a population of pairs of values for which the actual correlation is 0. The null hypothesis states that there is 0 correlation between these two variables in the population. If the correlation coefficient that is obtained from the sample data is too high to have come from a population in which the correlation is 0, the null hypothesis is rejected, and the conclusion is made that the two variables are correlated at a level that is significantly higher than 0.

If a correlation of .80 is obtained between two variables, it is quite probable that the variables are actually related. However, if a correlation coefficient such as .15 or .20 is obtained, there is a possibility that this value occurred as a result of sampling error or chance.

To determine if a correlation coefficient is significant, a *t*-test may be calculated or a table of significant values may be consulted. The degrees of freedom for the Pearson product-moment correlation are equal to the number of subjects minus 2 (N − 2). When the sample contains a large number of subjects, the size of the correlation coefficient may be quite small and still be significant. For example, with 20 degrees of freedom (22 subjects), an $r = .42$ is significant at the .05 level. If the degrees of freedom are increased to 80 (82 subjects), a correlation of $r = .22$ is significant at the .05 level. When interpreting the significance of correlation coefficients, it is important to examine the sample size.

As mentioned in Chapter 13, rather than using an inferential procedure to determine the statistical significance of a correlation coefficient, a more accurate interpretation of a correlation coefficient is obtained by squaring the coefficient (r^2), thereby determining the percentage of variance shared by the two variables. The r^2 for the first example, $r = .42$, would be .18 ($.42 \times .42 = .1764$). This means that these two variables share a common variance or overlap of 18%. If you knew the value of one variable, you would possess 18% of the knowledge you needed to be able to predict the value of the other variable. A correlation coefficient of .42 may not sound significant to you now, even though it might have been determined to be statistically significant. Remember, when a correlation coefficient is determined to be statistically significant, it only means that it is significantly different from 0. It does not take a very large correlation for it to be larger than 0! It is hoped that this information will help you to understand why some small correlations that are reported in research articles are said to be statistically significant. Occasionally you will see correlation coefficients as small as .15 or even .09 reported in the literature, and they will be starred (*) as being significant at the .05 level (or even doubled starred [**] for the .01 level).

ADVANCED STATISTICAL TESTS

Many advanced statistical tests are available for the researcher who wishes to study more than two variables in one study. One frequently used inferential procedure is multiple regression. **Multiple regression** is the procedure that is used when the researcher wishes to determine the influence of more than one independent variable on the dependent variable. For example, a researcher might want to determine what factors would most accurately predict a woman's decision to perform breast self-examination. A number of factors might be examined, such as history of breast cancer in the family, fear of cancer, and type of teaching received concerning the performance of breast self-examination.

Another frequently used test is the **analysis of covariance** (ANCOVA). ANCOVA is a powerful statistical test that is used when the researcher wishes to statistically control for some variable that may have an influence on the dependent variable. This test may also be used to statistically make two groups equal on some variable for which they are quite different before the experimental treatment is administered. For example, suppose a researcher wishes to determine if the anxiety levels of open-heart surgery patients will be lower postoperatively in the group that receives explicit pictorial information about postoperative procedures than in the group that receives verbal information about these procedures. It is self-evident that the preoperative anxiety levels of patients will influence their postoperative anxiety levels, regardless of the intervention they receive. Therefore, the researcher needs to measure the preoperative anxiety levels of both groups. Even if subjects are randomly assigned to the experimental and control groups, it is possible that the average anxiety levels of one group, just by chance, will be much higher than the other group. ANCOVA allows the researcher to make the two groups statistically similar. You might consider it like a golf game where an average player is given a handicap to allow him to have a chance of winning against a great player.

Two other advanced statistical tests that you may read about in research reports are canonical correlation and multivariate analysis of variance. **Canonical correlation** examines the correlation between two or more independent variables and two or more dependent variables. **Multivariate analysis of variance** (MANOVA) examines the difference between the mean scores of two or more groups on two or more dependent variables that are examined at the same time.

Researchers are beginning to examine the results of several research studies simultaneously, using statistical measures. **Meta-analysis** is a technique that combines the results of several studies that have been conducted on the same topic. The results of a large number of different studies are combined and statistically analyzed as if only one study had been conducted with one large group of subjects.

A meta-analysis study of age-related sleep variables was conducted by Floyd, Medler, Ager, and Janisse (2000). They examined 41 published studies (combined N = 3293) that contained 99 correlational effect sizes. Floyd et al. found that the amount of nighttime sleep and the ability to initiate sleep decreased with age. When sleep variables were measured using polysomnography rather than self-report, age-related associations were found to be even greater. They remarked that few of the researchers studied women or controlled for health variables that might have affected sleep.

CRITIQUING INFERENTIAL STATISTICS IN RESEARCH REPORTS

As mentioned in Chapter 13, readers are quite often intimidated by the statistics of a research report. The inferential statistics are even more intimidating than the descriptive statistics to many consumers of research. Although a thorough background in statistics is necessary to understand each and every statistical test that is discussed in research reports, a minimal understanding of inferential statistics is sufficient for the reader to understand the majority of the study results. Some guidelines for critiquing inferential statistics are presented in Box 14–1.

First, the reader searches the report for any indications that inferential statistics were used in data analysis. Then a determination must be made if there is enough information to make a decision about the appropriateness of each test that was used. For example, the level of measurement of the variables, the number of groups that were tested, and the sample size should be presented in the research report.

The reader should be provided with the value of the statistical test that was obtained, the degrees of freedom, and the significance level that was reached when each hypothesis was tested. The main concern of the reader is to be able to determine if each of the researcher's hypotheses were supported. Therefore, every research report should clearly present the results of hypothesis testing. These results should be presented both in the text of the report and in tables.

> ## Box 14–1.   Guidelines for Critiquing Inferential Statistics
>
> 1. Are inferential statistics presented in the research report?
> 2. If inferential statistics are presented, is enough information presented for the reader to determine whether the appropriate tests were used?
> 3. Is the reader provided with the calculated value of the inferential statistic, the degrees of freedom, and the level of significance that was obtained?
> 4. Were parametric or nonparametric tests used when the other type would have been more appropriate?
> 5. Are the chosen tests appropriate considering the level of measurement of the variables, the number of groups that were tested, the size of the sample, etc.?
> 6. Are inferential statistics presented for each hypothesis stated in the study?
> 7. Are the results of inferential tests clearly and thoroughly discussed?
> 8. Are the results presented both in the text and in tables?

SUMMARY

There are two broad purposes of inferential statistics: (a) estimating population parameters from sample data, and (b) testing hypotheses. The second purpose has been of more interest to nurse researchers.

When a sample is chosen to represent a population, there is some likelihood that the sample will not accurately reflect the population. The phenomenon in which sample values tend to be normally distributed around the population value is known as the **central limit theorem.** A frequency distribution based on an infinite number of samples is called a **sampling distribution.** Theoretical sampling distributions are used to estimate population characteristics. The standard deviation of the sampling distribution of the mean is called the **standard error of the mean** ($s_{\bar{x}}$).

A **confidence interval** is a range of values that, with a specified degree of probability, is thought to contain the population value. The researcher might establish a 95% confidence interval or a 99% confidence interval, for example.

Steps in hypothesis testing include (a) stating the study hypothesis, (b) choosing an appropriate statistical test, (c) deciding on the level of significance, (d) deciding if a one-tailed or a two-tailed test will be used, (e) calculating the test statistic, (f) comparing the calculated value to the critical value, (g) rejecting or failing to reject the null hypothesis, and (h) determining support or lack of support for the research hypothesis.

Although the study hypothesis (generally a directional research hypothesis) is of primary interest to an investigator, the null hypothesis (H_0) is the one that is subjected to statistical analysis.

Some of the questions that need to be answered when choosing a statistical procedure include these: Are you comparing groups? Are you correlating variables? What is the level of measurement of the variables? How large are the groups? How many groups are being compared? Are the observations dependent or independent? How many observations are available on each group?

The **level of significance,** also called alpha (α), is defined as the probability of rejecting a null hypothesis when it is true. The most common level of significance used is .05. This means that the researcher is willing to risk being wrong 5% of the time or 5 times out of 100 when rejecting the null hypothesis. More stringent levels of significance are .01 and .001.

If the researcher has stated a directional research hypothesis, it is appropriate to use a one-tailed test of significance. If a **one-tailed test of significance** is used, values will be sought in only one tail of the theoretical sampling distribution. A **two-tailed test of significance** is used to determine significant values in both ends of the sampling distribution.

A **critical value** is a cutoff point that denotes the place in a theoretical distribution at which all obtained values from a sample that are equal to or beyond that point are said to be statistically significant. Values beyond the critical value are said to lie in the **critical region** or **region of rejection.** If the computed value of a statistic is equal to or greater than the critical value, the null hypothesis is rejected.

The interpretation of a statistical test is dependent on the degrees of freedom (df). **Degrees of freedom** concern the number of values that are free to vary.

If the null hypothesis is actually true and it is rejected, a **Type I error** is made. If the null hypothesis is actually false and is not rejected, a **Type II error** is made. The level of significance set for the study determines the probability of a Type I error. Power analysis will help prevent a Type II error.

Inferential statistical tests may be classified as parametric and nonparametric. **Parametric tests** require interval or ratio data and make the assumption that the sample data have been taken from populations that are normally distributed and have equal variances. **Nonparametric tests** may be used with nominal and ordinal data and make no assumptions about the distribution of the population. Nonparametric tests are sometimes called distribution-free statistics.

The **power of a statistical test** is the ability of the test to reject a null hypothesis when it is false. The power of a test is dependent on the sample size and the level of significance chosen.

The **t-test** is a parametric test that examines the difference between the means of two groups. The *t*-test uses the *t*-distribution. There are two forms of the *t*-test. One form is used with independent samples and is called the **independent *t*-test** or *independent samples t-test*. The **dependent *t*-test,** also called *correlated samples t-test* and *paired t-test,* is used when scores or values are associated.

Analysis of variance (ANOVA) is used to compare the difference among more than two means. The ANOVA is a parametric test that uses the *F*-distribution.

The **chi-square test** is a nonparametric inferential technique that is appropriate for comparing sets of data that are in the form of frequencies or percentages. The frequencies that are obtained or observed are compared to the expected frequencies. The chi-square distribution is the theoretical sampling distribution used when the chi-square (χ^2) statistic is calculated.

An inferential procedure is necessary to determine if a correlation coefficient is statistically significant. The researcher may determine the significance of a correlation coefficient using a *t*-test or by consulting a table of significant values.

Advanced statistical tests include **multiple regression, analysis of covariance (ANCOVA), canonical correlation,** and **multivariate analysis of variance** (MANOVA). **Meta-analysis** combines the results of several similar studies.

NURSING RESEARCH ON THE WEB

For additional online resources, research activities, and exercises, go to www.prenhall. com/nieswiadomy. Select Chapter 14 from the drop down menu.

✖ GET INVOLVED ACTIVITIES

1. Write down all of the different kinds of inferential statistics found in this chapter and any others that you may recall from any statistics course that you may have taken. Leave space for adding other inferential tests that you may locate that are not on your list. Take this sheet of paper to the library. Examine three nursing research articles that were published in the 1980s, three nursing research articles that were published in the 1990s, and three recent nursing research articles. Place a check mark beside each type of inferential statistic that is mentioned in the articles. Write in any other tests that are mentioned that you do not have on your list. Additionally, write down as many levels of significance (p values) as you find.

2. Bring your list to class and compare it with the lists compiled by your classmates or colleagues. Determine the most common inferential statistic that is reported in nursing research articles. Make a tally of the number of times each type of inferential statistic was mentioned in the nursing research literature. Make a comparison among the articles published in the 1980s, the 1990s, and those published in recent years. Have the numbers and types of tests changed in recent years?

3. Compare the probability values (p values) that you located in the literature. Were most of them significant ($< .05$)? How many articles published results that were not significant?

4. Divide into groups. Propose an idea for a study and determine the type of descriptive statistic(s) that your group would use to report data on subjects and the type of inferential statistics that you would use to report the results of hypothesis testing or to present the answers to research questions.

✖ SELF-TEST

Circle the letter before the *best* answer.

1. Statistical significance means that the study findings:
   A. are important to the nursing profession.
   B. apply to a large target population.

C. are not likely to be the result of sampling error.

D. have proven the study hypothesis.

2. If study findings are statistically significant, this implies that the:

   A. null hypothesis should be rejected.

   B. research hypothesis should be rejected.

   C. null hypothesis should not be rejected.

   D. research hypothesis should not be rejected.

3. Parametric statistical tests would be appropriate for which of the following types of data?

   A. weight to nearest pound

   B. religion

   C. gender

   D. patients' room numbers

4. Which of the following is true concerning nonparametric statistical tests?

   A. should always be used with interval/ratio data

   B. estimate population parameters

   C. are generally used with large sample sizes

   D. none of the above

5. A research hypothesis states: "Male appendectomy patients ask for more pain medication on the first postoperative day than female appendectomy patients." When the data are analyzed, the mean number of requests for pain medication is 3.5 for males and 2.3 for females. The p value is calculated to be .04. What decision should be made about the findings of this study?

   A. Male appendectomy patients asked for significantly more pain medication on the first postoperative day than did female appendectomy patients.

   B. Female appendectomy patients asked for significantly more pain medication on the first postoperative day than did male appendectomy patients.

   C. There was no statistically significant difference in male and female patients' requests for pain medication on the first postoperative day after an appendectomy.

   D. No decision can be made about the difference in male and female appendectomy patients' requests for pain medication on the first postoperative day.

A researcher is trying to determine if type of educational preparation is associated with level of professional commitment. The mean scores on the *Commitment to the Nursing Profession* instrument are obtained for 30 diploma school graduates, 30 associate degree graduates, and 30 baccalaureate graduates. The probability level associated with the obtained F-value is .03. (Questions 6 through 10 pertain to this situation.)

6. What is the level of measurement of the dependent variable?

   A. nominal

   B. ordinal

   C. interval/ratio

7. How many sets of scores are being compared?

   A. one

   B. two

    C. three

    D. four

8. The scores on the dependent variable are:

    A. dependent.

    B. independent.

9. What inferential statistic was calculated?

    A. dependent *t*-test

    B. analysis of variance

    C. independent *t*-test

    D. chi-square test

10. Which of the following decisions concerning scores on the *Commitment to the Nursing Profession* instrument is correct, based on the probability level of .03 that was obtained when the data were analyzed?

    A. No significant difference exists among diploma, associate degree, and baccalaureate graduates' scores.

    B. A significant difference exists among diploma, associate degree, and baccalaureate graduates' scores.

    C. No decision can be made as to whether a significant difference exists among diploma, associate degree, and baccalaureate graduates' scores.

✖ REFERENCES

Bliss, D. Z., Johnson, S., Savik, K., Clabots, C. R., & Gerding, D. N. (2000). Fecal incontinence in hospitalized patients who are acutely ill. *Nursing Research, 49,* 101–108.

Defloor, T. (2000). The effect of position and mattress on interface pressure. *Applied Nursing Research, 13,* 2–11.

Elzey, F. (1974). *A first reader in statistics* (2nd ed.). Monterey, CA: Brooks/Cole.

Floyd, J. A., Medler, S. M., Ager, J. W., & Janisse, J. J. (2000). *Research in Nursing & Health, 23,* 106–117.

Polit, D. F. (1996). *Data analysis & statistics for nursing research.* Stamford, CT: Appleton & Lange.

Rothstein, H., & Tonges, M. C. (2000). Beyond the significance test in administrative research and policy decisions. *Journal of Nursing Scholarship, 32,* 65–70.

Shott, S. (1990). *Statistics for health care professionals.* Philadelphia: W. B. Saunders.

Spatz, C., & Johnston, J. (1984). *Basis statistics: Tales of distribution* (3rd ed.). Monterey, CA: Brooks/Cole.

CHAPTER 15

Presentation and Discussion of Study Findings

✺ OBJECTIVES

On completion of this chapter, you will be prepared to:

1. Describe the methods used to present research findings
2. Discuss the findings of research studies
3. Relate study findings to study hypotheses
4. Distinguish between statistical and clinical significance
5. Identify the conclusions of research studies
6. Determine the implications of research studies
7. Discuss the recommendations of research studies
8. Critique the findings, conclusions, implications, and recommendations of published research studies

✳ NEW TERMS DEFINED IN THIS CHAPTER

cells
columns
rows

We have reached the final steps in the research process. However, these final steps are very important. You might say that "the best has been saved for last."

The findings, discussion of findings, conclusions, implications, and recommendations of a research study may be placed under various headings in a research report. In theses and dissertations, you will probably find each of these sections under a separate heading. In research journal articles there is a great deal of variation. All of these elements of a report may be found under a section titled "Discussion of Findings" or there may be a section on "Findings" and another section for "Discussion." Some articles may have a section titled "Results and Conclusions." Regardless of the division of the material under various headings, each research report should contain the elements mentioned: findings, discussion of findings, conclusions, implications, and recommendations. Each of these areas are discussed individually.

FINDINGS OF THE STUDY

The findings of a study are the presentation of the results in the form of empirical data or facts. Do you remember the TV showed titled "Dragnet" in which Sergeant Friday would say, "Just the facts, ma'am, just the facts"? This holds true for the findings of a research study. This is not the place for the researcher to express opinions or reactions to the data.

Findings are written in the past tense, of course, because data are being reported that have already been gathered and analyzed before the writing of the report. A note of caution: DATA ARE PLURAL. Frequently, the word *data* is used incorrectly as a singular noun rather than a plural noun. *Datum* is the singular noun and is rarely used because the information that is gathered nearly always involves more than one item.

The findings come from the analysis of the data obtained in the study. Descriptive statistics are always used to describe the sample and to present the findings; inferential statistics are used to present the findings in studies where hypotheses are tested or research questions are posed.

PRESENTATION OF FINDINGS

Most research reports present the findings in both a narrative form and in tables. There is some disagreement about the function of the table in relation to the narrative presentation. Some people want to see all of the results in both places. Others contend that results presented in tables should not be reported in their entirety in the text; only highlights or important items from the table should be presented in the narrative. According to the publication manual of the American Psychological Association (1994), if the text discusses every item in the table, the table is unnecessary. Generally speaking, however, the table and the narrative should "stand alone," particularly when the results of hypothesis testing are presented. The reader should be able to obtain the results of hypothesis testing in both places.

Curran (1999) has published an interesting article in *Applied Nursing Research* that present tips on how to display data. She contended that the way data are displayed is as important as the data that are being displayed.

NARRATIVE PRESENTATION OF FINDINGS

The findings of a study should be clearly and concisely presented in the text. As much attention should be paid to data that fail to support a particular study hypothesis as is given to data that support a hypothesis.

Certain information should always be included in the text when discussing the study hypothesis(es). The statistical test that was used, the test results, degrees of freedom, and the probability value should be listed. Two common methods of reporting the same information are:

$$t\,(30) = 2.75; p = .01$$
$$t = 2.75; df = 30; p = .01$$

In the past, the probability value was frequently reported with a "less than" symbol in front of it ($p = < .05$) to indicate that the actual probability level was less than the given figure. Today, with the use of computers, the exact probability value should be reported. The computer printout will usually provide the probability value to four or more decimal places. Usually the probability value is then listed in a research report as two decimal places. So, if the probability level was .0212, it would be reported as .02 and not as <.05, as was common in years past.

In qualitative research studies, hypotheses are rarely tested and, therefore, inferential statistics are not included in these reports. The narrative presentation frequently contains many direct quotes made by the subjects. Then the researcher may present a summary of the findings by discussing patterns and themes found in the data.

TABLES

Tables are a means of organizing data so that they may be more easily understood and interpreted. The discussion of the table should be as clear as possible in the text. However, some of the responsibility for understanding the table is left with the reader. If a table is being used to present the results of hypothesis testing, a footnote should provide the test results, degrees of freedom, and the probability level. This information would be presented in the format described under the narrative type of presentation. For example, the following might be found under a table:

$$\chi^2 = 13.39; df = 5; p = .02$$

Some general guidelines concerning tables include the following:

1. Tables should appear as soon as possible in the report after they have been referred to in the text.

2. Information presented in tables should also be discussed in the narrative of the report.

3. Titles should be clear, concise, and contain the variables that are presented in the data. The name of the statistical test should not be used. For example, the following would be an inappropriate title for a table: "T-Test for Difference Between Means." An appropriate title might be "Guided Relaxation and Anxiety Levels of Cardiac Patients."

4. All data entries should be rounded to the same number of decimal places (one or two decimal places is common).

5. The decimal points, if present, should be lined up under each other in the data columns.

6. If data are not available for a section of the table, a dash (—) should be entered, rather than leaving a blank space, to make it clear that no data have accidentally been omitted from the table.

Some tables contain rows, some contain columns, and some contain both rows and columns. The vertical entries in a table are referred to as **columns,** and the horizontal entries are called **rows. Cells** are the boxes that are formed where rows and columns intersect.

Columns

		Cell			

Rows

FIGURES

The word *figure* is the term used to indicate any type of visual presentation other than a table. Figures include graphs, diagrams, line drawings, and photographs. Figures may help to enliven a narrative presentation and should be considered as a valuable means of displaying research results. These methods are particularly useful in presenting demographic data about subjects. See Chapter 13 for examples of various types of figures.

DISCUSSION OF FINDINGS

The discussion of the findings is a much more subjective section of a research report than the presentation of the findings. The "Discussion" section of a study report allows the researcher to make interpretations of the findings. The findings are interpreted in light of the theoretical framework and within the context of the literature review. No literature should be cited in the discussion of the findings section that has not been referred to in the review of the literature section of the report. When new literature sources are cited, it appears as if the investigator went back to the library after the data were collected to search for a source or sources that would be in agreement with the study findings.

In the discussion of the findings, the researcher discusses aspects of the results that are in agreement and those that are not in agreement with previous research and theoretical explanations. The researcher also reports study limitations.

Barroso (1999) conducted a study to describe the perceptions of people who had been diagnosed with HIV disease for at least 7 years. These individuals were labeled as "long-term nonprogressors." The researcher was trying to determine why these people thought their disease had not progressed. Participants had to self-report a CD4 count of at least 500. The researcher suggested that the self-report CD4 count might not have been accurate and called for longitudinal studies that would follow this group over time and include biomedical markers of disease progression.

Although study limitations should be discussed, this is not the time for "true confessions." A beginning researcher will frequently list all of the weaknesses and problems of the study and appear to ask the reader to disregard the findings of the present study when they are not in agreement with the theoretical framework or past research results. Experienced investigators are able to interpret findings within the context of the strengths and weaknesses of their studies.

DISCUSSION OF STUDY HYPOTHESES

The most important aspect of the findings in studies where hypotheses have been formulated is the presentation of inferential statistics used to test the hypotheses. As discussed in Chapter 14, the null hypothesis is subjected to statistical analysis, and the results allow the researcher to reject or fail to reject the null hypothesis. If the null hypothesis is rejected, support is provided for the research hypothesis. Remember, the research hypothesis predicts study results based on the theoretical framework or on previous research studies.

Results of hypothesis testing fall into one of three categories: (a) the null hypothesis is not rejected, (b) the null hypothesis is rejected and the research hypothesis is supported, and (c) the null hypothesis is rejected and the results are in the opposite direction from the prediction of the research hypothesis.

When the study results are congruent with the study prediction found in the research hypothesis, the researcher is overjoyed, and the task of describing the results of the study is relatively easy. The explanation for the findings will have already been discussed in the section on the theoretical framework or in the review of the literature section where previous research results were presented. Although the researcher should never say that the results "proved" the study hypothesis, the findings of a study provide empirical support for the hypothesis, and the investigator asserts with a degree of certainty (probability level) that the results were not due to chance. When significant results are found, the researcher will feel like celebrating and may begin to think about publishing the results.

When the null hypothesis is not rejected, the researcher may become discouraged and start trying to determine "what went wrong." Beginning researchers are particularly prone to start picking apart their studies when the null hypothesis is not rejected. They discuss the small sample size and the inadequate instrument and all the other limitations that can be identified. It is not uncommon for a graduate student who is writing a thesis to become upset after discovering nonsignificant study results. The student may put all material away and never complete the writing of the thesis. Researchers must be objective when considering negative results (those not in agreement with the prediction). Negative results may be as important as positive results.

Some researchers think that the only studies that are published are those in which the findings are in agreement with the study predictions. Many of the published research studies do report positive findings. However, a recent review of the research journals revealed that studies are being published in which nonsignificant results were found.

Although the discovery of nonsignificant results is disheartening, the discovery of results that are in the opposite direction of the study prediction is even more devastating and puzzling. These types of results are not supportive of the study's theoretical framework. These results may also be incongruent with previous research results. For an investigator faced with this dilemma, the best thing that can be done is to try to make some sense out of the findings and give some tentative explanations for the results. Recommendations may then be made for further research based on the explanations.

> Coronary artery bypass graft surgery patients and their family member caregivers were studied by Lenz and Perkins (2000). The experimental group in the study received a psychoeducational intervention delivered over 12 weeks. Their hypothesis predicted that the experimental group would have more favorable outcomes than the control group. Data revealed that the number of complications and adverse symptoms reported was in the opposite direction from the prediction. They suggested, "the treatment was apparently not sufficiently targeted or sustained to effect change in the chosen outcomes" (p. 148). They further asserted that unmeasured factors in the patients' home environments might have been more influential than the psychoeducational intervention.

STATISTICAL AND CLINICAL SIGNIFICANCE

It is important to distinguish between statistical and clinical significance. Statistical significance means that the null hypothesis has been rejected and that the differences found between groups on the variable of interest, or the correlations found between two variables, are not likely to be a chance occurrence. The differences or correlations are probably real. These real differences or correlations, however, may not be clinically important. Clinical significance means that the findings may be useful in the clinical setting with patients.

The significance of a correlation coefficient is dependent on the sample size. As the sample size increases, the size of the correlation needed to reach significance decreases. For example, with a sample size of 15, a correlation coefficient of .48 is needed to be statistically significant at the .05 level. With a sample of 100 subjects, a correlation of .19 is statistically significant. Remember, a statistically significant correlation only means that you are reasonably sure that the actual correlation between these two variables in the population from which the sample was obtained is greater than 0. Sometimes the difference between groups (experimental and control) on the dependent variable does not have to be very large to decide that a significant difference exists.

> Norman, Gadaleta, and Griffin (1991) evaluated three methods of measuring blood pressure in a stabilized acute trauma population. The three methods were two indirect methods—the bell and diaphragm components of the stethoscope—and one direct arterial method. Data were collected using a sphygmomanometer for indirect blood pressure and radial intraarterial cannula for direct blood pressure measurement. K1, K4, and K5 measurements (Korotkoff sounds) were compared among the three methods. A significant difference was found in K1 (systolic) readings between diaphragm and bell values. However, the difference was only 3.8 mm Hg. The authors cited critical care experts' opinion that a disparity of 5 mm Hg or less was not considered clinically significant. The investigators noted the need to distinguish between statistical and clinical significance.

There are instances where no statistical significance is found, but the researcher believes that the findings have some clinical significance. Sometimes the researchers find that an intervention has no significant effect for the experimental group as a whole, but that the intervention is effective for certain subgroups within the larger group.

> The quick relaxation technique (QRT) was used on 24 primary aorta-coronary bypass surgical patients to help prepare them for chest tube removal (Houston & Jesurum, 1999). Subjects rated their pain on a visual analogue scale immediately after chest tube removal and 30 minutes later. The experimental group received analgesia plus the QRT, while the control group received analgesia only. Although there was not a statistically significant difference between the two groups, the results approached significance ($p = .062$). The researchers suggested that the results were "clinically intriguing." When they examined the data closely, they found that elderly men reported much lower pain intensity ratings following chest tube removal when QRT was used, whereas elderly women reported higher pain ratings when QRT was used. Therefore, the researchers suggested further investigation of the use of QRT with elderly men.

CONCLUSIONS

The study conclusions are the researcher's attempt to show what knowledge has been gained by the study and are also an attempt to generalize the findings. In writing conclusions, the researcher returns to the study problem, purpose, hypothesis, and theoretical framework. Was the study problem answered? The research purpose met? The research hypothesis supported? The theoretical framework supported? The researcher should leave no doubt in the reader's mind about what the study has demonstrated in these areas. On the other hand, it is probably wise to be somewhat conservative in drawing conclusions from the findings.

In formulating conclusions, the researcher must consider the sample size and the population from which the sample was drawn. An example of a study conclusion that was generalized beyond the findings of the study is found in Jones' (1981) report. Theft behavior among 33 nurses in one hospital was examined. The investigator revealed that theft behavior was fairly prevalent among this group and concluded: "These figures suggest that employee theft among nursing personnel is widespread and needs to be reduced" (p. 35). Do you agree that this is an example of overgeneralization? A sample size of 33 nurses in one hospital does not warrant the use of the word "widespread." Although this study is now 20 years old, I continue to include this example because it is so awful!

The findings of a study are concrete and tied into the specific data of the study. The conclusions are more abstract and use more general terms. Conclusions are not just a restatement of the findings. It is not uncommon to find a conclusion in a student's research report that states, "There is a significant relationship between anxiety and test scores among nursing students." This is a finding and not a conclusion. The conclusions should go beyond the findings. For example, a study finding might be, "There is a significant increase in the exercise performance of a group of senior citizens who have used mental practice to increase their performance." A conclusion based on this finding would be, "Mental practice appears to be an effective means of increasing exercise performance in the elderly." You may think that these two statements are quite similar, but examine them more closely and you will see that the conclusion goes beyond the finding. The finding addresses the difference in exercise performance of one group of people from the pretest to the posttest. The conclusion generalizes the results to other subjects and to other points in time. Remember, the purpose of scientific quantitative research is to be able to generalize results to the broad population, not just to the study sample. In some types of research, such as phenomenological studies, nurses may be as interested in the responses of individuals as in the responses of groups, but in the traditional scientific method the interest is in populations rather than in samples or in individuals. The generalization of findings is, therefore, of great interest to study investigators.

Generalizations are risky business, however. The study design and sampling procedures must always be considered. If the senior citizens in the previous example had consisted of 10 volunteers who said before the study that they enjoyed exercising, there would be no basis for making the conclusion that mental practice was the reason for the increase in exercise performance. There would be too many threats to the validity of the study because of the design used and the sampling technique. You would have no way of knowing if the group changed because of the treatment or because of other factors, such as the Hawthorne effect. Because the subjects were volunteers who said that they enjoyed exercising, they may have been more motivated to increase their exercise performance.

IMPLICATIONS

The implications section of the research report gives the researcher an opportunity to be creative. Imagine that you have the power to make changes in the way certain courses are taught in your curriculum or in the way certain procedures are carried out in the hospital where you work. Based on the conclusions of your study, what changes would you suggest?

The implications of a study contain the "shoulds" that result from the study. "Nurse educators should…" or "nurse clinicians should…" are the types of statements that are found in the implications section of a research report. Based on the conclusions of the study, what changes, if any, should be considered?

The implication may be that no change is needed, that more research is called for to further verify the study results, or that changes need to be made based on the study conclusions. Although it is possible that no change is deemed necessary and that nurses should continue with their practices, it is more common to see implications that call for more research in the subject area or for certain changes to be made based on the conclusions of the study.

For every conclusion of a study, there should be at least one implication. Implications may be addressed to any or all of the following: educators, clinicians, researchers, administrators, or theorists.

Consider the following conclusion: Guided relaxation is an effective means of controlling anxiety in a patient about to undergo a proctoscopic examination. An implication of this conclusion might be this: Nurses should consider using guided relaxation techniques with patients about to undergo proctoscopic examinations. Although this implication may seem to be quite simple and to be derived from common sense, the implications of a study may be very challenging to write.

RECOMMENDATIONS

It has often been said that every research study raises more questions than it answers. The last section of every research report should contain recommendations for further research. This section should discuss logical extensions and replication of the study. In the recommendations section, other research studies are suggested that consider the limitations of the present study.

EXTENSIONS OF THE RESEARCH STUDY

Recommendations concerning extension of the research study should answer the question, "What comes next?" After completing a study, the investigator should be in a good position to determine the next step that needs to be taken to examine the subject area under consideration. It is important to distinguish extensions of the study from the common recommendations that are often found in research studies. These recommendations suggest a larger sample or a different setting or more reliability studies on the instrument. Although the limitations of a study need to be discussed, this is not the most important function of the recommendations section. In this section of the report, the researcher has the opportunity to make suggestions for future research that are based on the findings of this particular study, the findings of previous research, and the current state of the theoretical framework that was used in the study. This is a great challenge.

REPLICATION OF THE RESEARCH STUDY

Replication of a study involves carrying out a study similar to one that has previously been done. Only minor changes are made from the previous study, such as using a different type of sample or setting. Partial replication studies are probably more common than exact replications. If an instrument is changed or a new tool is added, it is probably more accurate to call this type of study a partial replication study.

Nurses have appeared to be reluctant to replicate the studies of other investigators. Beck (1994) decried the small number of replication studies. She contended that the lack of replication studies has seriously hampered the implementation of research findings. Beck conducted a computerized search and a hand search for replication studies published between 1983 and 1992. She located 49. Of these 49 studies, 27 were replicated by the original nurse researchers and 22 were replicated by other nurses. Beck admonished nurses who consider replication studies as "simple, dull, and repetitive" (p. 193). She asserted that this type of research takes "considerable imagination and skill" (p. 191).

Research studies published in *Nursing Research* and *Applied Nursing Research* during 2000 were examined to determine the number of replication studies that are being conducted. It appears that none of these studies would be considered replication studies.

As a result of nurses' reluctance to replicate studies, many isolated pieces of nursing research exist. Researchers must become convinced of the value of replication. The body of nursing knowledge needs to be based on research findings. Hypotheses must be tested over and over on different samples and in different settings to build confidence in research results.

Replication studies are appropriate for beginning researchers. This type of research is an excellent means of gaining research experience. Experienced researchers must also be willing to conduct replications to verify or repudiate previous research results.

CONSIDERATION OF STUDY LIMITATIONS IN FUTURE RESEARCH

When recommending future research studies, the limitations of the present study are considered. Some of the most common recommendations that are made concerning limitations are (a) alteration in the sample (different age group or educational level of the subjects), (b) alteration in the instrument (either a change in an existing instrument or use of another instrument), (c) control of variables (taking only a certain age group in the sample or selecting a random sample instead of using a convenience sample), and (d) change in methodology (providing 6 weeks of the experimental treatment instead of 4 weeks or using structured observations to collect data rather than self-report measures from the subjects).

ETHICAL ISSUES IN PRESENTING RESEARCH FINDINGS

When presenting the results of research studies, the rights of subjects must be considered. The researcher has the responsibility of ensuring that no subjects can be identified. The names of subjects should never be reported. Generally, only group data are presented in a report.

The name of the agency in which the study took place should never be mentioned, unless this agency has specifically agreed to be identified in the final report. The agency should be described in general terms such as "a large public teaching hospital in the northeastern United States."

CRITIQUING THE PRESENTATION OF STUDY FINDINGS

When presenting the findings of a study, the investigator must be objective. None of the investigator's personal opinions should be included. However, in discussing the study results, the researcher has an opportunity to interject some subjective interpretation of the data. For example, the researcher might mention some environmental factor that was thought to affect the study results. In one study, a group of subjects were trying to improve the time needed to complete a run around a track. Subjects had been taught the use of guided imagery to help them run faster. During the time the subjects were running the track, a dust storm came up. The researcher proposed that this might have been the reason for the nonsignificant study findings.

The discussion section of a research report should discuss the findings of each hypothesis that was tested or each research question that was answered. The findings should be interpreted in light of the study framework and previous literature on the topic. If the study hypotheses were not supported, the researcher should give the reader some idea about why these findings may have occurred. If these findings were thought to be related to the limitations of the study, the researcher should acknowledge these limitations and make suggestions for how these problems could be corrected in future studies. The study conclusions should be presented; implications for nursing practice, nursing education, and nursing research should be indicated; and recommendations for replication or extension of the study should be suggested. Some guidelines for critiquing the presentation and discussion of study findings are presented in Box 15–1.

Box 15.1 Guidelines for Critiquing the Presentation of Study Findings

1. Is the information concerning the study findings presented clearly and concisely?
2. Are the findings presented in an objective manner?
3. Is each study hypothesis or research question addressed separately?
4. Are the findings described in relation to the study framework?
5. Are the findings compared to those of other studies discussed in the literature review section of the report?
6. Does the investigator discuss the limitations that may have influenced the findings of the study?
7. Are both statistical and clinical significance discussed?
8. Are study conclusions clearly stated?
9. Are generalizations made that are based on the data and that take into consideration the sample size and sampling method, or does it appear that the investigator has overgeneralized the findings of the study?
10. Are implications suggested for nursing practice, nursing education, and nursing research?
11. Are recommendations made for future research studies? If so, do these recommendations take into consideration the limitations of the present study?

SUMMARY

Each research report should contain the findings, discussion of findings, conclusions, implications, and recommendations for future research. These elements of a research report may be found under various types of headings.

The findings of a study are the presentation of the study results in the form of empirical data. Methods of presenting findings include narrative presentations, tables, and figures.

The findings of a study should be clearly and concisely presented in the narrative text of the study report. Results of hypothesis testing should contain the statistical test used, test results, degrees of freedom, and the obtained probability level.

Tables are a means of organizing data to make study findings more easily understood and interpreted. Tables should never appear in a report unless they have been discussed in the text and should appear as soon as possible in the report after they have been referred to in the text. The vertical entries in a table are the **columns,** and the horizontal entries are called **rows. Cells** are the boxes that are formed where rows and columns intersect.

The word *figure* is the term used to indicate any visual presentation of data, other than a table. Figures include graphs, diagrams, line drawings, and photographs.

The discussion of findings is a more subjective section of a research report than the presentation of findings. The researcher interprets the findings in light of the theoretical framework and in the context of the literature review. The researcher also discusses any problems that may have occurred while conducting the study.

An important aspect of the findings of a study is the discussion of the hypotheses testing. Results fall into one of three categories: (a) the null hypothesis is not rejected and, therefore, the research hypothesis is not supported; (b) the null hypothesis is rejected and the research hypothesis is supported; and (c) the null hypothesis is rejected, and the results are in the opposite direction from the prediction of the research hypothesis.

It is important to distinguish between statistical and clinical significance. Statistical significance means that the null hypothesis has been rejected and that the study findings are probably not due to chance. Clinical significance means that the findings may be useful in the clinical setting.

The study conclusions are the researcher's attempt to generalize the findings. Conclusions are based on the findings and take into consideration the study problem, purpose, hypothesis, and theoretical framework. The population, sample, and sampling method must also be considered when trying to generalize study results.

The implications of a study contain the "shoulds" that result from the study. Appropriate changes are recommended that should be carried out by nurses in any of the following roles: educator, clinician, researcher, administrator, and theorist.

Recommendations for further research should be contained in each research report. Recommendations concern extensions of the study, replication of the study, and suggestions for additional studies that take into consideration the limitations of the present study.

When presenting research results, the rights of subjects must be protected. Names of subjects should never be reported, and, generally, only group data are presented.

NURSING RESEARCH

For additional online resources, research activities, and exercises, go to www.prenhall. com/nieswiadomy. Select Chapter 15 from the drop down menu.

✖ GET INVOLVED ACTIVITIES

1. Try to find study conclusions in three published research articles. Peruse the final section or sections of research articles (these sections are usually labeled "Discussion of Findings," "Discussion and Conclusions," or some similar heading). Search for the sentence or sentences in which the researcher attempts to generalize the results of the study. What word or words indicated to you that you had located the conclusion(s)? When meeting with your classmates or colleagues after this exercise, share with them any difficulty you had in finding conclusions in the research articles that you reviewed.

2. In these same research articles that you have reviewed, determine if the researcher presented any implications. If implications were found, did they appear to be aimed at clinicians, educators, administrators, researchers, or theorists?

3. Visit your library and locate the section that contains theses and dissertations written by nurses. Read the recommendations sections of these research reports. Write down two recommendations that are most appealing to you for future studies. Bring these suggestions to class. Share them with your colleagues. Determine, by vote, the single most worthwhile recommendation for a nursing study.

4. Locate a replication study in the nursing research literature. Did the original researcher conduct the replication? Was the study an exact replication or a partial replication? How long after the original study was the replication done? Did the researcher obtain similar results to those found in the original study?

5. Discuss the need for replication studies among your classmates or colleagues who are meeting together. Make suggestions for areas of research for which replication studies seem to be the most critical in nursing's attempt to develop a body of knowledge for the profession.

✖ SELF-TEST

Circle the letter before the *best* answer.

1. The conclusions of a study are based on the:
   A. findings of the study.
   B. review of the literature.
   C. implications of the study.
   D. recommendations for future research.

2. Which of the following statements is true concerning statistical and clinical significance?

   A. Statistical significance is necessary for clinical significance.
   B. Findings may be both statistically and clinically nonsignificant.
   C. If findings are said to be clinically significant, they must also be statistically significant.
   D. Findings must be either statistically significant or clinically significant.

3. Which of the following methods is appropriate for the presentation of research findings?

   A. narrative presentations
   B. tables
   C. figures
   D. all of the above

4. Guidelines for the use of tables in research studies include which of the following?

   A. A table should appear in the report immediately before the narrative discussion of the table.
   B. If data are missing, a blank space should appear in the table to indicate missing data.
   C. Titles should include the name of the statistical test used to analyze the data.
   D. All of the above.
   E. None of the above.

5. Consider the following conclusion: "There is a positive relationship between children's anxiety levels and their failure to cooperate with physical examinations." Determine an appropriate implication derived from this conclusion.

   A. Nurses must discover why high anxiety levels cause children to be uncooperative during physical examinations.
   B. Nurses should try to assess the anxiety levels of children before physical examinations.
   C. Physical examinations should be conducted infrequently with small children.
   D. A parent should be instructed to remain in the room with the child during a physical examination.

6. The recommendations of a study might contain which of the following?

   A. a discussion of the study findings
   B. suggestions for extension of the study
   C. comparisons of results with previous research findings
   D. a means of implementing the study findings

Write true (T) or false (F) beside the following statements:

_____ 7. The names of subjects are listed in a research report unless the subjects specifically ask not to be identified.

_____ 8. The implications of a study are based on the recommendations of the study.

_____ 9. The most important recommendations of a research report are those that suggest a larger sample size or a different type of sample.

_____ 10. The most puzzling finding of a research report is one that is directly opposite to the study prediction.

_____ 11. Conclusions are a restatement or rewording of the study findings.

_____ 12. Study generalizations should consider the sampling method used in the study.

✖ REFERENCES

American Psychological Association. (1994). *Publication manual* (4th ed.). Washington, D.C.: Author.

Barroso, J. (1999). Long-term nonprogressors with HIV disease. *Nursing Research, 48,* 242–249.

Beck, C. T. (1994). Replication strategies for nursing research. *Image: Journal of Nursing Scholarship, 26,* 191–194.

Curran, C. R. (1999). Data display techniques. *Applied Nursing Research, 12,* 153–158.

Houston, S., & Jesurum, J. (1999). The quick relaxation technique: Effect on pain associated with chest tube removal. *Applied Nursing Research, 12,* 196–205.

Jones, J. (1981). Attitudinal correlates of employee theft of drugs and hospital supplies among nursing personnel. *Nursing Research, 30,* 349–351.

Lenz, E. R., & Perkins, S. (2000). Coronary artery bypass graft surgery patients and their family member caregivers: Outcomes of a family-focused staged psychoeducatonal intervention. *Applied Nursing research, 13,* 142–150.

Norman, E., Gadaleta, D., & Griffin, C. C. (1991). An evaluation of three blood pressure methods in a stabilized acute trauma population. *Nursing Research, 40,* 86–89.

PART VI

Research Findings and Nursing Practice

CHAPTER 16

Communication and Utilization of Nursing Research

OUTLINE

Communication of Nursing Research Findings

- Preparing a Research Report
- Presenting Research Results at Professional Conferences
  - Presenting a Research Paper
  - Presenting a Research Poster
- Publishing a Journal Article
  - Preparing the Article
  - Selecting a Journal
  - Choosing Between Refereed and Nonrefereed Journals
  - Sending Query Letters
  - Reasons for Manuscript Rejection
- Preparing Research Reports for Funding Agencies
- Preparing Theses and Dissertations

Utilization of Nursing Research Findings

- Barriers to Nursing Research Utilization
  - Nurses' Lack of Knowledge
  - Nurses' Negative Attitudes
  - Inadequate Dissemination of Research Findings
  - Lack of Institutional Support
  - Findings Are Not Ready for Use in Practice
- Bridging the Gap Between Research and Practice

Summary

Nursing Research on the Web

Get Involved Activities

Self-test

OBJECTIVES

On completion of this chapter, you will be prepared to:

1. Discuss the preparation of a research report
2. Describe two means of presenting research results at professional meetings
3. Explore the steps in publishing a journal article
4. Recognize the responsibility for preparing a research report for an agency that has provided funds for a study
5. Discuss theses and dissertations as means of presenting research results
6. Elaborate on the need for utilization of nursing research findings
7. Recognize the barriers to nursing research utilization
8. Discuss measures that have been taken to facilitate nursing research utilization
9. Recall the Stetler criteria for determining if nursing research findings are ready for use in practice

NEW TERMS DEFINED IN THIS CHAPTER

blind review
call for abstracts
galley proofs
nonrefereed journal
peer review
query letters
refereed journal
research report

Your research project has been completed, and you have been asked to present your study results at a national research conference. Do these sound like delusions of grandeur? Maybe so, but it is hoped that some day you will present, to your colleagues, the results of a study you have conducted. Once a researcher has completed a study, plans should be made to communicate or disseminate the results. In fact, these plans should be made before the beginning of the project. The final step in a nursing research project is to communicate the findings to other nurses when the study is completed.

Winslow (1996) has made a plea for nurses to publish the findings of their studies. She wrote that failure to publish study findings is a form of scientific misconduct. Those are strong words! Patricia Grady, Director of the National Institute of Nursing Research, referred to the old saying that "research not published is research not done" (Grady, 2000, p. 54). She reported that reviewers of research applications are looking harder at the number and type of publications that have emerged from an applicant's previous funding before considering awarding funds for another study by this investigator.

Although the communication of research findings is the last formal step in the research process, it is only the beginning of the most important phase of research—the utilization of research findings. If research findings are not used, the conduct of research becomes a wasted effort. Nurse researchers need to exert as much effort in implementing research findings as they do in conducting research in the first place. This chapter discusses various means of communicating and promoting the utilization of nursing research findings.

COMMUNICATION OF NURSING RESEARCH FINDINGS

There are two major ways for researchers to communicate the results of their studies. They can talk about them or write about them. A researcher might begin by presenting the results to peers at school or in the agency where she or he works. Next, the researcher might attend a research conference at which study results are discussed in an oral presentation or in a poster session. As a next step, study results might be published in a journal article. If funding was received for a research project, the researcher probably will be required to submit a written report of the study to the funding agency. Finally, many researchers are pursuing advanced degrees and will present their research results in the form of theses and dissertations. The research report and the various methods used to communicate study findings are discussed in the next section of this chapter.

Although researchers have the prime responsibility of communicating the findings of their studies, other nurses and nursing organizations also bear the responsibility of seeing that research findings are distributed inside the nursing profession, to other health care disciplines, and even to the general public.

A framework for disseminating research findings has been developed at the Frances Payne Bolton School of Nursing (Brooten et al., 1999). The project identified several types of target audiences: scientific, clinical, academic, and business communities; the lay public; print, broadcast, and electronic media; and local, state, and national officials. The next crucial step in the framework is the development of the necessary infrastructure to facilitate the preparation of publications and presentations. For example, the Center for Research and Scholarship (CFRS) at the School of Nursing keeps an up-to-date file of author guidelines for more than 150 journals in nursing and allied health disciplines. Another means of assistance is the Writer's Club, which meets once or twice a month. Another step in the dissemination process involves the identification of the most appropriate means of communicating research findings to the target audiences. For example, calls for abstracts and manuscripts are posted for all faculty and students to see. Procedures have been established for the communication of findings to agencies from which funding was received. Also, three strategies have been identified for disseminating research findings to the media, the public, the government, and business communities: press releases, media contacts, and "student power." Brooten et al. asserted that if only 25% of the schools, colleges and departments of nursing used "student power" to disseminate research findings, there would be more than 1000 new messages distributed each year, or almost 3 messages per day, about nursing research. I would like to ask you, the reader of this textbook, "Have you thought about the 'power' you have to disseminate research findings?"

PREPARING A RESEARCH REPORT

A **research report** is a written or oral summary of a study. No research project is complete until the final report has been written. Even when a verbal presentation is planned, the research report should be written out in its entirety.

Writing is not easy. Dougherty (2000) wrote in an editorial in *Nursing Research,* "Writing is learned by imitation and practice" (p. 121). Effective writing is the result of planning and organization before writing is begun. Good writing should be clear, accurate, and concise. Technical or scientific writing is not meant to be humorous or entertaining. It is also not meant to be dull. The results of a study should be presented in an interesting and informative manner.

The research report should be presented in the order of the research process, beginning with the problem of the study and ending with conclusions, implications, and recommendations for future studies. The major part of the research report is written in the past tense because the study has already occurred. Hypotheses and conclusions are written in the present tense, and the implications and recommendations are directed toward the future.

PRESENTING RESEARCH RESULTS AT PROFESSIONAL CONFERENCES

Many nurse researchers give first consideration to nursing journals as a publication medium for their research results. However, the time lag for publication of a report in a journal may be two or more years. Presentations of research findings at local, regional, and national conferences promote more rapid distribution of study results.

Nurses should present their research results at nursing conferences as well as at interdisciplinary conferences. In an editorial in *Clinical Nursing Research,* Hayes (1995) said that the value of nursing research must be recognized "outside the supportive walls of the profession" (p. 356). She proposed interdisciplinary presentations as the best way to share our knowledge and be able to take our rightful place as a recognized health care discipline.

There are two ways to present research results at professional conferences: oral and poster presentations. Traditionally, oral presentations have been used most frequently, but in the last decade poster presentations have become popular.

Many opportunities exist for nurses to present their study results at research conferences and seminars. Nursing organizations such as the American Nurses Association and Sigma Theta Tau sponsor research seminars. Many nursing schools and regional nursing associations sponsor research conferences. Some organizations make special provisions for presentations by students.

Potential participants are contacted through a "call for abstracts." The **call for abstracts** is a request for a summary of a study that the researcher wishes to present at a conference. These requests are published in professional journals and distributed to educational institutions, health care agencies, and potential participants whose names have been obtained through the mailing lists of professional organizations. Notices of research conferences are generally distributed 6 to 12 months before the event.

Each conference or seminar will provide special guidelines for presenters and deadlines for submission of abstracts. The required length of the abstract varies from 50 to 1000 words, but many have a 200- to 300-word limitation. Abstracts should contain the purpose, research question(s) or hypothesis(es), design, methodology, major findings, and conclusions. If the research is still in progress, the last two items are not required. Abstracts are evaluated, and participants are notified about the selection decisions.

Generally, those people who are selected to participate receive no pay and are required to cover their own travel expenses. Sometimes, the conference registration fee is waived or reduced for participants. A commitment to nursing research is a prime motivator for participants. Of course, personal recognition is also a reward.

Presenting a Research Paper. The oral presentation of a research report is usually referred to as a paper presentation. The word *paper* is used because the report of the study has been written out on paper and is read to the audience by the investigator. Guidelines for paper presentations are found in the literature. In an article in *Applied Nursing Research,* Miracle and King (1994) presented guidelines for both paper and poster presentations.

If the principal investigator is unable to attend the conference, a co-investigator or another person familiar with the study presents the paper. A written report of the study is necessary if the proceedings of the conference are to be published.

Presenting research results at a conference has advantages over publishing the findings in a journal article. First, the investigator has the opportunity to present findings that are recent. Because of the time lag in publishing, research presented in journals may be outdated when it is printed. Second, the researcher will have the opportunity to interact with those people who are interested in the study and will be able to locate other researchers who are studying the same or similar phenomena.

Although many presentations are read directly from the research paper, more interest is created when an outline is used, and the presenter communicates with the audience in an informal manner. The use of audiovisual aids, such as slides and PowerPoint displays, greatly enhance a presentation. Audiences usually appreciate written handouts in the form of abstracts or summaries of the study.

A presenter is usually allotted 15 to 30 minutes. At some conferences, additional time is allotted for questions. At other conferences, the presenter will have to allow time for questions, if questions are desired. Even when no time remains for questions or certain members of the audience do not get a chance to ask their questions, presenters are usually willing to respond to questions during break times or when the conference has ended.

The format of the oral presentation is similar to that of a journal article or other written presentation of the study, in that the steps of the research process are usually presented in chronological order. The main difference lies in the condensation of the material to fit the time constraints of the conference. Some presenters prefer to attract the attention of the audience by reporting the findings first, proceeding with the other parts of the study, and then returning to discuss the findings in more detail later in the presentation. The review of the literature is usually not discussed in detail, with only pertinent studies being mentioned.

Generally, conference organizers will distribute evaluation sheets on which the audience may rate each presenter. The presenter should try to read the evaluations with an open mind. Although 99 of 100 comments may be favorable, the presenter probably will react most strongly to that one unfavorable comment. One colleague was devastated when reading a comment given to her after a presentation. The comment read, "You forgot to take the price tag off your dress sleeve." She was able to laugh about it later, but she was thoroughly embarrassed at the time.

Presenting a Research Poster. An increasingly popular way to present research results is through poster presentations. This visual method of presentation may be seen by a large number of people in a short time period.

At a poster session, the presenters usually remain with their posters and interact with the viewers. Posters appeal to those who want to get a general, overall view of the many research studies that are being conducted by nurses. Because of time constraints, a research conference participant can only attend a few oral presentations in a 1- or 2-day research conference. It is possible to view a fairly large number of posters in an hour or two.

Poster sessions generally are held during research conferences where oral presentations are also given. Usually, 1 or 2 hours of the conference will be devoted to posters. Occasionally, educational institutions and clinical agencies hold research conferences in which the only method of presentation is through posters. Godkin (1999) asserted that if a poster is placed in a hallway in a clinical setting, patients and their visitors, as well as the nursing staff, can view the material at their leisure.

Research poster sessions are an excellent way for beginning researchers to "get their feet wet." This type of presentation does not seem to be as scary as the idea of standing up in front of an audience and orally discussing a study.

The size of the posters varies according to different research conference requirements. Many conferences are held in hotels, and the size of the assigned rooms may dictate the number and size of the posters. A common poster size is 4 feet by 8 feet. If a poster will be displayed on a table, some type of support will be needed to make the poster stand erect. Commercial products may be purchased or a support can be built out of materials such as Styrofoam blocks or wooden wall moldings.

Careful consideration should be given to the construction of posters. Technical help may be sought from a graphic artist, or researchers may design and construct their own posters. The poster should not appear as if it had been thrown together at the last minute or constructed by a group of cub scouts who were "all thumbs." The initial view of the poster is important. Color combinations should be used that are attractive. Some examples that have been found to be eye catching are black on tan, white on blue, and white on black. Size, thickness, and color of the poster board may be determined after visiting an art store.

Posters should contain the research problem statement, hypothesis(es) or research question(s), a description of the sample, the methods, the findings, and major conclusions. Diagrams, graphs, and tables are effective means of presenting certain aspects of the study, such as the findings.

It is better not to place too much material on a poster. A cluttered poster will distract the viewers or, worse yet, cause them to pass by the poster because they think it will take too long to decipher the meaning of all of the material. The major titles on the poster should be in large letters—at least 1 inch high. Viewers will need to be able to see these letters from about 3 feet away. Typed material should be prepared with large letters. Many computer software programs have this capability. Letters also may be prepared freehand, with the use of a stencil or vinyl adhesive letters.

When posters must be transported long distances, such as by airplane, care should be taken that the poster does not get dirty or bent. Many excellent sources in the literature discuss the process of constructing a poster (Fowles, 1992; Kleinbeck, 1988; Lippman & Ponton, 1989; Miracle & King, 1994; Rempusheski, 1990; Ryan, 1989; Sexton, 1984; Taggart & Arslanian, 2000).

Make it a point to attend poster sessions. These sessions are an excellent source of research information for beginning researchers. In an article in *Applied Nursing Research,* Martin (1994) presents tips to nurses who will be viewing poster presentations. Also, tips for viewers of posters, called "poster etiquette," are presented by Brooks-Brunn (1996).

PUBLISHING A JOURNAL ARTICLE

The growth of the nursing profession depends on the ability of its members to build and share a body of knowledge. Nursing research is the method of building the knowledge, and publications are the major medium for sharing this knowledge. Research should always be conducted with the idea of publication in mind. Emphasis will be placed on writing an article for a journal because this communication medium has the potential for reaching the largest percentage of nurses.

The preparation of an article for a journal is a service to the profession as well as a means of obtaining recognition for the author or authors. A few journals pay authors an honorarium or a per-page fee. Generally, authors do not receive any compensation. Authors may actually have to pay for any revisions they wish to have made after the galleys are received. **Galley proofs** are sheets of paper showing how the article will appear in typeset form. When the author receives the galleys (about 2 months before the publication date), these sheets must be proofread for errors. No charge will be made to correct typographical or grammatical errors. If, however, the author wishes to delete a paragraph or add a paragraph, for example, a charge may be assessed by the journal for each line that is revised. This assessment discourages a lot of last minute changes by the author.

Some journals provide an author with several complimentary copies of the issue in which the article appears. Other journals send the author a number of complimentary reprints of the article. Additional reprints may usually be obtained at a reduced rate.

When an author receives an acceptance letter from a journal, an approximate date or month of publication is usually included. In 1991 Swanson et al. reported that the average waiting period, or lag time, between acceptance of an article and its publication varied from 1 month to 3 years, with an average wait of 7 months.

The number of nursing journals in the United States continues to grow. The exact number of these journals in existence at the present time could not be determined through a published source. However, the Web page of the ONLINE Nursing Editors, sponsored by *Nurse Author & Editor* publication, listed the Web pages for 136 editors of nursing journals (http://members.aol.com/suzannehj.naed.htm). The Web site for science.komm (www.sciencekomm.at/journals/medicine/nurse.html) indicates that there are 174 nursing journals. It appears that some journals are included on one list and not on the other and vice versa.

Six surveys concerning nursing journals have been published in the last 25 years. The sources for these studies are listed below in chronological order:

McCloskey, J. C. (1977). Publishing opportunities for nurses: A comparison of 65 journals. *Nurse Educator, 2*(4), 4–13.
McCloskey, J., & Swanson, E. (1982). Publishing opportunities for nurses: A comparison of 100 journals. *Image, 14,* 50–56.
Swanson, E., & McCloskey, J. (1986). Publishing opportunities for nurses. *Nursing Outlook, 34,* 227–235.
Swanson, E. A., McCloskey, J. C., & Bodensteiner, A. (1991). Publishing opportunities for nurses: A comparison of 92 U.S. journals. *Image: Journal of Nursing Scholarship, 23,* 33–38.
McConnell, E. A. (1995). Journal and publishing characteristics for 42 nursing publications outside the United States. *Image: Journal of Nursing Scholarship, 27,* 225–229.
McConnell, E. A. (2000). Nursing publications outside the United States. *Journal of Nursing Scholarship, 32,* 87–92.

The first three surveys concerned journals published in both the U.S. and in other countries. The fourth survey, conducted in 1991, examined only journals published in the U.S. The last two surveys focused on English-language journals that were published outside the United States. The authors of the first four surveys stated that the number of nursing journals in the surveys was probably 80 to 90% of the actual number of U.S. nursing journals in existence at the time of each survey.

Preparing the Article. Because of space constraints, journal articles provide somewhat brief coverage of research reports. The length of journal articles varies a great deal, but most editors prefer articles of 10 to 15 typed pages. The sections of the article and the format will vary according to the journal. Most articles contain these parts: introduction, review of literature, methods, findings, and discussion. It is important for the researcher to examine the target journal carefully for style and format.

Selecting a Journal.   Selecting an appropriate journal for an article is an important decision. With each passing year, more nursing and allied health journals are coming into existence. Before 1978, *Nursing Research* was the only journal devoted to the publication of nursing research studies. Since that time, the journals *Applied Nursing Research, Biological Research for Nursing, Clinical Nursing Research, Research in Nursing and Health,* and *Western Journal of Nursing Research* have been initiated. Additionally, *Advances in Nursing Science* devotes a large percentage of space to coverage of research studies. Many of the other journals contain research reports. In Swanson et al.'s (1991) survey, 25 out of 92 journals (27%) reported that 50% or more of their published manuscripts were research reports.

The *Journal of Undergraduate Nursing Scholarship* (juns.nursing.arizona.edu) is an online publication sponsored by the University of Arizona. This journal provides an opportunity for students in baccalaureate nursing programs to submit reports of original research investigations and papers on current issues in health care or the nursing profession.

McConnell (1995) surveyed 109 English-language nursing journals published outside the United States during 1992 and 1993. Of the 42 replies from publishers, nearly all of them indicated that their journals published research reports, with two of the journals, *The Canadian Journal of Nursing Research* and *Curationis,* being strictly research publications. The number of research journals had increased from two to eight when McConnell (2000) reported the results of her replication study that was conducted in 1996–1997. Approximately 91% of the 82 responding journal editors indicated that research reports were published in their journals.

The choice of a journal may be made before or after a manuscript is prepared. If the manuscript is written first, the author then seeks a journal that is appropriate for the proposed article as written. Another option is to determine the journal most appropriate for the content of the article and then prepare the manuscript according to the guidelines of that particular journal and the needs of that journal's readers. A manuscript that does not meet the needs of the journal's audience will not be accepted for publication in that particular journal.

An important source for nurses wishing to publish an article in a journal is the *Writer's Guide to Nursing & Allied Health Journals* written by Bradigan, Powell, and Van Brimmer (1998). This book discusses more than 500 nursing and allied health journals. Information is provided about the focus of the journal, desired writing style, readership, acceptance rate, and whether the manuscript should be sent in hard copy form or on a floppy disk.

Important information on how to get a manuscript published is found in an article by Nemcek in the July 2000 issue of the *AAOHN Journal.* This journal is the official publication of the American Association of Occupational Health Nursing. Nemcek discusses both print and online publications.

The nurse author should not forget magazines designed for the general public. Although the format would need to be simple and the content would need to be presented in easily understood terms, nurses will reach a wide section of health consumers by publishing study results in appropriate lay magazines.

Choosing Between Refereed and Nonrefereed Journals.   A choice must be made by an author to publish in a refereed or nonrefereed journal. Although there is no consensus on the definition of a refereed journal, generally speaking a **refereed journal** is one in which subject experts, chosen by the journal's editorial staff, evaluate manuscripts. A **nonrefereed journal** uses editorial staff members or consultants to review manuscripts. The issue of publication in refereed versus nonrefereed journals seem to be almost a moot issue. In Swanson et al.'s (1991) survey, 94% of the editors indicated that their journals were refereed publications. In both refereed and nonrefereed journals, the journal editor makes the final decision about the publication of an article.

Panels of experts evaluate each manuscript submitted to peer-reviewed journals. The review of manuscripts by professional colleagues who are content or methodological experts is called **peer review.** In a **blind review,** the reviewers are not aware of the author's identity before the manuscript is evaluated. This process is very important to a writer with a limited publication record. An unknown writer would have an equal chance with a well-known author.

In its February 2000 issue, *Applied Nursing Research* thanked its panel of almost 250 reviewers. Each manuscript submitted to this journal is sent to two teams of reviewers. Each team consists of a clinician and a researcher (who is frequently in an academic setting). These individuals have expertise in the content area or in the research methods presented in the manuscript. Each team member individually writes a review of the manuscript, and then the two team members write a joint review of the manuscript.

Sending Query Letters.   Before submitting an article to a journal, it may be wise for the author to first determine the journal's interest in the manuscript. This is done through a letter of inquiry called a query letter. A **query letter** contains an outline of a manuscript and important information about the manuscript that an author sends to an editor to determine the editor's interest in publishing the material. The letter should be addressed to the editor by name. It is never wise to address a query letter to "The Editor of…" or to "Dear Sir." The time should be taken to review a copy of the latest issue of that journal to obtain the name of the editor.

Approximately 60% of the editors of the nursing journals surveyed by Swanson et al. (1991) preferred a query letter before the submission of a manuscript. This preference for query letters has risen as the number of submitted manuscripts has increased. Editors may save a great deal of editorial review time by discouraging manuscripts that do not fit the needs of the journal. In response to query letters, editors usually provide helpful hints to authors about possible revisions of manuscripts that have not yet been submitted.

Query letters may be sent to several journals at the same time. Responses fall into three categories: (a) request for submission of the manuscript as outlined in the query letter, (b) suggestions for revisions in the manuscript and then submission, and (c) discouragement of submission of the manuscript. If the author receives positive responses from more than one journal, a decision must then be made as to which journal to choose for the submission of the manuscript. A manuscript should be sent to only one journal at a time. Many journals require a signed statement that the manuscript is not being considered by any other journal.

Reasons for Manuscript Rejection. Swanson et al.'s (1991) survey revealed that the highest ranked reason for rejection of manuscripts by editors of nursing journals was that the manuscript was poorly written. A poorly written manuscript continued to be the highest ranked reason for rejection reported in McConnell's (2000) survey of English-language journals published outside the U.S. Downs (1991a) reported that over 25% of the manuscripts submitted to *Nursing Research* are never sent for review because they are poorly written. She stated even in this day when spelling errors can be corrected automatically and paragraphs can be moved from here to there, technology cannot correct "slipshod expression of ideas" (p. 4). Other reasons for rejection determined by Swanson et al. (1991) in descending rank order were poorly developed idea, not consistent with purpose of journal, term paper style, methodology problems, content undocumented, content inaccurate, content not important, clinically not applicable, statistical problems, data interpretation problems, subject covered recently, content scheduled for future, and too technical.

When the editor sends a letter to the author concerning the evaluation of a manuscript, suggestions for revision may be made and the author asked to resubmit a revised manuscript. If a letter is received asking for revisions, the changes should be made and the manuscript resubmitted to the journal. If an article is rejected outright, the reasons for the rejection will be indicated. The critique may be quite terse. *Nursing Research* editor Florence Downs (1985) apologized for the tone of rejection letters and stated that "time and reviewer availability preclude the construction of polished essays that might soften the blow" (p. 3).

Rejection of an article does not necessarily mean that it is not a good article. There is a lot of competition for the limited space in the nursing and allied health journals. Swanson et al. (1991) reported that the average acceptance rate of manuscripts was 41%. The acceptance rate is probably lower today because of the increase in the number of manuscripts that are submitted to nursing journals. Seven of the journals included in McConnell's (2000) survey of non-U.S. nursing journals reported acceptance rates of less than 25%.

When a rejection letter is received, the manuscript may or may not be returned, according to the policy of the journal. In either case, the author should consider submitting a copy of the manuscript to another journal.

Preparing Research Reports for Funding Agencies

Research projects cost money, and researchers frequently seek funding sources. Many organizations provide funds for nursing research. Some public organizations that might be approached for support are the National Institute of Nursing Research, National Institute of Mental Health, Veterans Administration, and the U.S. Public Health Service. Although public sources have provided most of the funding for nursing research, nurses are increasingly seeking funds from private foundations. Some of these private foundations are Robert Wood Johnson, Kellogg, Alcoa, and Lilly. Voluntary health organizations such as the American Cancer Society and the American Heart Association have supported nursing research. Businesses and corporations such as Apple Computer Corporation and Del Monte Foods have provided funds for nurse researchers. Charitable organizations, including churches and sororities, as well as individual philanthropists, may be approached for funding. Intramural funding is available in many universities and health care agencies. Finally, various groups within the nursing profession, such as Sigma Theta Tau and the American Nurses' Foundation, make funds available for research.

If funding is received for a study, the researcher is nearly always expected to provide a final report at the completion of the project. This report may be a brief summary or a lengthy report. As with other research reports, the steps in the research process are followed in the report.

PREPARING THESES AND DISSERTATIONS

Theses and dissertations are an important means of communication for research studies that are conducted to fulfill educational requirements. Because these documents serve a dual purpose of communicating research findings and providing educators with evidence of the students' ability to perform scholarly work, theses and dissertations are usually lengthy documents that may contain 100 pages or more and are divided into several chapters. Dissertations contain more in-depth investigations than theses and provide new knowledge for the profession. Theses are usually concerned with testing existing theory, whereas dissertations focus on refining existing theories or generating new theories.

UTILIZATION OF NURSING RESEARCH FINDINGS

Now that you are near the end of this text, recall the first goal for conducting nursing research: to promote evidence-based nursing practice. Therefore, for nursing research to be useful to the profession, study findings must be implemented in nursing practice.

The use of research findings in nursing practice is called research utilization. It means going beyond the somewhat artificial research setting to the "real world" of nursing. In the past, many actions of nurses have been based on tradition or authority. This is no longer acceptable in this day of evidence-based practice. Nurses should be able to justify the decisions they make and the care that they give.

Many nursing leaders have indicated the high priority that should be placed on the utilization of research findings in nursing practice. However, they have pointed out the gap between nursing research and nursing practice (Bircumshaw, 1990; Bock, 1990; Brett, 1987; Dufault & Sullivan, 2000; Gennaro, 1996; Lewis et al., 1998; Sparkman, Quigley, & McCarthy, 1991).

Barriers to the utilization of nursing research have been identified in many studies. Various means to bridge the gap between research and practice have also been identified.

BARRIERS TO NURSING RESEARCH UTILIZATION

Many articles have been published that list barriers to the utilization of research findings by nurses in this country and around the world. These include articles by Carroll et al. (1997), Funk, Champagne, Weiss, & Tornquist (1991a), Funk, Champagne, Weiss, & Tornquist (1991b), Funk, Champagne, Weiss, & Tornquist (1995), Kajermo, Nordström,

Krusebrant, and Björvell (1998), Lewis, Prawant, Cooper, and Bonner (1998), Retsas (2000).

There are many barriers to the utilization of nursing research findings in nursing practice. Five of the most common barriers will be discussed: (a) nurses' lack of knowledge of nursing research, (b) nurses' negative attitudes toward nursing research, (c) inadequate means of disseminating nursing research findings, (d) lack of institutional support, and (e) study findings that are not ready for use in nursing practice.

Nurses' Lack of Knowledge.   There is a great deal of evidence to indicate that nurses are unaware of many research findings. Funk, Champagne, Wiese, and Tornquist (1991b) sent a survey concerning barriers to research utilization to 5000 nurses selected from the American Nurses Association membership roster. Returns were received from 1989 individuals (40%). The third most important barrier listed was that the nurse is unaware of research findings. Of the 600 respondents who provided suggestions for facilitating research utilization, the second highest ranked suggestion concerned improving availability and accessibility of research reports, and the third ranked suggestion proposed advanced education and increasing the research knowledge base. Specific suggestions included use of research role models for less experienced staff, creation of a nursing research department, establishment of a formal nursing research committee, presentation of research grand rounds, participation in informal research interest groups and research journal clubs, and establishment of collegial relationships with university faculty. In 1995, these same authors published the findings from the sample of nurse administrators who responded to their 1991 survey. Nurses' lack of awareness of research was listed by 77.2% of the administrator respondents as the greatest barrier to research utilization. An almost identical percentage (76.5) of the 1100 respondents in Carroll et al.'s (1997) study identified lack of awareness of research findings as a barrier to research utilization. In a study by Lewis et al. (1998) of nephrology nurses, lack of awareness of research findings was the third highest ranked barrier to the use of research in practice.

Nurses' Negative Attitudes.   Champion and Leach (1989) found that nurses' attitudes toward research were related to research utilization ($r = .55$). Attitude was more strongly correlated with research utilization than the other two variables that were considered: institutional support and availability of research findings. The authors suggested strategies to help nurses develop positive attitudes toward research. These strategies included role models in the clinical area who value research, research courses at the undergraduate level that help the student develop enthusiasm for research, and faculty with positive attitudes who help students, early in their careers, develop positive attitudes toward research. Champion and Leach called for more emphasis to be placed on research and statistics in baccalaureate nursing programs.

In Funk et al.'s (1991b) study, approximately 35% of the respondents did not see the value of research for practice. A similar percentage (34.1) of nephrology nurses in Lewis et al.'s (1998) study did not value the use of research in practice. Approximately 31% of Australian nurses in a study by Retsas (2000) did not recognize the value of research findings.

Funk, Champagne, Wiese, and Tornquist (1991a) discussed the persuasion stage of research utilization that occurs before a nurse adopts an innovation that is based on research. Knowledge of the innovation is acquired first. Then persuasion occurs when the nurse forms a favorable or unfavorable attitude toward the new research finding. This persuasion is influenced by interactions with colleagues or with a person who is knowledgeable about the new innovation. The next step is called the decision stage, where the nurse decides to try out the innovation. Implementation then occurs when the innovation is actually put to use. Finally, confirmation is the last step in research utilization. The nurse seeks reinforcement that the decision to implement the innovation was correct.

Inadequate Dissemination of Research Findings.

Inadequate dissemination of nursing research findings involves two areas. First, most nursing research studies are never published or presented at research meetings or workshops. Second, those that are published or presented are often not written or verbally presented at a level where the practicing nurse can understand the findings.

Many references are found in the literature that attest to practicing nurses' unhappiness with the dissemination of nursing research findings (Bock, 1990; Carroll et al., 1997; Funk et al., 1991b; Gennaro, 1996; Kajermo et al., 1998; Retsas, 2000). Swedish nurses in Kajermo et al.'s (1998) study ranked the lack of availability of research findings as the greatest barrier to the use of these findings.

Practicing nurses complain about their inability to understand articles in the research journals. The language is technical and the articles are often lengthy. Research reports are frequently written for researchers rather than for clinicians. In Funk et al.'s (1991b) study, respondents suggested that research be reported in the journals that are read most frequently by clinicians and that these reports be more readable and contain clinical implications. Nurse researchers tend to present their research findings in very formal research meetings and in research publications. Researchers in academic settings are sometimes rewarded more (promotions, salary raises, tenure) for publications in prestigious research journals rather than for publications in practice journals.

Nurses need to make an effort to publish in the popular clinical journals. This does not mean that nurse researchers should not prepare publications for the scholarly journals but that there is also an obligation to disseminate the findings in a manner understandable to the nurse in practice; this usually means publishing findings in practice journals. Nurse researchers also should consider publications and presentations for the lay media. Back in 1991, Downs (1991b) called for readers of *Nursing Research* to send in suggestions for how to relay the outcomes of nursing research to the public. Brooten et al. (1999) asserted, "The lay public in general is woefully uninformed of the research conducted by nurses" (p. 133). It appears that we have made very little progress in communicating the results of nursing research to nurses, much less to the general public!

Lack of Institutional Support.

Nurses frequently perceive that there is little institutional support for nursing research. Lack of institutional support has been identified as a barrier to research utilization in all of the published studies.

Champion and Leach (1989) proposed methods that could be used by administrators to indicate support. These included providing time off for nurses to attend nursing conferences, making current journals available in the institution's library, and allocating time for nurses to read research reports during the workday.

Edwards-Beckett (1990) cited the necessity of research sources being provided by institutions. She mentioned helpful suggestions that she found in the literature, such as adequate library facilities, photocopying equipment, typing, software and computers, statistical help, and data analysis help.

In Funk et al.'s (1991b) study of approximately 2000 nurses, the two greatest barriers to research utilization were the nurses' report that they did not have "enough authority to change patient care procedures" and "insufficient time on the job to implement new ideas." The authors considered both barriers to be related to the setting (institution). Nurse administrators in this same survey ranked "insufficient time on the job to implement new ideas" as the second highest barrier to research (Funk et al., 1995). More than 600 of the staff nurse respondents gave suggestions for facilitating research findings (Funk et al., 1991b). One of the most frequent suggestions concerned increasing administrative support and encouragement. Funk et al. proposed that nursing staff must believe the environment is conducive for the use of research findings before they will believe that they have the authority to change their practice based on research results.

One of the most effective facilitators of research utilization identified by nephrology nurses in Lewis et al.'s (1998) study was increased administrative support and encouragement. These researchers called for administrators to allow nurses time to read and participate in discussions of research articles. Lewis et al. also called for administrators to find ways to recognize and reward the use of research in practice.

Tsai (2000) surveyed 382 staff nurses and nurse managers in the Republic of China. The main barriers to research utilization identified by these nurses were lack of time and lack of staff. The respondents called for role models, consultation, and guidance in locating useful research.

Findings Are Not Ready for Use in Practice.   In a 1981 editorial in *Nursing Research,* Downs asserted, "Research is not something that can be brewed over night and ingested the next morning" (p. 322). She warned against the "premature consumption" of research findings. She stated that this practice might be "hazardous to someone's health" (p. 322). In a 1996 editorial, Downs continued to call for caution in regard to research findings. She contended that much of the material that is published in *Nursing Research* is not ready for immediate use.

No study findings should be implemented if the study has not been replicated in several clinical settings, with similar results being found. Often research is carried out with "normal" subjects, rather than with hospitalized patients. The findings may be quite different between the two types of subjects.

Bock (1990) contended that replication studies should be respected as a legitimate scholarly activity. One of the most recent nursing research journals to be published, *Clinical Nursing Research,* indicated its intent to publish replication studies (Hayes, 1993). Martin (1995) wrote that a single study is seldom a sufficient foundation for making decisions about practice or about policies. Polit (1996) agreed that replication studies are needed because nurse researchers use nonrandom samples so frequently. Deets (1998) called for replication studies to be conducted by master's students. In turn, Deets asserted that journals would have to be willing to publish the results of these replication studies.

For research to be ready for use in practice, the findings must have been replicated at least *once* and demonstrated to be true with "real" patients as well as with "normal" subjects. When trying to help students decide if research results are ready for use in practice, this author has two initials that are used—NR. I tell students if it is *Not Replicated*, it is *Not Ready* for practice.

BRIDGING THE GAP BETWEEN RESEARCH AND PRACTICE

In the past few years, the nursing literature has shifted some of the emphasis from research utilization (RU) to evidence-based practice (EBP) (Omery & Williams, 1999). Although these terms sometimes are used interchangeably, Omery and Williams have made a distinction between these two concepts. They described EBP as broader in scope than RU in that EBP encompasses not only evidence based on scientific findings but also evidence that is based on expert clinical opinion. Estabrooks (1999) also described evidence-based practice as a more general term that encompasses research utilization as well as other factors. DiCenso and Williams (1998) have included patient preferences and existing resources as part of evidence-based practice. Omery and Williams (1999) wrote that the impact of the shift from the strict interpretation of research utilization to the broader interpretation of evidence-based practice has yet to be appraised.

Many nursing research utilization projects have been described in the literature, beginning in the 1970s. Two widely known projects that have fostered research utilization are the Western Council on Higher Education for Nursing (WCHEN) Regional Program for Nursing Research Development project conducted in the early 1970s and the Conduct and Utilization of Research in Nursing (CURN) project conducted in the late 1970s. Both projects received funding from the Division of Nursing.

In the research utilization aspect of the WCHEN project, nurses from various settings attended 3-day workshops in which they were taught how to use the change process to bring about research utilization. The nurses came in pairs from the same geographic location but worked in different settings. For example, a school nurse and a community health nurse who came from a rural community developed together a plan to provide nursing interventions for elementary school students who had high rates of absenteeism (Elliott, 1977). Although the WCHEN project was considered to be successful, one major problem encountered was the lack of reliable nursing studies that were appropriate for implementation in nursing practice.

The most well-known nursing research utilization project is the CURN project, a 5-year project sponsored by the Michigan Nurses Association. The two major goals of this project were to stimulate the conduct of research in clinical settings and to increase the use of research findings in the daily practice of nurses. The steps to be carried out, according to Horsley, Crane, Crabtree, and Wood (1983), were as follows:

1. Identify specific clinical nursing practice problems.
2. Assess the existing knowledge base on the issue.
3. Design a nursing practice innovation based on a scientific research base.
4. Implement clinical trials and evaluation of the innovation.
5. Decide to adopt, revise, or reject the innovation.
6. Develop strategies to extend the innovation to other settings.
7. Determine means of continuing the innovation over time.

As a result of this project nursing innovations (protocols) were developed for nine practice problems. The titles of the nine published volumes covering these areas are:

- *Mutual Goal Setting in Patient Care*
- *Closed Urinary Drainage Systems*
- *Distress Reduction Through Sensory Preparation*
- *Pain*
- *Intravenous Cannula Change*
- *Preventing Decubitus Ulcers*
- *Preoperative Sensory Preparation to Promote Recovery*
- *Reducing Diarrhea in Tube-fed Patients*
- *Structured Preoperative Teaching*

Other individual projects have been reported in the literature that describes nurses' attempts to incorporate new research-based knowledge into their clinical practice. Goode, Lovett, Hayes, and Butcher (1987) used the CURN model to promote the use of nursing research findings in clinical practice in a small, rural, 42-bed acute care hospital. A research committee was established to serve as change agents to facilitate the utilization process. The goals of the committee were (a) to learn to read reports of research, (b) to review and discuss findings from current research, and (c) to evaluate the research and make recommendations regarding its use. The committee chose three areas to study: temperature measurements, breastfeeding, and preoperative teaching. As a result of the review of research literature and the efforts of the research committee to implement research findings, several changes were instituted at the hospital. The nurses began to take oral temperatures on patients receiving oxygen, the obstetric nurses gave all breastfeeding mothers the same information, and a structured preoperative teaching program was developed.

Funk, Tornquist, and Champagne (1989) developed a nursing research dissemination model. The model has three mechanisms that facilitate utilization of research: (a) topic-focused, practice-oriented research conferences; (b) related, broadly distributed, carefully edited volumes based on the conference presentations; and (c) an information center to provide ongoing dialogue, support, and consultation. They described their first application of the model in their article published in 1989. They planned a conference titled "Key Aspects of Comfort: Management of Pain, Fatigue, and Nausea." They sent out a call for conference presenters to submit a comprehensive summary of their work rather than the usual short abstract that is called for. The purpose of asking for the comprehensive summary was to obtain sufficient detail about the study to determine its value and relevance for practice. The potential presenters were told that the conference would discuss applications of the research to practice, implementation of the study in health care settings, and the study limitations that would be of concern for practitioners. Submissions were received from 137 potential presenters. Funk, Tornquist, and Champagne were disappointed that technical language was used in a number of the summaries that they received. Each summary was edited, and feedback was provided in preparing a presentation for clinical audiences. Researchers and clinicians alike were very positive in their evaluations of the conference. However, 20% of the conference attendees indicated that the implications for practice were not made clear. Only a small majority (57%) indicated that conflicting findings had been adequately addressed, and only 68% thought that methods for implementing findings had been suggested. When some of the presenters were asked why they had aimed their presentations more at their research peers than at the clinicians in the audience, the most frequent answer was that they "felt compelled to convince those researchers of the value and rigor of their work. They felt that they were walking a tightrope between two audiences, and the researcher audience won out" (pp. 490–491). The research conference organizers thought that the conference had gone a long way toward effectively communicating with a clinical audience, but that much more work was needed in this area.

Sparkman, Quigley, and McCarthy (1991) described a project at the James A. Haley Veterans' Hospital in Tampa, Florida. The CURN model was used to reach the goals of encouraging nurses to conduct research and to enhance staff nurses' application of research-based knowledge to clinical practice. The authors discussed the success achieved on one rehabilitation unit where nurses examined (a) medication administration, (b) nutritional support, and (c) goal clarification among the nurse, patient, and family. The project was not nearly so successful on a general medicine unit where the focus was placed on collaboration between physicians and nurses. The authors proposed that the difference in level of success might have been related to the type of problem that was studied. The medicine unit focused on a multidisciplinary, organizational problem as opposed to a patient care problem that was specific to nursing. The CURN model was designed specifically for nursing practice issues. It appeared that the physician-nurse collaborative issue was beyond the intended use of the CURN model.

Nolan, Larson, McGuire, Hill, and Haller (1994) described two other research utilization models, one by the American Association of Critical Care Nurses (AACN) and another at the University of North Carolina (UNC). The AACN evaluated their AACN Scope of Practice and their Standards of Care. A demonstration project was conducted to see whether the values and practices of AACN members resulted in positive outcomes. The outcomes of the demonstration project were evaluated to see if AACN values and practices brought about results that were consistent with existing literature findings on the same outcome variables.

The UNC model involved six steps. First, research topics were selected from the literature and surveys of nurses. Next, a call for abstracts on these topics was sent out. In the third step, an expert panel selected abstracts. The fourth step involved the provision of editorial, methodological, and statistical help for participants. After the conference, a monograph was published and disseminated. Finally, an information center was set up, which published a newsletter and set up a referral service.

The Stetler model for research utilization (Stetler, 1994) was first described 25 years ago. In 1976, Stetler and Marram wrote a classic article about the steps to be taken before the nurse decides research findings are applicable for nursing practice. The authors contended that numerous guidelines have been proposed to help consumers critique the strength of the research design but that no systematic criteria have been established that help carry the consumer from the critiquing stage to the application stage. Stetler and Marram listed three phases of critical thinking: (a) validation, (b) comparative evaluation, and (c) decision making. In Stetler's revised model there are six phases: (a) preparation, (b) validation, (c) comparative evaluation, (d) decision making, (e) translation/application, and (f) evaluation. The validation phase is called "research utilization critique" (Stetler, 1994, p. 20), and during this phase the decision is made to accept or reject a particular study.

Validation concerns the overall examination of the strengths and weaknesses of a study. The consumer must question every step of the research process that was carried out. A traditional research critique is done. If a biased sample was used, operational definitions were not provided, or invalid statistical procedures were used, the findings would be questionable for application in practice. If the study design and procedures were determined to be valid, nurse consumers also should search for findings and conclusions that might be valid in their clinical settings. Stetler and Marram (1976) wrote that the consumer should search for "what was found, about whom or what, under what conditions, by whom, when, where, and how" (p. 560).

If the nurse determines that the study is valid, then a comparative evaluation should be done. What variables would affect the decision to change practice based on research findings? Would it be possible to implement the findings in the nurse's practice? The nurse would want to know how similar the research setting was to her or his own setting and how similar the study sample was to patients/clients with whom the nurse works. Finally, in doing a comparative evaluation, the nurse must determine the feasibility of implementing the findings based on the constraints of the particular practice setting. Are there any legal or ethical risks to the involved clients, nurses, or the institution? Would applying the findings involve a major organizational change? Are the resources available (time, money, equipment)?

Once the nurse has examined the feasibility, the decision about application is made. The nurse may decide against application or make a cognitive or a direct application of the findings. Cognitive application means that the nurse is not yet ready to apply the findings in practice but will use the information to enhance her or his knowledge base and may consider moving to a direct application in the future. Direct application of research findings means that the nurse chooses to test out the findings in practice. This does not mean that the nurse will not continue to check the validity of the findings, but it means that this validity check will now be done directly rather than cognitively.

Many research utilization studies and projects have been discussed in recent literature. Three of these are presented.

Radjenovic and Chally (1998) described the use of the Stetler model in a research utilization component of a senior-level maternity/pediatrics clinical course. Students were guided through all of the six phases, from the preparation phase to the evaluation phase. Students critiqued articles on a topic chosen by their instructor. Each student critiqued a different article. At the end of the semester poster presentations were made. The faculty expressed the hope that the project helped students to develop "an appreciation of the need for searching beyond a single report, critically summarizing a body of literature, and applying elements of the change process to support nursing practice" (p. 29).

Omery and Williams (1999) conducted a survey of research utilization (RU) among nurses across the United States. Telephone interviews were conducted with a convenience sample of 19 doctorally prepared nurses who were thought to be involved in RU. Results showed that RU is occurring in medical centers throughout the country. Many different types of projects were identified, such as those on pain management and infection control. Few facilities had a formal RU process in place. Barriers and facilitators were the same as those previously discussed in the literature. According to the respondents, nurses must be educated about and understand the research process for RU to be successful (I hope you read that sentence several times!).

Dufault and Sullivan (2000) conducted a study to evaluate a collaborative research utilization model for pain management. Multidisciplinary academic scientists were paired with clinicians and undergraduate and graduate nursing students. This group (a) evaluated the existing research on pain management, (b) generated a research-based standard for pain management, and (c) evaluated the effectiveness of the standards on four patient outcome variables. Results showed that subjects whose caregivers used the new standards had less pain, less interference by pain with their quality of life, and greater satisfaction with the interventions used and the caregivers' responses to their pain.

SUMMARY

A **research report** is a written or spoken communication of the findings of a study. The report should be presented in the order of the research process. Research reports may be presented as (a) oral presentations, (b) poster presentations, (c) journal articles, (d) written reports for funding agencies, and (e) in theses and dissertations.

Research conferences are sponsored by many nursing organizations. Participants are contacted through a **call for abstracts,** which is a request for summaries of research studies that researchers wish to present.

An oral presentation of a research report at a conference is referred to as a paper presentation. The researcher may also present research results in the form of a poster.

Research is generally published in journal articles. A **refereed journal** is one that uses subject experts to review manuscripts. **Nonrefereed journals** use editorial staff members or consultants to review manuscripts.

The **peer review** process involves the review of a manuscript by professional colleagues who have content and methodological expertise in the area of the study discussed in the manuscript. Frequently, journals use a **blind review** process in which no authors' names are included on the manuscripts.

Before submitting an article, a letter of inquiry, called a **query letter,** should be sent to determine the editor's interest in reviewing a certain manuscript. A manuscript, however, must never be sent to more than one journal at a time.

About 2 months before an article is published, the author will receive the galleys. **Galley proofs** are sheets of paper containing the article as it will appear in typeset form.

If funding is received for a study, the researcher is usually expected to provide a final report at the completion of the project. This report may be a brief summary or a lengthy report.

Theses and dissertations are a means of communicating results of research studies that are conducted in conjunction with educational requirements. These documents are generally quite long and are divided into several chapters.

Five common barriers to utilization of nursing research findings are (a) nurses' lack of knowledge of research findings, (b) nurses' negative attitudes toward nursing research, (c) inadequate means of disseminating nursing research findings, (d) lack of institutional support, and (e) study findings that are not ready for use in nursing practice.

Two widely known nursing research utilization projects are the Western Council on Higher Education for Nursing (WCHEN) Regional Program for Nursing Research Development project conducted in the early 1970s and the Conduct and Utilization of Research in Nursing (CURN) project conducted in the late 1970s.

Nurses should use traditional research critique methods before determining that research results are ready for practice. Also, nurses must evaluate research findings for applicability to their particular clinical settings. If the study findings are determined to be valid, both in design and procedures and in applicability to the clinical setting, the feasibility of implementing the findings must be determined. Many nursing research findings are not yet ready for use in practice.

NURSING RESEARCH ON THE WEB

For additional online resources, research activities, and exercises, go to www.prenhall. com/nieswiadomy. Select Chapter 16 from the drop down menu.

✳ GET INVOLVED ACTIVITIES

1. Determine an area in which you might like to conduct research in the future. Choose a funding source that you might approach to gain support for your project.

2. Discuss with your colleagues various methods that might be used to ensure that nurses at each of the hospitals where you work or where you are receiving clinical experiences are aware of the importance of research findings (consider the principles of change theory when determining approaches to use).

3. Locate a nursing study that you believe has very important findings but that needs to be replicated before the findings are implemented in nursing practice.

4. Identify a finding of a nursing study that you think is ready for implementation at your work or clinical site but for which you believe there would be resistance.

✳ SELF-TEST

1. What communication medium is most likely to reach the largest percentage of nurses?

   A. dissertation
   B. journal article
   C. conference oral presentation
   D. poster

2. The communication medium for research findings that is probably most appropriate for a beginning researcher is a:

   A. journal article.
   B. thesis.
   C. research paper.
   D. poster.

3. Which of the following is a reason for the rejection of a manuscript that has been submitted to a journal?

    A. manuscript is poorly written
    B. content of manuscript is inaccurate
    C. content of manuscript is not appropriate for the journal's readers
    D. all of the above
    E. none of the above

4. Which of the following is true concerning journal articles?

    A. Revisions are generally not needed in manuscripts that are submitted to journals.
    B. Many journals prefer that a query letter be sent before a manuscript is submitted.
    C. There is a general agreement among nursing journals about the format for research articles.
    D. Journals do not accept manuscripts from beginning researchers.

5. Support for nursing research has been furnished primarily by:

    A. public sources.
    B. private foundations.
    C. businesses.
    D. individual philanthropists.

6. A researcher will probably receive a monetary reward for which of the following methods of presenting research?

    A. journal article
    B. thesis
    C. research paper
    D. poster
    E. none of the above

7. Which of the following statements is true?

    A. Most nurses have adequate knowledge of nursing research findings.
    B. Many nursing research findings are never published.
    C. Inadequate research skills of nurses is the most frequently cited reason for lack of utilization of research findings.
    D. Most nursing research findings are ready for use in practice.

8. Research studies have demonstrated which of the following?

    A. Nurses' attitudes toward research are negatively correlated with research utilization.
    B. Nurses are more influenced by research findings in journals than by those that they learned about in their basic nursing educational programs.
    C. Nurses prefer published findings that are written in a technical manner.
    D. All of the above.
    E. None of the above.

Write true (T) or false (F) beside the following statements:

_____ 9. If a study has been replicated at least once, there is no need for further research in the same area of study.

_____ 10. The Conduct and Utilization of Research in Nursing (CURN) is one of the most well-known nursing research utilization projects.

_____ 11. Replication studies are the most common type of nursing research studies.

_____ 12. Surveys of nurses have found that most nurses have positive attitudes toward the utilization of research findings.

✖ REFERENCES

Bircumshaw, D. (1990). The utilization of research findings in clinical nursing practice. *Journal of Advanced Nursing, 15,* 1271–1280.

Bock, L. R. (1990). From research to utilization: Bridging the gap. *Nursing Management, 21,* 50–51.

Bradigan, P. S., Powell, C. A., & Van Brimmer, B. (1998). *Writer's guide to nursing and allied health journals.* Washington, DC: American Nurses Association.

Brett, J. L. L. (1987). Use of nursing practice research findings. *Nursing Research, 36,* 344–349.

Brooks-Brunn, J. (1996). Poster etiquette. *Applied Nursing Research, 9,* 97–99

Brooten, D., Youngblut, J. M., Roberts, B. L., Montgomery, K., Standing, T., Hemstrom, M., Suresky, J., & Polis, N. (1999). Disseminating our breakthrough: Enacting a strategic framework. *Nursing Outlook, 47,* 133–137.

Carroll, D. L., Greenwood, R., Lynch, K. E., Sullivan, J. K., Ready, C. H., & Fitzmaurice, J. B. (1997.) Barriers and facilitators to the utilization of nursing research. *Clinical Nurse Specialist, 11,* 207–212.

Champion, V. L., & Leach, A. (1989). Variables related to research utilization in nursing: An empirical investigation. *Journal of Advanced Nursing, 14,* 705–710.

Deets, C. (1998). When is enough, enough? *Journal of Professional Nursing, 14,* 196.

DiCenso, A., Cullum, N., & Ciliska, D. (1998). Implementing evidence-based nursing: Some misconceptions. *Evidence-Based Nursing, 1*(2), 38–40.

Dougherty, M. C. (2000). On writing (editorial). *Nursing Research, 49,* 121.

Downs, F. (1981). Soap (editorial). *Nursing Research, 30,* 322.

Downs, F. (1985). News from the fourth estate (editorial). *Nursing Research, 34,* 3.

Downs, F. (1991a). A construction report (editorial). *Nursing Research, 40,* 4.

Downs, F. (1991b). Informing the media (editorial). *Nursing Research, 40,* 195.

Downs, F. S. (1996). On clinical interpretation of research findings (editorial) *Nursing Research, 45,* 195.

Dufault, M. A., & Sullivan, M. (2000). A collaborative research utilization approach to evaluate the effects of pain management standards on patient outcomes. *Journal of Professional Nursing, 16,* 240–250.

Edwards-Beckett, J. (1990). Nursing research utilization techniques. *Journal of Nursing Administration, 20,* 25–30.

Elliott, J. E. (1977). Research programs and projects of WCHEN. *Nursing Research, 26,* 277–280.

Estabrooks, C. A. (1999). The conceptual structure of research utilization. *Research in Nursing & Health, 22,* 203–216.

Fowles, E. R. (1992). Poster presentations as a strategy for evaluating nursing students in a research course. *Journal of Nursing Education, 31,* 287.

Funk, S. G., Champagne, M. T., Wiese, R. A., & Tornquist, E. M. (1991a). Barriers: The barriers to research utilization scale. *Applied Nursing Research, 4,* 39–45.

Funk, S. G., Champagne, M. T., Wiese, R. A., & Tornquist, E. M. (1991b). Barriers to using research findings in practice: The clinician's perspective. *Applied Nursing Research, 4,* 90–95.

Funk, S. G., Champagne, M. T., Tornquist, E. M., & Wiese, R. A. (1995). Administrators' views on barriers to research utilization. *Applied Nursing Research, 8,* 44–49.

Funk, S. G., Tornquist, E. M., & Champagne, M. T. (1989). Application and evaluation of the dissemination model. *Western Journal of Nursing Research, 11,* 486–491.

Gennaro, S. (1996). Research utilization: An overview. *Journal of Gynecological and Neonatal Nursing, 23,* 313–319.

Godkin, M. E. (1999). Posters meet clinical news needs. *Reflections, 25,* 31.

Goode, C. J., Lovett, M. K., Hayes, J. E., & Butcher, L. A. (1987). Use of research based knowledge in clinical practice. *Journal of Nursing Administration, 17,* 11–17.

Grady, P. A. (2000). News from NINR. *Nursing Outlook, 48,* 54.

Hayes, P. (1993). Replication studies (editorial). *Clinical Nursing Research, 2,* 243–244.

Hayes, P. (1995). Expanding the horizon of nursing research (editorial). *Clinical Nursing Research, 4,* 355–356.

Horsley, J. A., Crane, J., Crabtree, M., & Wood, D. (1983). *Using research to improve nursing practice: A guide.* New York: Grune & Stratton.

Kajermo, K. N., Nordström, G., Krusebrant, Å., & Björvell, H. (1998). Barriers to and facilitators of research utilization, as perceived by a group of registered nurses in Sweden. *Journal of Advanced Nursing, 27,* 798–807.

Kleinbeck, S. V. M. (1988). Poster sessions bring research to the OR. *AORN Journal, 47,* 1299–1304.

Lewis, S. L., Prowant, B. F., Cooper, C. L., & Bonner, P. N. (1998). Nephrology nurses' perceptions of barriers and facilitators to using research in practice. *ANNA Journal, 25,* 397–405.

Lippman, D. T., & Ponton, K. S. (1989). Designing a research poster with impact. *Western Journal of Nursing Research, 11,* 477–485.

McCloskey, J. C. (1977). Publishing opportunities for nurses: A comparison of 65 journals. *Nurse Educator, 2*(4), 4–13.

McCloskey, J., & Swanson, E. (1982). Publishing opportunities for nurses: A comparison of 100 journals. *Image, 14,* 50–56.

McConnell, E. A. (1995). Journal and publishing characteristics for 42 nursing publications outside the United States. *Image: Journal of Nursing Scholarship, 27,* 225–229.

McConnell, E. A. (2000). Nursing publications outside the United States. *Journal of Nursing Scholarship, 32,* 87–92.

Martin, P. A. (1994). Poster session tips for the novice viewer. *Applied Nursing Research, 7,* 208–210.

Martin, P. A. (1995). More replication studies needed. *Applied Nursing Research, 8,* 102–103.

Miracle, V. A., & King, K. C. (1994). Presenting research: Effective paper presentations and impressive poster presentations. *Applied Nursing Research, 7,* 147–151.

Nemcek, M. A. (2000). Getting published online and in print. *AAOHN Journal, 48,* 344–348.

Nolan, M. T., Larson, E., McGuire, D., Hill, M. N., & Haller, K. (1994). A review of approaches to integrating research and practice. *Applied Nursing Research, 7,* 199–207.

Omery, A., & Williams, R. P. (1999). An appraisal of research utilization across the United States. *Journal of Nursing Administration, 29,* 50–56.

Polit, D. F. (1996). *Data analysis & statistics for nursing research.* Stamford, CT: Appleton & Lange.

Radjenovic, D., & Chally, P. S. (1998). Research utilization by undergraduate students. *Nurse Educator, 23,* 26–29.

Rempusheski, V. (1990). Resources necessary to prepare a poster for presentation. *Applied Nursing Research, 3,* 134–137.

Retsas, A. (2000). Barriers to using research evidence in nursing practice. *Journal of Advanced Nursing, 31,* 599–606.

Ryan, N. M. (1989). Developing and presenting a research poster. *Applied Nursing Research, 2,* 52–55.

Sexton, D. (1984). Presentation of research findings: The poster session. *Nursing Research, 33,* 374–375.

Sparkman, E. D., Quigley, P., & McCarthy, J. (1991). Putting research into practice. *Rehabilitation Nursing, 16,* 12–14.

Stetler, C. B. (1994). Refinement of the Stetler-Marram Model for Application of Research Findings to Practice. *Nursing Outlook, 42,* 15–25.

Stetler, C. B., & Marram, G. (1976). Evaluating research findings for applicability in practice. *Nursing Outlook, 24,* 559–563.

Swanson, E., & McCloskey, J. (1986). Publishing opportunities for nurses. *Nursing Outlook, 34,* 227–235.

Swanson, E. A., McCloskey, J. C., & Bodensteiner, A. (1991). Publishing opportunities for nurses: A comparison of 92 U.S. Journals. *Image: Journal of Nursing Scholarship, 23,* 33–38.

Taggart, H. M., & Arslanian, C. (2000). Creating an effective poster presentation. *Orthopaedic Nursing, 19,* 47–52.

Tsai, S. (2000). Nurses' participation and utilization of research in the Republic of China. *International Journal of Nursing Studies, 37,* 434–444.

Winslow, E. H. (1996). Failure to publish research: A form of scientific misconduct? (editorial) *Heart & Lung, 25,* 169–171.

CHAPTER 17

Critique of Research Reports

✖ OBJECTIVES

On completion of this chapter, you will be prepared to:

1. Discuss the guidelines for critiquing a research study
2. Critique selected research studies

With the increased emphasis on evidence-based practice, Downs (1999) pointed out the increased need for nurses to be able to evaluate research findings. She also contended that neither educators nor practitioners have critique skills that are as sharp as they need to be. As a reader of this book, you may take some consolation in knowing that you are not the only one who is not an expert in critiquing research articles. If you have made it all the way to this page in the book, I hope you have gained some knowledge that will help you to critique published research articles.

You may believe that the only research articles that are published report on "good" research. Unfortunately, this is not always true. Although the review process that is used by most nursing journals helps to ensure the publication of valid research, some published studies contain serious flaws.

All studies have strong and weak points. The word *critique* is often equated with the word *criticism.* This is unfortunate because the purpose of a research critique is to assess the strengths as well as the weaknesses of a study.

Critiquing research articles is particularly helpful to the beginning researcher because the critiquing process aids in the development of research skills. As the reader assesses the parts of a published study, ideas come to mind for the development of future research projects or for improvements in studies that have already been conducted or those that are in progress.

The research critique involves a thorough examination of all the parts of the study. Generally, the best way to conduct a critique is to read the entire study and make an initial evaluation of the report. Then each part of the study should be subjected to an in-depth evaluation.

Most research articles contain an abstract that is placed either at the top of the article or down along the left margin on the first page of the article. The body of the article begins with an introductory section that has no heading preceding the material. Generally there are four headings in a research article. The first heading, which follows the introduction, is generally labeled "Literature Review," "Relevant Literature," or "Background." The second heading is titled "Methods." Next, a heading identifies the "Results" section. Finally, the last heading is labeled "Discussion." There are variations to these four headings. Some articles contain additional headings for "Theoretical Framework" and for "Conclusions." Even though the research article may contain only four or five headings, all of the parts of the research study should be included within these sections. For example, the "Methods" section generally contains information about the study design, setting, population, sample, data-collection methods, and data-collection instruments.

Probably the most important part of a research article to focus on, after a cursory review, is the area where the design is discussed. As mentioned, information on the design will usually be found in a section titled "Methods." After you determine how the researcher actually carried out the study, then you can go back to see if the other parts of the study are congruent. For example, if the design is described as a pretest-posttest design, two groups should show up in the problem or purpose statement, two groups should be listed in the hypothesis, and two groups should be mentioned when the population and sample are being discussed.

Beginning researchers frequently take pride in the ability to find faults in the research reports that they read. This success in uncovering the errors in published reports often results in questions such as, "How could this study have been published?" It is well to remember that the author of the published report has had the courage and motivation to become involved in nursing research, whereas many other nurses have not. This is not to say that critiquers should be lenient in their evaluation of published research, but it is important that nursing research be conducted, and severe criticism of their work may dim the enthusiasm of nurse researchers. This is especially true for those who are just beginning to become involved in nursing research. Keep in mind that it is much easier to evaluate the research of others than to conduct research yourself.

Some guidelines for evaluating research reports follow. These guidelines are certainly not an exhaustive list. Many other guidelines could be used and questions posed when reading research. As ideas come to mind while you are critiquing research reports, jot them down. In this way, you will be able to develop your own research critique assessment tool to use in the future.

Frequently, there are no "right" or "wrong" answers when evaluating research reports. Even experts may disagree about certain aspects of a particular study. In evaluating research, reviewers should be as objective as possible and present sound rationale for their judgments.

Several articles containing guidelines for critiquing quantitative research reports have been published in nursing journals (Beck, 1990; Carlson, Kruse, & Rouse, 1999; Fosbinder, & Loveridge, 1996; Giuffre, 1998; Grant, Davis, & Kinney, 1993; Ryan-Wenger, 1992). An article published in the January/February 2000 issue of *The Journal of Continuing Education in Nursing* contained the most recent set of guidelines that could be located (Rasmussen, O'Conner, Shinkle, & Thomas, 2000). A few articles have addressed critiques of qualitative research articles (Cobb, & Hagemaster, 1987; Molzahn, & Sheilds, 1997; Morse, 1991).

Although sets of critiquing guidelines may be helpful, Downs (1999) cautioned that their use might fragment the overall meaning of the research study. She contended that it is the entire report that must ultimately be evaluated. As mentioned previously, read the entire report before you begin picking apart the pieces of the study.

GUIDELINES FOR USE IN CRITIQUING RESEARCH REPORTS

RESEARCHER QUALIFICATIONS

The first question to ask about research studies concerns the persons who conducted the research and their qualifications regarding that particular study. Many nursing studies have been conducted by nonnurses. As nurses have become more qualified to conduct research, the majority of these studies are now being conducted by nurses.

Authorities in a certain subject area are generally more qualified than other people to conduct research in that particular area. Frequently, there is a brief biographical sketch that will assist the reader in evaluating the qualifications of the author or authors. If this information is not provided, the initials after the name, such as M.S. or Ph.D., will inform the reader of the educational background of the researcher. If the research has been funded by a reputable organization, such as the American Nurses' Foundation, the reader of the report could have more confidence in the study results.

TITLE

Clarity and conciseness are the major considerations in evaluating the title of a research article or report. The focus of the research should be apparent in the study title. It should contain the population and the major variable(s). The title should be brief, containing no more than 15 words, if possible. Extraneous words such as "A study of...," "The relationship between...," or "The effects of..." should be avoided. Nouns serve as the key words in the title.

One of the most important determinants of the use of research findings is the ability of the research consumer to obtain the study findings in the literature. Today, a literature review is often accomplished through a computerized search process. This search process uses the words or phrases in the title to locate studies of interest to the research consumer. It is very important that the title contain the critical words or phrases that describe the research project.

ABSTRACT

Research reports, particularly those published in journals, frequently contain an abstract or summary of the study. Because the abstract may be the only section of the article that is read, the researcher should present the essential components of the study in the abstract. Typically, abstracts are 100 to 200 words and contain the hypothesis(es) or research question(s), methods, description of subjects, and the major findings.

INTRODUCTION

Although a research report is not meant to be a literary work of art, there is no reason to write the report in a dull and uninteresting fashion. The introduction should catch the interest of the reader and set the stage for the presentation of the research report. The best way to accomplish this is through a brief exploration of the study area. Background information on the problem and the significance of this problem to nursing should be included. The study purpose may also be included in this section.

PURPOSE

The author should leave no doubt in the reader's mind about the purpose of the study. The reason or reasons for undertaking the study should have been clearly formulated before the research was begun, and the researcher should convey this information to the reader in the form of the study purpose. The broad purpose of the study may be made more specific in the form of objectives or goals.

PROBLEM STATEMENT

The problem of the study should be clearly identified. This is best accomplished through a formal and concise statement of the problem in one sentence. This sentence may be declarative or interrogative, but the interrogative form is preferable. The problem statement should contain the population and the major variable(s) and be empirically testable. The ethical nature of the study should be clear. The feasibility and significance of the study can be evaluated through reading the problem statement. Sometimes it may appear that a researcher has made the focus of his or her study too broad and tried to examine too many variables in one study.

Although few research articles follow this format, a formal heading should precede the statement of the problem or the purpose. This heading would call attention to the exact nature of the investigation early in the report of the study. Frequently, the research consumer must read the hypothesis(es) to determine the explicit nature of the study because the purpose or problem statement is not clearly identified.

The purpose and problem statement are separate entities; however, many research reports identify only one of these aspects of the research process. In many published reports, the purpose of the study may be identified more clearly than the specific statement of the problem.

Review of the Literature

The most important consideration in the review of the literature section of a research report is the relevance of the sources to the research under consideration. Other important considerations are the conciseness and comprehensiveness of the review. Both classic sources and current sources need to be included, and primary sources should be used when possible. If most of the references are from journals, you will have more confidence that primary sources were used.

A comprehensive literature review presents theory and research that both support and oppose the expected study results. Frequently, the reader is not made aware of opposing ideas until the discussion section of the research report. When this occurs, it appears as if the researcher conducted another literature review to help explain the study findings that are counter to the expected results.

The literature review should flow logically. Generally, classic sources are presented, and then current sources are discussed. Key sources should be critically compared and appraised, rather than simply being alluded to. Paraphrasing is preferred rather than the use of large numbers of direct quotations. Finally, the review should conclude with a sentence or two that indicates how the present study will contribute to the existing body of knowledge in that subject area.

The reader of a research report published in a journal article must keep in mind that the review of the literature section may have been reduced to meet the requirements for article length. If the research consumer is seriously interested in the study topic, it may be possible to obtain a copy of the complete research report by contacting the author.

Theoretical/Conceptual Framework

Many nursing study reports published today are based on a theoretical or conceptual framework. As the nursing profession tries to build a knowledge base for practice, research with a sound theoretical base will be the greatest means of achieving the desired nursing knowledge.

The most critical point to assess in the evaluation of the framework used in a study is whether a theoretical or conceptual framework is actually identifiable. If a framework is identified, is it the most appropriate one for the study? Is the framework based on a nursing theory or a theory from another discipline? With the great emphasis on theoretically based nursing research, researchers are becoming aware of the need for a framework but may not choose the most appropriate one for the study.

In searching for the study framework, the reader may find a clearly identified section for the framework, or this information may be found in the introductory section or the literature review section of the research article or report. When a theoretical or conceptual framework is included in a research report, the reader should then evaluate the thoroughness of the presentation. Concepts should be clearly defined, and the relationship between concepts should be indicated and explained.

Assumptions

All studies are based on assumptions. These assumptions may be of the universal type, such as "all human beings need to feel loved." Assumptions also come from theory and previous research. Finally, the researcher may make some commonsense assumptions that are necessary to proceed with the research. Such an assumption might be, "The respondents will answer the questions honestly."

Explicit assumptions are those that are asserted by the researcher and are clearly identifiable by the reader. Implicit assumptions are those that are made by the researcher but are not clearly identified in the research report.

The reader should search for the researcher's explicit assumptions but should also try to identify assumptions that it appears were made by the researcher but were never stated specifically. For example, if the study sought to determine if giving a back rub at bedtime would decrease patients' requests for sleeping medications, the researcher has made at least three assumptions: adequate sleep is necessary for patients, sleeping medications are not the most healthful type of sleep enhancer, and one of the roles of nurses is to try to assist patients in obtaining adequate sleep.

Limitations

Uncontrolled variables may affect research results. The researcher should clearly identify those aspects of the research situation over which no control has been exercised. In experimental studies, internal and external threats to validity should be listed under the section on limitations.

The reader should not have to search out the limitations of a study. Frequently, the first mention is found in the discussion section, where the author will comment on the inappropriateness of the instrument or the small sample size. These limitations should be openly and honestly stated in the early part of a research report.

As is the case with the assumptions of a study, many research reports do not contain a separate section on the study limitations. Because the researcher frequently acknowledges some of the study limitations in the discussion section, study limitations may be easier to identify than the assumptions on which the study was based. Readers frequently are able to identify additional limitations of a study other than those acknowledged by the researcher.

HYPOTHESIS(ES)

All studies that examine relationships between variables should contain hypotheses. Many nursing studies contain hypotheses. Studies of a purely descriptive nature and methodological studies are types of research that usually do not contain hypotheses. When hypotheses are not needed for a study, research questions may be used.

Hypotheses should be clearly and concisely stated in a declarative sentence and in the present tense. Hypotheses should be based on theory or research findings. Directional research hypotheses, rather than null or nondirectional hypotheses, are the preferred type. The exception is those situations where there is no available research or theory that predicts the relationship between the variables that are being examined.

The hypothesis should contain the population and the variables and reflect the problem statement. Sometimes it appears as if one person wrote the problem statement and another person wrote the hypothesis because different terms are found in the problem statement and the hypothesis. For example, if the variable *depression* is used in the problem statement, this word should also appear in the hypothesis rather than a similar word such as *despair*.

Hypotheses should be empirically testable and should contain only one prediction. To be testable, it must be possible to gather empirical or objective data on the variables of interest. Single predictions are necessary in a hypothesis to avoid the "partial support" crisis that occurs when two predictions are made and only one is supported. An error that sometimes is detected in published hypotheses is the multiple predictions they contain.

DEFINITION OF TERMS

A section on definition of terms may not be included in a journal article because of space constraints. Definitions of key terms in a research report are necessary, however, to make explicit what is being studied. Replication of studies is aided by clear definitions of terms. The key terms generally reflect the theoretical or conceptual framework for the study; therefore, some of the definitions of the terms may be derived from the study framework.

Terms should be defined both conceptually and operationally. A conceptual definition presents an overall meaning of a word. This definition may be a dictionary definition or may be derived from a theory. Operational definitions indicate the observable, measurable phenomena associated with the study variables. Frequently, operational definitions are provided through the research instruments that are being used to gather data.

RESEARCH DESIGN

The research design should be clearly identified and adequately described. The reader can then determine the appropriateness of the design for the study under consideration. Quantitative designs and qualitative designs are evaluated with different criteria.

In experimental studies, the research consumer is concerned with the experimental treatment. Is the treatment adequately described and appropriate for the particular study? The method of assigning subjects to groups, if there is more than one group, should be discussed. Means to control threats to internal and external validity should be included in the section on research design.

In nonexperimental quantitative studies, the means of selecting study participants should be discussed. Any extraneous variables that have been controlled, such as age and educational background of the respondents, should be identified.

Qualitative research reports may be difficult to critique. Guidelines are not clear-cut, and each qualitative study is unique. The main task for the reader is to try to determine if the particular qualitative approach that was used was appropriate to obtain data to answer the research questions. Also, the data-collection process needs to be fully discussed in the research report, as well as how the researcher was able to keep personal bias from influencing data collection and analysis.

SETTING

The setting for the research project needs to be described. Many agencies do not want to be identified in research reports. The description of the setting is usually of a general nature. This description might be "a small, private psychiatric institution in the southeastern United States." The reader must then determine if the setting seems appropriate for the particular study.

POPULATION AND SAMPLE

Generally, the study sample is easily identified. The target population and the accessible population may not be as easily identified. The author has the responsibility to mention the broad group of interest as well as that available group from which the sample was selected.

The section on the sample should include the identification and description of the sampling method. The reader has the right to know the specific type of probability or non-probability sampling method that was used. Then the appropriateness of the sampling method can be determined.

A description of the demographic characteristics of the sample and the sample size should be included. The percentage of the population represented by the sample should be listed. Acknowledgment must be made of any dropout of subjects that occurred during the study and any other potential sampling biases that may have been recognized by the researcher. Finally, the section on population and sample should discuss the methods taken to protect subjects' rights. Generally, little information is provided about ethical issues because of space limitations in published articles. Most research articles contain only one or two sentences on this aspect of a study. Anonymity or confidentiality should be discussed and the permissions that were obtained to conduct the study should be mentioned.

DATA-COLLECTION METHODS

The data-collection section would need to be very long and explicit to allow exact replication of a study. Space limitations, particularly in journal articles, require the deletion of many of the details of the data-collection procedures.

Five general questions asked in evaluating the data-collection section concern "what, how, who, where, and when." What data will be collected? How will the data be collected? Who will collect the data? Where will the data be collected? When will the data be collected?

The specific data-collection method(s) dictate additional questions that need to be asked. For example, if questionnaires were used, the research report should provide enough information for the reader to determine if a questionnaire was the most appropriate method to collect data. If interviews were used, the interviewer training process should be explained. Observation research requires that the reader be told how observations were made, who made the observations, and how data were recorded. If physiological instruments were used, the means of assessing the accuracy of these instruments needs to be addressed.

DATA-COLLECTION INSTRUMENTS

All of the data-collection instruments used in a study should be clearly identified and described. Scoring procedures and the range of possible scores on the instrument should also be included, where appropriate.

Many studies make use of several data-collection instruments. The characteristics of each instrument should be discussed. If an instrument has been used in previous research, the results of this use should be presented in the discussion of the instrument.

The most important characteristics of an instrument concern its reliability and validity. The reader must determine if the appropriate types of reliability and validity have been reported and if the evidence of the reliability and validity is adequate for use of the instrument in the present study. Pilot study results should be included for any newly developed or revised instrument.

DATA ANALYSIS

Many research consumers cringe when reading the data analysis section of a research report because they are fearful of the statistics that are discussed in this section. A beginning knowledge of statistics will be sufficient, however, to evaluate the majority of the published research findings. The research consumer must decide if appropriate statistical tests were selected and if the results are presented accurately and completely.

Descriptive statistics on the characteristics of the study sample should be presented first. Next, the subjects' scores on the various instruments need to be reported. Finally, inferential statistics should be presented, if the study tested a hypothesis. The author should state whether the study hypothesis was supported or not supported. The results of the statistical test, the degrees of freedom, and the probability value should be given. These findings should be clearly presented in both the text and tables.

The results section of a qualitative research report is quite different from that of a quantitative research report. Rather than presenting statistics, the researcher usually reports results as themes that have been discovered in the data. Each theme may have its own separate heading.

DISCUSSION OF FINDINGS

Research reports vary in the material presented in the discussion of findings section. In some reports, data analysis, interpretation of findings, conclusions, implications, and recommendations are all included in this section. Each of these areas is considered separately here.

The findings, or facts of the study, should be presented in a completely objective fashion. In the discussion of findings section of a research report, the author interprets the study results. This material may be more subjective than the information in the findings section.

The author should compare the present study findings with those of other studies discussed in the literature review. No new literature sources should be introduced in the discussion of the findings that were not referred to in the review of literature section of the report.

Study findings should also be discussed in light of the theoretical or conceptual framework that was tested. The author must make it clear that the findings either supported or failed to support the framework of the study.

Both statistical and clinical significance should be discussed. These two types of significance are not always congruent. Findings that are statistically significant may have little or no clinical significance. Results that were determined to be statistically nonsignificant could, in fact, have clinical significance.

The researcher should discuss the study limitations and how these limitations are thought to have affected the study results. This is not the time for "true confessions," however. Frequently, the discussion section will contain the author's apologies for all of the "bad" things about the study. The author may convince the reader that any findings that do not support a given theory are strictly the result of mistakes on the part of the researcher. Although study limitations need to be identified and discussed, readers should be allowed to come to their own decisions about the worth of the findings.

CONCLUSIONS

Conclusions answer the "so what?" question that might be posed to a researcher at the end of a study. Through the conclusions, the author demonstrates the meaning and worth of the research. The study conclusions are the author's attempt to make generalizations based on the study findings. Conclusions are often difficult to write, and many authors merely restate the findings or go to the other extreme and make overgeneralizations.

The findings are *bound* to the data; the conclusions are *based* on the data. Therefore, the researcher has some freedom to go beyond the data when presenting the conclusions. Although subjectivity may enter into the author's formulation of the study conclusions, personal experiences and opinions should not influence the conclusions.

IMPLICATIONS

Implications need to be explicitly identified by the researcher for nursing practice, nursing education, and nursing research. The implications section of a research report contains the "shoulds" that result from the research findings. For example, nurse educators *should* include material in nursing curriculums on the topic of the study or nurse researchers *should* conduct more research in the area of interest. When the study findings are not statistically or clinically significant, the implications of the study may be that no changes are recommended as the result of the present study.

RECOMMENDATIONS

Although recommendations may be made for nursing practice and nursing education, recommendations generally concern future research that is needed. A suggestion may be made that the study be replicated. Another suggestion may concern further development of the instrument or use of a larger sample size. Recommendations should consider the limitations of the present study and the findings of previous studies. Nursing can ill afford to conduct impractical or irrelevant research or to "reinvent the wheel."

OTHER CONSIDERATIONS

Although the most important areas to evaluate in a research report are the components of the research process, there are other areas to be evaluated. Correct grammar, sentence structure, and punctuation are essential. The research consumer may have difficulty evaluating the merits of the research report if structural errors are found. The author's writing style and use of words are also important to the reader. If too many complex words or technical terms are used, the reader may become discouraged and never finish reading the report.

Another important area to evaluate is the accuracy and completeness of the reference list. It is discouraging to the reader to discover a source of interest in the literature review section and then be unable to find this source listed in the reference section. It is not uncommon to find sources in the reference section that were never referred to in the research report.

SUMMARY

Most research studies have both strong and weak points. A critical evaluation of all the sections of a research report is essential in determining the usefulness of the research results. Although many additional questions may be raised when examining research reports, this chapter has presented some guidelines that will be useful to the beginning researcher as she or he appraises published research reports.

✖ REFERENCES

Beck, C. T. (1990). The research critique: General criteria for evaluating a research report. *JOGNN: Journal of Gynecological and Neonatal Nursing, 19,* 18–22.

Carlson, D. S., Kruse, L. K., & Rouse, C. L. (1999). Critiquing nursing research: A user-friendly guide for the staff nurse. *Journal of Emergency Nursing, 25,* 330–332.

Downs, F. S. (1999). How to cozy up to a research report. *Applied Nursing Research, 12,* 215–216.

Fosbinder, D., & Loveridge, C. (1996). Cover to cover: How to critique a research study. *Advanced Practice Nursing Quarterly, 2,* 68–71.

Giuffre, M. (1998). Critiquing a research article. *Journal of Perianesthesia Nursing, 13,* 104–108.

Grant, J. S., Davis, L. L., & Kinney, M. R. (1993). Criteria for critiquing clinical nursing research reports. *Journal of Post Anesthesia Nursing, 8,* 163–171.

Molzahn, A., & Sheilds, L. (1997). Qualitative research in nephrology nursing. *AANA Journal, 24*, 13–21.

Morse, J. M. (1991). Evaluating qualitative research. *Qualitative Health Research, 1,* 283–286.

Rasmussen, L., O'Conner, M., Shinkle, S., & Thomas, M. K. (2000). The basic research review checklist. *Journal of Continuing Education in Nursing, 31,* 13–17.

Ryan-Wenger, N. M. (1992). Guidelines for critique of a research report. *Heart & Lung: Journal of Critical Care, 21,* 394–401.

Answers to Self-Test

CHAPTER 1

1. C
2. C
3. A
4. B
5. A
6. A
7. E
8. A
9. E
10. C

CHAPTER 2

1. D
2. B
3. A
4. A
5. A
6. C
7. A
8. D
9. D
10. E

CHAPTER 3

1. D
2. A
3. C
4. B
5. B
6. F
7. F
8. T
9. F
10. T

CHAPTER 4

1. D
2. D
3. A
4. A
5. D
6. B
7. D
8. A
9. B
10. C

CHAPTER 5

1. B
2. C
3. A
4. D
5. D
6. C
7. D
8. B
9. B
10. B

CHAPTER 6

1. B
2. A
3. D
4. C
5. E
6. C
7. A
8. A
9. C
10. D

CHAPTER 7

Identification of independent and dependent variables.

Independent Variable(s)	**Dependent Variable(s)**
1. gender of patients	requests for pain medications
2. number of prenatal classes	fear concerning labor and delivery
3. marital status	body image
4. anxiety	requests for pain medication
5. high school grade level	marijuana usage
6. retirement	self-image
7. length of employment	a. job turnover rate
	b. job dissatisfaction levels

Evaluation of hypotheses.

8. One level of the independent variable is missing. To what group is the baccalaureate-prepared nurse group being compared?
9. Did you notice the question mark at the end of the sentence? This statement is not a hypothesis.
10. The population is not identified.
11. Watch those value words like "better."
12. This one looks good.

CHAPTER 8

1. E
2. A
3. D
4. B
5. C
6. C
7. D
8. B
9. A
10. B
11. B

CHAPTER 9

1. F
2. F
3. T

4. T
5. F
6. F
7. B
8. B
9. B
10. A

CHAPTER 10

1. F
2. F
3. T
4. T
5. convenience sampling
6. cluster sampling
7. systematic sampling
8. quota sampling
9. simple random sampling
10. B

CHAPTER 11

1. stability reliability
2. face validity
3. construct validity
4. predictive validity
5. equivalence reliability
6. F
7. T
8. T
9. T
10. F

CHAPTER 12

1. Answers are not mutually exclusive. There is overlapping of categories. A person who is 20, 25, or 30 years old might check two of the categories.
2. B
3. C
4. C
5. C
6. B
7. D
8. A
9. C
10. B

CHAPTER 13

1. A
2. B
3. C
4. D
5. B
6. D
7. B
8. D
9. C
10. E

CHAPTER 14

1. C
2. A
3. A
4. D
5. A
6. C
7. C
8. B
9. B
10. B

CHAPTER 15

1. A
2. B
3. D
4. E
5. B
6. B
7. F
8. F
9. F
10. T
11. F
12. T

CHAPTER 16

1. B
2. D
3. D
4. B
5. A
6. E
7. B
8. E
9. F
10. T
11. F
12. F

APPENDIX A

Consent Form

CONSENT TO ACT AS A SUBJECT FOR RESEARCH AND INVESTIGATION

I. I hereby authorize _____ to perform the following investigation:
   The study will involve my 4-year-old child participating in an experiment. The investigation will consist of a physical examination of the eyes, ears, throat, elbow, and knee reflexes. Blood pressure and temperature by mouth will also be checked. The physical examination will require about 15 minutes. The child will receive a play session before the physical examination, or not, depending on the group to which he (she) is randomly assigned. If the child does not receive the play session before the physical examination, he (she) will receive the same play session after the physical examination. The physical examination and the play sessions will be conducted by registered nurses. The examining nurse will be experienced in the examination of children. The play sessions will be conducted by the researcher, who is experienced in working with children and with play techniques. Another registered nurse will observe the child during the physical examination.

II. The procedure or investigation listed in Paragraph I has been explained to me by _____.

III. I understand that the procedures or investigations described in Paragraph I involve the following possible risks or discomforts:
   1. Confidential information from the study results might be accidentally released.
   2. The child may feel anxious about the physical examination procedure.

IV. I understand that my child's rights and welfare will be protected as follows:
   1. Safeguards against the accidental release of data will include the use of a code number, and only the investigator will know the name and the code number of each child. No names or code numbers will be used in the final research report. Only statistics by groups will be reported. There will be no way a reader of the final report can identify any of the participants. Any information pertaining to the identity of the participants will be destroyed when the study is completed.

2. The child will not be pressured into participating in the physical examination procedure. If the child does not want to participate in the activity, the child will not be examined.
3. The participation or nonparticipation of the child in the study will not influence care received at the day-care center. The child's participation in the study is strictly voluntary. The child may be withdrawn from the study at any time, without any penalty.
4. Participants who do not receive the play session before the physical examination will be given the play session in small groups after their physical examinations are done. The registered nurse conducting the play periods with the physical examination equipment is experienced in working with children and various play techniques.

V. I understand that the procedures and investigations described in Paragraph I have the following potential benefits to myself and others:
1. By participation in this study, the child will become more familiar with possible frightening equipment that is routinely used during physical examinations.
2. Because the child is more familiar with the equipment used, the child may be less anxious and more cooperative during the examination.
3. The results of physical examinations are more accurate if the child is not resistive during the procedures.
4. The child may have increased self-esteem because the child is better able to control behavior during the examination.
5. Participation in this study will help to produce new knowledge that will assist child-care workers in dealing with young children.

VI. I understand that no medical service or compensation is provided to the subjects by the University as a result of injury from participation in research.

VII. An offer has been made to answer all of my questions regarding the study. If alternative procedures are more advantageous to me, they have been explained. I understand that I may terminate my child's participation in the study at any time. The subject is a minor (age ____).

Signatures (One Required)

_____   _____
Father   Date

_____   _____
Mother   Date

_____   _____
Guardian   Date

APPENDIX B

Sources of Research Instruments

Chun, K.T., Cobb, S., & French, J. R., Jr. (1975). *Measures for psychological assessment: A guide to 3,000 original sources and their applications.* Ann Arbor, MI: Institute for Social Research, University of Michigan.

Comrey, A. L., Backer, T. E., & Glaser, E. M. (1973). *A sourcebook for mental health measures.* Los Angeles: Human Interaction Research Institute.

Conoley, J. C., & Kramer, J. J. (Eds.). (1989). *The tenth mental measurement yearbook.* Lincoln, NE: University of Nebraska Press.

Frank-Stromborg, M., & Olson, S. (Eds.). (1997*). Instruments for clinical health-care research* (2nd ed.) Boston: Jones & Bartlett.

Goldman, B. A., & Saunders, J. L. (1974). *Directory of unpublished experimental mental measures.* New York: Behavioral Publications.

Impara, J.C., & Plake, B. S. (Eds.). (1998). *The thirteenth mental measurements yearbook.* Lincoln, NE: The University of Nebraska Press.

Johnson, O. G. (1976). *Test and measurements in child development: Handbooks I and II.* San Francisco: Jossey-Bass.

Mangen, D., & Peterson, W. (Eds.). (1982). *Research instruments in social gerontology: Vol. 1. Clinical and social psychology.* Minneapolis: University of Minnesota Press.

Mangen, D., & Peterson, W. (Eds.). (1982*). Research instruments in social gerontology: Vol. 2. Social roles and social participation.* Minneapolis: University of Minnesota Press.

Mangen, D., & Peterson, W. (Eds.). (1984). *Research instruments in social gerontology: Vol. 3. Health, program evaluation and demography.* Minneapolis: University of Minnesota Press.

Mitchell, J. V. (Ed.). (1983). *Tests in print III.* Lincoln, NE: University of Nebraska Press.

Reeder, L. G., Ramacher, L., & Gorelnik, S. (1976). *Handbook of scales and indices of health behavior.* Pacific Palisades, CA: Goodyear.

Robinson, J. P., & Shaver, P. R. (1973). *Measures of social psychological attitudes.* Ann Arbor, MI: Institute for Social Research, University of Michigan.

Sawin, K. J., & Harrigan, M. P. (1994). *Measures of family functioning for research and practice.* New York: Springer.

Shaw, M. E., & Wright, J. M. (1967). *Scales for the measurement of attitudes.* New York: McGraw-Hill.

Steiber, S. R., & Krowinsik, W. J. (1990). *Measuring and managing patient satisfaction.* Chicago: American Hospital Publishing.

Strauss, M. A., & Brown, B. W. (1978*). Family measurements techniques: Abstract of published instruments. 1935-1974* (rev. ed.). Minneapolis: University of Minnesota Press.

Strickland, O. L., & Waltz, C. F. (Eds.). (1988). *Measurement of nursing outcomes (Vol. 1). Measuring client outcomes.* New York: Springer.

Strickland O. L., & Waltz, C. F. (Eds.). (1988). *Measurement of nursing outcomes (Vol. 2). Measuring nursing performance: Practice, education, and research.* New York: Springer.

Strickland, O. L., & Waltz, C. F. (Eds.). (1990). *Measurement of nursing outcomes (Vol. 3). Measuring clinical skills and professional development in education and practice.* New York: Springer.

Strickland, O. L., & Waltz, C. F. (Eds.). (1990*). Measurement of nursing outcomes (Vol. 4). Measuring client self-care and coping skills.* New York: Springer.

Sweetland, R., & Keyser, D. (Eds.). (1983). *Tests: A comprehensive reference for assessments in psychology, education and business.* Kansas City, MO: Test Corporation of America.

Sweetland, R., & Keyser, D. (Eds.). (1984). *Test critiques. (Vols. I, II, III, IV, V, VI).* Kansas City, MO: Test Corporation of America.

Toulistos, J., Perlmutter, B. F., & Strauss, M.A. (1990). *Handbook of family measurement.* Newbury Park, CA: Sage.

Ward, M. J., & Lindeman, C. A. (Eds.). (1979). *Instruments for measuring nursing practice and other health care variables* (DHEW Publication No. HRA 78-53, Vol. 1). Washington, DC: U.S. Government Printing Office.

Ward, M. J., & Lindeman, C. A. (Eds.). (1979). *Instruments for measuring nursing practice and other health care variables* (DHEW Publication No. HRA 78-54, Vol. 2). Washington, DC: U.S. Government Printing Office.

Glossary

abstracts. (research abstracts). Brief summaries of research studies; generally contain the purpose, methods, and major findings of the study.

accessible population. The group of people or objects that is available to the researcher for a particular study.

alpha (α). See level of significance.

alternate forms reliability. Results are compared using two forms or versions of the same instrument.

alternative hypothesis. See research hypothesis.

ambiguous questions. Questions that contain words that may be interpreted in more than one way.

analysis of covariance (ANCOVA). A statistical test that allows the researcher to statistically control for some variable(s) that may have an influence on the dependent variable.

analysis of variance (ANOVA). A parametric statistical test that is used to compare the difference between the means of two or more groups or sets of values.

anonymity. The identity of research subjects is unknown, even to the study investigator.

applied research. Research that is conducted to find a solution to an immediate practical problem.

assumptions. Beliefs that are held to be true but have not necessarily been proven; assumptions may be explicit or implicit.

attitude scales. Self-report data collection instruments that ask respondents to report their attitudes or feelings on a continuum.

attribute variables. See demographic variables.

bar graph. A figure used to represent a frequency distribution of nominal or ordinal data.

basic research (pure research). Research that is conducted to generate knowledge rather than to solve immediate problems.

beta (β). See Type II error.

bimodal. A frequency distribution that contains two identical high frequency values.

bivariate study. A research study in which the relationship between two variables is examined.

blind review. Manuscript reviewers are not made aware of the author's identity before the manuscript is evaluated.

bracketing. A process in which qualitative researchers put aside their own feelings or beliefs about a phenomenon that is being studied to keep from biasing their observations.

call for abstract. A request for a summary of a study that the researcher wishes to present at a research conference.

canonical correlation. Examines the correlation between two or more independent variables and two or more dependent variables.

case studies. Research studies that involve an in-depth examination of a single person or a group of people. A case study might also examine an institution.

cells. Boxes in a table that are formed by the intersection of rows and columns.

central limit theorem. The phenomenon in which sample values tend to be normally distributed around the population value.

chi-square test (χ^2). A nonparametric statistical test that is used to compare sets of data that are in the form of frequencies or percentages (nominal level data).

class interval. A group of scores in a frequency distribution.

clinical nursing research. Nursing research studies involving clients or that have the potential for affecting clients.

close-ended questions. Questions that require respondents to choose from given alternatives.

cluster random sampling. A random sampling process that involves two or more stages. The population is first listed by clusters or categories (e.g., hospitals) and then the sample elements (e.g., hospital administrators) are randomly selected from these clusters.

coefficient of determination (r^2, R^2). A statistic obtained by squaring a correlation coefficient and is interpreted as the percentage of variance shared by two variables.

cohort study. A special type of longitudinal study in which subjects are studied who have been born during one particular period or who have similar backgrounds.

collectively exhaustive categories. Categories are provided for every possible answer.

columns. Vertical entries in a table.

comparative studies. Studies in which intact groups are compared on some dependent variable. The researcher is not able to manipulate the independent variable, which is frequently some inherent characteristic of the subjects, such as age or educational level.

comparison group. A group of subjects in an experimental study that does not receive any experimental treatment or receives an alternate treatment such as the "normal" or routine treatment.

complex hypothesis. A hypothesis that concerns a relationship where two or more independent variables, two or more dependent variables, or both are being examined.

computer-assisted literature searches. The use of a computer to obtain bibliographic references that have been stored in a database.

computerized database. A compilation of information that can be retrieved by computer.

concept. A word picture or mental idea of a phenomenon.

conceptual framework. A background or foundation for a study; a less well-developed structure than a theoretical framework; concepts are related in a logical manner by the researcher.

conceptual model. Symbolic presentation of concepts and the relationships between these concepts.

concurrent validity. A type of criterion validity in which a determination is made of the instrument's ability to obtain a measurement of subjects' behavior that is comparable to some other criterion used to indicate that behavior.

confidence interval. A range of values that, with a specified degree of probability, is thought to contain the population value.

confidentiality. The identity of the research subjects is known only to the study investigator(s).

confounding variable. See extraneous variable.

construct. A highly abstract phenomenon that cannot be directly observed but must be inferred by certain concrete or less abstract indicators of the phenomenon.

construct validity. The ability of an instrument to measure the construct that it is intended to measure.

content analysis. A data collection method that examines communication messages that are usually in written form.

content validity. The degree to which an instrument covers the scope and range of information that is sought.

contingency questions. Questions that are relevant for some respondents and not for others.

contingency table. A table that visually displays the relationship between sets of nominal data.

control group. A group of subjects in an experimental study that does not receive the experimental treatment (see comparison group).

convenience sampling (accidental sampling). A nonprobability sampling procedure that involves the selection of the most readily available people or objects for a study.

correlation. The extent to which values of one variable (X) are related to the values of a second variable (Y). Correlations may be either positive or negative.

correlation coefficient. A statistic that presents the magnitude and direction of a relationship between two variables. Correlation coefficients range from −1.00 (perfect negative relationship) to +1.00 (perfect positive relationship).

correlational studies. Research studies that examine the strength of relationships between variables.

criterion validity. The extent to which an instrument corresponds or correlates with some criterion measure of the information that is being sought; the ability of an instrument to determine subjects' responses at present or predict subjects' responses in the future.

critical region (region of rejection). An area in a theoretical sampling distribution that contains the critical values, which are values that are considered to be statistically significant.

critical value. A scientific cut-off point that denotes the value in a theoretical distribution at which all obtained values from a sample that are equal to or beyond that point are said to be statistically significant.

cross-sectional study. A research study that collects data on subjects at one point in time.

data. The pieces of information or facts collected during a research study.

database. See computerized database.

deductive reasoning. A reasoning process that proceeds from the general to the specific, from theory to empirical data.

degrees of freedom (df). A concept in inferential statistics that concerns the number of values that are free to vary.

Delphi technique. A data collection method that uses several rounds of questions to seek a consensus on a particular topic from a group of experts on the topic.

demographic questions. Questions that gather data on characteristics of the subjects (see demographic variables).

demographic variables. Subject characteristics such as age, educational levels, and marital status.

dependent *t*-test. A form of the *t*-test that is used when one set of scores or values is associated or dependent on another set of scores or values.

dependent variable. The "effect"; a response or behavior that is influenced by the independent variable; sometimes called the criterion variable.

descriptive statistics. That group of statistics that organizes and summarizes numerical data obtained from populations and samples.

descriptive studies. Research studies in which phenomena are described or the relationship between variables is examined; no attempt is made to determine cause-and-effect relationships.

design. See research design.

directional research hypothesis. A type of hypothesis in which a prediction is made of the type of relationship that exists between variables.

disproportional stratified sampling. Random selection of members from population strata where the number of members chosen for each stratum is not in proportion to the size of the stratum in the total population.

double-barreled questions. Questions that ask two questions in one.

element. A single member of a population.

empirical data. Objective data gathered through the sense organs.

empirical generalization. A summary statement about the occurrence of phenomena that is based on empirical data from a number of different research studies.

equivalence reliability. The degree to which two forms of an instrument obtain the same results or two or more observers obtain the same results when using a single instrument to measure a variable.

ethnographic studies. Research studies that involve the collection and analysis of data about cultural groups.

event sampling. Observations made throughout the entire course of an event or behavior.

experimental design. See quasiexperimental, preexperimental, and true experimental designs.

experimenter effect. A threat to the external validity of a research study that occurs when the researcher's behavior influences the subjects' behavior in a way that is not intended by the researcher.

explanatory studies. Research studies that search for causal explanations; usually experimental in nature.

exploratory studies. Research studies that are conducted when little is known about the phenomenon that is being studied.

ex post facto studies. Studies in which the variation in the independent variable has already occurred in the past, and the researcher, "after the fact," is trying to determine if the variation that has occurred in the independent variable has any influence on the dependent variable that is being measured in the present.

external criticism (external appraisal, external examination). A type of examination of historical data that is concerned with the authenticity or genuineness of the data. External criticism might be used to determine if a letter was actually written by the person whose signature was contained on the letter.

external validity. The degree to which study results can be generalized to other people and other research settings.

extraneous variable. A type of variable that is not the variable of interest to a researcher but that may influence the results of a study. Other terms for extraneous variable are *intervening variable* and *confounding variable.*

face validity. A subjective determination that an instrument is adequate for obtaining the desired information; on the surface or the "face" of the instrument it appears to be an adequate means of obtaining the desired data.

factor analysis. A type of validity used to identify clusters of related items on an instrument or scale.

field studies. Research studies that are conducted "in the field" or real-life setting.

filler questions. Questions used to distract respondents from the purpose of other questions that are being asked.

focus group. A small group of individuals who meet together and are asked questions by a moderator about a certain topic or topics.

framework. See conceptual framework and theoretical framework.

frequency distribution. A listing of all scores or numerical values from a set of data and the number of times each score or value appears; scores may be listed from highest to lowest or lowest to highest.

frequency polygon. A graph that uses dots connected with straight lines to represent the frequency distribution of interval or ratio data. A dot is placed above the midpoint of each class interval.

galley proofs. Sheets of paper that show how an article or book will appear in typeset form.

generalization. See empirical generalization.

grand theories. Theories that are concerned with a broad range of phenomena in the environment or in the experiences of humans.

grounded theory studies. Research studies in which data are collected and analyzed and then a theory is developed that is "grounded" in the data.

Hawthorne effect. A threat to the external validity of a research study that occurs when study participants respond in a certain manner because they are aware that they are involved in a research study.

histogram. A graph used to represent the frequency distribution of variables measured at the interval or ratio level.

historical studies. Research studies that are concerned with the identification, location, evaluation, and synthesis of data from the past.

history. A threat to the internal validity of an experimental research study; some event besides the experimental treatment occurs between the pretreatment and posttreatment measurement of the dependent variable, and this event influences the dependent variable.

hypothesis. A statement of the predicted relationship between two or more variables.

independent *t*-test. A form of the *t*-test that is used when there is no association between the two sets of scores or values that are being compared.

independent variable. The "cause" or the variable that is thought to influence the dependent variable; in experimental research it is the variable that is manipulated by the researcher.

indexes. Compilations of reference materials that provide information on books and periodicals.

inductive reasoning. A reasoning process that proceeds from the specific to the general, from empirical data to theory.

inferential statistics. That group of statistics concerned with the characteristics of populations and uses sample data to make an "inference" about a population.

informed consent. A subject voluntarily agrees to participate in a research study in which he or she has full understanding of the study before the study begins.

instrumentation change. A threat to the internal validity of an experimental research study that involves changes from the pretest measurements to the posttest measurements as a result of inaccuracy of the instrument or the judges' ratings rather than as a result of the experimental treatment.

interaction effect. The result of two variables acting in conjunction with each other.

internal consistency reliability (scale homogeneity). The extent to which all items of an instrument measure the same variable.

internal criticism. A type of examination of historical data that is concerned with the accuracy of the data. Internal criticism might be used to determine if a document contained an accurate recording of events as they actually happened.

internal validity. The degree to which changes in the dependent variable (effect) can be attributed to the independent or experimental variable (cause) rather than to the effects of extraneous variables.

interobserver reliability. See interrater reliability.

interquartile range. Contains the middle half of the values in a frequency distribution.

interrater reliability (interobserver reliability). The degree to which two or more independent judges are in agreement about ratings or observations of events or behaviors.

interval level of measurement. Data can be categorized and ranked, and the distance between the ranks can be specified; pulse rates and temperature readings are examples of interval data.

intervening variable. See extraneous variable.

interview. A method of data collection in which the interviewer obtains responses from a subject in a face-to-face encounter or through a telephone call.

interview schedule. An instrument containing a set of questions, directions for asking these questions, and space to record the respondents' answers.

known-groups procedure. A research technique in which a research instrument is administered to two groups of people whose responses are expected to differ on the variable of interest.

laboratory studies. Research studies in which subjects are studied in a special environment that has been created by the researcher.

level of significance (probability level). The probability of rejecting a null hypothesis when it is true; symbolized by lowercase Greek letter alpha (α); also symbolized by p.

Likert scale. An attitude scale named after its developer, Rensis Likert. These scales usually contain five or seven responses for each item, ranging from "strongly agree" to "strongly disagree."

limitations. Weaknesses in a study; uncontrolled variables.

longitudinal study. Subjects are followed during a period in the future; data are collected at two or more different time periods.

manipulation. The independent or experimental variable is controlled by the researcher to determine its effect on the dependent variable.

maturation. A threat to the internal validity of an experimental research study that occurs when changes that take place within study subjects as a result of the passage of time (growing older, taller) affect the study results.

mean (M). A measure of central tendency; the average of a set of values that is found by adding all values and dividing by the total number of values. The population symbol is μ and the sample symbol is $\bar{x}$.

measurement. A process in scientific research that uses rules to assign numbers to objects.

measures of central tendency. Statistics that describe the average, typical, or most common value for a group of data.

measures of relationship. Statistics that present the correlation between variables.

measures of variability. Statistics that describe how spread out values are in a distribution of values (e.g., range, standard deviation).

measures to condense data. Statistics that are used to condense and summarize data.

median (Md, Mdn). A measure of central tendency; the middle score or value in a group of data.

meta-analysis. A technique that combines the results of several similar studies on a topic and statistically analyzes the results as if only one study had been conducted.

methodological studies. Research studies that are concerned with the development, testing, and evaluation of research instruments and methods.

middle-range theories. Theories that have a narrow focus; they are concerned with only a small area of the environment or of human experiences.

modal class. The category with the greatest frequency of observations; used with nominal and ordinal data.

mode (Mo). A measure of central tendency; the category or value that occurs most often in a set of data.

model. A symbolic representation of some phenomenon or phenomena.

mortality. A threat to the internal validity of an experimental research study that occurs when the subject drop-out rate is different or characteristics are different between those who drop out of the experimental group and those who drop out of the comparison group.

multimodal. A frequency distribution in which more than two values have the same high frequency.

multiple regression. A statistical procedure used to determine the influence of more than one independent variable on the dependent variable.

multivariate analysis of variance (MANOVA). A statistical test that examines the difference between the mean scores of two or more groups on two or more dependent variables that are measured at the same time.

multivariate study. A research study in which more than two variables are examined.

mutually exclusive categories. Categories are uniquely distinct; no overlap occurs between categories.

negative relationship (inverse relationship). A relationship between two variables in which there is a tendency for the values of one variable to increase as the values of the other variable decrease.

negatively skewed. A frequency distribution in which the tail of the distribution points to the left.

network sampling. See snowball sampling.

nominal level of measurement. The lowest level of measurement; data are "named" or categorized, such as race and marital status.

nondirectional research hypothesis. A type of research hypothesis in which a prediction is made that a relationship exists between variables, but the type of relationship is not specified.

nonequivalent control group design. A type of quasiexperimental design; similar to the pretest-posttest control group experimental design, except that there is no random assignment of subjects to groups.

nonparametric tests (distribution-free statistics). Types of inferential statistics that are not concerned with population parameters, and requirements for their use are less stringent; can be used with nominal and ordinal data and small sample sizes.

nonparticipant observer-covert. Research observer does not identify herself or himself to the subjects who are being observed.

nonparticipant observer-overt. Research observer openly identifies that she or he is conducting research and provides subjects with information about the type of data that will be collected.

nonprobability sampling. A sampling process in which a sample is selected from elements or members of a population through nonrandom methods; includes convenience, quota, and purposive.

nonrefereed journal. A journal that uses editorial staff members or consultants to review manuscripts.

nonsymmetrical distribution (skewed distribution). Frequency distribution in which the distribution has an off-center peak. If the tail of the distribution points to the right, the distribution is said to be positively skewed; if the tail of the distribution points to the left, the distribution is said to be negatively skewed.

normal curve. A bell-shaped curve that graphically depicts a normally distributed frequency distribution (see normal distribution).

normal distribution. A symmetrical, bell-shaped theoretical distribution; has one central peak or set of values in the middle of the distribution.

null hypothesis (H_o). A statistical hypothesis that predicts there is no relationship between variables; the hypothesis that is subjected to statistical analysis.

nursing research. A systematic, objective, process of analyzing phenomena of importance to nursing.

observation research. A data-collection method in which data are collected through visual observations.

one-group pretest-posttest design. A type of preexperimental design; compares one group of subjects before and after an experimental treatment.

one-shot case study. A type of preexperimental design; a single group of subjects is observed after a treatment to determine the effects of the treatment. No pretest measurement is made.

one-tailed test of significance. A test of statistical significance in which the critical values (statistically significant values) are sought in only one tail of the theoretical sampling distribution (either the right or the left tail); used when a directional research hypothesis has been formulated for a study.

open-ended questions. Questions that allow respondents to answer in their own words.

operational definition. The definition of a variable that identifies how the variable will be observed or measured.

ordinal level of measurement. Data can be categorized and placed in order; small, medium, and large is an example of a set of ordinal data.

outcomes research. Research that examines the outcomes or results of patient care interventions.

parallel forms reliability. See alternate forms reliability.

parameter. A numerical characteristic of a population (e.g., the average educational level of people living in the United States).

parametric tests. Types of inferential statistics that are concerned with population parameters. When parametric tests are used assumptions are made that (a) the level of measurement of the data is interval or ratio, (b) data are taken from populations that are normally distributed on the variable that is being measured, and (c) data are taken from populations that have equal variances on the variable that is being measured.

participant observer-covert. Research observer interacts with subjects and observes their behavior without their knowledge.

participant observer-overt. Research observer interacts with subjects openly and with the full awareness of those people who will be observed.

peer review. The review of a research manuscript by professional colleagues who have content or methodological expertise concerning the material that is presented in the manuscript.

percentage (%). A statisic that represents the proportion of a subgroup to a total group, expressed as a % ranging from 0 to 100%.

percentile. A data point below which lies a certain percentage of the values in a frequency distribution.

personality inventories. Self-report measures used to assess the differences in personality traits, needs, or values of people.

phenomenological studies. Research studies that examine human experiences through the descriptions of the meanings of these experiences provided by the people involved.

pilot study. A small-scale, trial run of an actual research study.

population. A complete set of persons or objects that possess some common characteristic that is of interest to the researcher.

positive relationship (direct relationship). A relationship between two variables in which the variables tend to vary together; as the values of one variable increase or decrease, the values of the other variable increase or decrease.

positively skewed. A frequency distribution in which the tail of the distribution points to the right.

posttest-only control group design. True experimental design in which subjects in the experimental and comparison groups are given a posttest after the experimental group receives the study treatment.

power analysis. A procedure that is used to determine the sample size needed to prevent a Type II error.

power of a statistical test. The ability of a statistical test to reject a null hypothesis when it is false (and should be rejected).

predictive validity. A type of criterion validity of an instrument in which a determination is made of the instrument's ability to predict behavior of subjects in the future.

preexisting data. Existing information that has not been collected for research purposes.

preexperimental design. A type of experimental design in which the researcher has little control over the research situation; includes the one-shot case study and the one-group pretest-posttest design.

pretest-posttest control group design. True experimental design in which subjects in the experimental and comparison groups are given a pretest before and a posttest after the administration of the study treatment to the experimental group.

primary source. In the research literature, it is an account of a research study that has been written by the original researcher(s); in historical studies, primary sources consist of firsthand information or direct evidence of an event.

probability level (*p*). See level of significance.

probability sampling. The use of a random sampling procedure to select a sample from elements or members of a population; includes simple, stratified, cluster, and systematic random sampling techniques.

probes. Prompting questions that encourage the respondent to elaborate on the topic that is being discussed.

projective technique. Self-report measure in which a subject is asked to respond to stimuli that are designed to be ambiguous or to have no definite meaning. The responses reflect the internal feelings of the subject that are projected on the external stimuli.

proportional stratified sampling. Random selection of members from population strata where the number of members chosen from each stratum is in proportion to the size of the stratum in the total population.

proposition. A statement or assertion of the relationship between concepts.

prospective studies. Studies in which the independent variable or presumed cause (use of birth control pills, for example) is identified at the present time and then subjects are followed for some time in the future to observe the dependent variable or effect (thrombophlebitis or myocardial infarctions, for example).

purposive sampling (judgmental sampling). A nonprobability sampling procedure in which the researcher uses personal judgment to select subjects who are considered to be representative of the population.

Q-sort (Q methodology). A data-collection method in which subjects are asked to sort statements into categories according to their attitudes toward, or rating of, the statements.

qualitative research. Research that is concerned with the subjective meaning of an experience to an individual.

quantitative research. Research that is concerned with objectivity, tight controls over the research situation, and the ability to generalize findings.

quasiexperimental design. A type of experimental design in which there is either no comparison group or no random assignment of subjects to groups; includes the non-equivalent control group design and time-series design.

query letter. A letter of inquiry sent to a journal to determine the editor's interest in publishing a manuscript. The letter usually contains an outline of the manuscript and important information about the content of the manuscript.

questionnaire. A paper-and-pencil, self-report instrument used to gather data from subjects.

quota sampling. A nonprobability sampling procedure in which the researcher selects the sample to reflect certain characteristics of the population.

random assignment. A procedure used in an experimental study to ensure that each study subject has an equal chance of being placed into any one of the study groups.

random sampling. See probability sampling.

range. A measure of variability; the distance between the highest and lowest value in a group of values or scores.

ratio level of measurement. Data can be categorized and ranked, the distance between ranks can be specified, and a "true" or natural zero point can be identified; the amount of money in a checking account and the number of requests for pain medication are examples of ratio data.

reactive effects of the pretest. A threat to the external validity of a research study that occurs when subjects are sensitized to the experimental treatment by the pretest.

refereed journal. A journal that uses experts in a given field to review manuscripts.

region of rejection. See critical region.

reliability. The consistency and dependability of a research instrument to measure a variable; types of reliability are stability, equivalence, and internal consistency.

replication study. A research study that repeats or duplicates an earlier research study, with all of the essential elements of the original study held intact. A different sample or setting may be used.

research design. The overall plan for gathering data in a research study.

research hypothesis (H_1). An alternative hypothesis to the statistical null hypothesis; predicts the researcher's actual expectations about the outcome of a study; also called scientific, substantive, and theoretical.

research instruments (research tools). Devices used to collect data in research studies.

research report. A written or oral summary of a research study.

retrospective studies. Studies in which the dependent variable is identified in the present (e.g., a disease condition) and an attempt is made to determine the independent variable (e.g., cause of the disease) that occurred in the past.

Rosenthal effect. The influence of interviewers on respondents' answers.

rows. Horizontal entries in a table.

sample. A subset of the population that is selected to represent the population.

sampling bias. (a) The difference between sample data and population data that can be attributed to a faulty selection process; (b) a threat to the external validity of a research study that occurs when subjects are not randomly selected from the population.

sampling distribution. A theoretical frequency distribution that is based on an infinite number of samples. Sampling distributions are based on mathematical formulas and logic.

sampling error. Random fluctuations in data that occur when a sample is selected to represent a population.

sampling frame. A listing of all the elements of the population from which a sample is to be chosen.

saturation. The researcher is hearing a repetition of themes or ideas as additional participants are interviewed in a qualitative study.

scatter plot (scatter diagram, scattergram). A graphic presentation of the relationship between two variables. The graph contains variables plotted on an X axis and a Y axis. Pairs of scores are plotted by the placement of dots to indicate where each pair of Xs and Ys intersect.

secondary source. In the research literature, it is an account of a research study that has been written by someone other than the study investigators; in historical studies, secondary sources are secondhand information or data provided by someone who did not observe the event.

selection bias. A threat to the internal validity of an experimental research study that occurs when study results are attributed to the experimental treatment when, in fact, the results may be due to pretreatment differences between the subjects in the experimental and comparison groups.

semantic differential. Attitude scale that asks subjects to indicate their position or attitude about some concept along a continuum between two adjectives or phrases that are presented in relation to the concept that is being measured.

semiquartile range. Determined by dividing the interquartile range in half (see interquartile range).

semistructured interviews. Interviewers ask a certain number of specific questions, but additional questions or probes are used at the discretion of the interviewer.

simple hypothesis. A hypothesis that predicts the relationship between one independent and one dependent variable.

simple random sampling. A method of random sampling in which each element of the population has an equal and independent chance of being chosen for the sample.

simulation studies. Laboratory studies in which subjects are presented with a description of a case study or situation that is intended to represent a real-life situation.

skewed distribution. A frequency distribution that is nonsymmetrical.

snowball sampling. A sampling method that involves the assistance of study subjects to help obtain other potential subjects.

Solomon four-group design. True experimental design that minimizes threats to internal and external validity.

stability reliability. The consistency of a research instrument over time; test-retest procedures and repeated observations are methods to test the stability of an instrument.

standard deviation (SD; s). A measure of variability; the statistic that indicates the average deviation or variation of all the values in a set of data from the mean value of that data.

standard error of the mean ($s_{\bar{x}}$). The standard deviation of the sampling distribution of the mean.

statistic. A numerical characteristic of a sample (e.g., the average educational level of a random sample of people living in the United States).

stratified random sampling. A random sampling process in which a sample is selected after the population has been divided into subgroups or strata according to some variable of importance to the research study.

structured interviews. Interviewers ask the same questions in the same manner of all respondents.

structured observations. The researcher makes the determination of behaviors to be observed before data collection. Usually some kind of checklist is used to record behaviors.

survey studies. Research studies in which self-report data are collected from a sample to determine the characteristics of a population.

symmetrical distributions. Frequency distributions in which both halves of the distribution are the same.

systematic random sampling. A random sampling process in which every *k*th (e.g., every fifth) element or member of the population is selected for the sample.

***t*-test (*t*).** A parametric statistical test that examines the difference between the means of two groups of values. Types of *t*-tests are the independent *t*-test (independent samples *t*-test) and the dependent *t*-test (paired *t*-test).

table of random numbers. A list of numbers that have been generated in such a manner that there is no order or sequencing of the numbers. Each number is equally likely to follow any other number.

target population. The entire group of people or objects to which the researcher wishes to generalize the findings of a study.

telephone interviews. Data are collected from subjects through the use of phone calls rather than in face-to-face encounters.

testing. A threat to the internal validity of a research study that occurs when a pretest is administered to subjects; the effects of taking a pretest on responses on the posttest.

test-retest reliability. See stability reliability.

theoretical framework. A study framework based on propositional statements from a theory.

theory. A set of related statements that describes or explains phenomena in a systematic way.

time sampling. Observations of events or behaviors that are made during certain specified time periods.

time-series design. Quasiexperimental design in which the researcher periodically observes subjects and administers an experimental treatment between two of the observations.

triangulation. Combining both qualitative and quantitative methods in one study.

true experimental design. An experimental design in which the researcher (a) manipulates the experimental variable, (b) includes at least one experimental and one comparison group in the study, and (c) randomly assigns subjects to either the experimental or comparison group; includes the pretest-posttest control group design, posttest-only control group design, and Solomon four-group design.

two-tailed test of significance. A test of statistical significance in which critical values (statistically significant values) are sought in both tails of the sampling distribution; used when the researcher has not predicted the direction of the relationship between variables.

Type I error (α). A decision is made to reject the null hypothesis when it is actually true; a decision is made that a relationship exists between variables when it does not.

Type II error (β). A decision is made not to reject the null hypothesis when it is false and should be rejected; a decision is made that no relationship exists between variables when, in fact, a relationship does exist.

unimodal. A frequency distribution that contains one value that occurs more frequently than any other.

univariate study. A research study in which only one variable is examined.

unstructured interviews. The interviewer is given a great deal of freedom to direct the course of the interview; the interviewer's main goal is to encourage the respondent to talk freely about the topic that is being explored.

unstructured observations. The researcher describes behaviors as they are viewed, with no preconceived ideas of what will be seen.

validity. The ability of an instrument to measure the variable that it is intended to measure.

variable. A characteristic or attribute of a person or object that differs among the persons or objects that are being studied (e.g., age, blood type).

variance (SD^2;s^2). A measure of variability; the standard deviation squared.

visual analogue scale. Subjects are presented with a straight line that is anchored on each end with words or phrases that represent the extremes of some phenomenon, such as pain. Subjects are asked to make a mark on the line at the point that corresponds to their experience of the phenomenon.

volunteers. Subjects who have asked to participate in a study.

z-score. A standard score that indicates how many standard deviations that a particular value is away from the mean of the set of values.

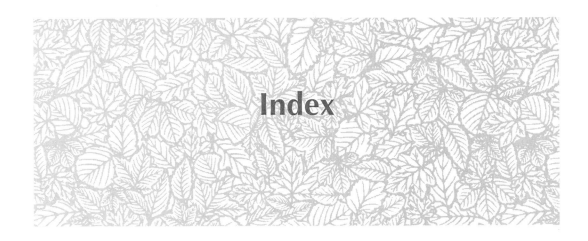

Index

Letters after page numbers represent boxes (*b*), figures (*f*), and tables (*t*). Italicized numbers represent glossary entries.